TREATING
SLEEP
DISORDERS

TREATING SLEEP DISORDERS

PRINCIPLES AND PRACTICE OF BEHAVIORAL SLEEP MEDICINE

Edited by

Michael L. Perlis
Kenneth L. Lichstein

WILEY

John Wiley & Sons, Inc.

Copyright © 2003 by John Wiley & Sons, Inc. All rights reserved.

Published by John Wiley & Sons, Inc., Hoboken, New Jersey.
Published simultaneously in Canada.

Library of Congress Cataloging-in-Publication Data:

Treating sleep disorders : principles and practice of behavioral sleep medicine / edited by
Michael L. Perlis & Kenneth L. Lichstein.
    p. cm.
  Includes bibliographical references and index.
  ISBN 0-471-44343-3 (cloth : alk. paper)
   1. Sleep disorders. I. Perlis, Michael L. II. Lichstein, Kenneth L.
  [DNLM: 1. Sleep Disorders—psychology. 2. Sleep Disorders—therapy. WM 188 T7834 2003]
  RC547.T745   2003
  616.8′498—dc21

                        2002191040

Printed in the United States of America.

10 9 8 7 6 5 4 3 2 1

*To Kenny, I thank you for lending your
seniority, sage advice, and guidance to this
(I know you told me so) Herculean project.*

*To Leisha Smith, I am grateful to you for your support
and hard work, especially in the closing months of this
project. Your influx of energy turned out to be
an essential "counterfatigue measure."*

*To my parents (Edie and Marvin Perlis), what can any son say
for a lifetime of support and love? "Thank you" is a small,
but heartfelt, payment . . . and "cya at the docks" . . .*

*To Donna, I thank you for providing so much. This book, my
research, and my career would have come to a grinding halt long
ago, but for your care, kindness, and generosity.*

M. L. P.

To the men in my life, David, Benjamin, Jeremy, and Noah.

K. L. L.

Contents

Preface

The youthfulness of the profession of psychology is fertile ground for exciting changes. In the past 40 years, we have witnessed two, and perhaps three, paradigm shifts of sub-Kuhnian proportion. Behavior modification burst on the scene in the 1960s and created no less than a clinical revolution. During the 1970s, the emergence of behavioral medicine and its formal christening at the Yale conference in 1977 created almost volcanic excitement. And now, many of us are both observer and participant in the blossoming of behavioral sleep medicine. These are wondrous times for those of us interested in the application of behavioral-cognitive science to sleep.

As exciting as the prospects are for our nascent field and as tempting as it is to include the birth of behavioral sleep medicine as a major event, it is important that we take into account the greater context and humbly appreciate that not all "revolutions" are the same. If the emergence of behavioral sleep medicine characterizes the 2000s, can we say that the 1960s, the 1970s, and the 2000s all had paradigm shifts of significant and/or equal proportion? The answer is probably no. Behavior modification and behavioral medicine were events that occurred virtually in a vacuum. Save for Rogerian psychology and murmurings by other small movements, the practice of clinical psychology during the first half of this century was mainly resigned to psychological testing and psychoanalytic aspirations. Against this background, the behavior modification movement created an extraordinary revision in theory and procedures and in the role of psychologists. This probably represented an unqualified paradigm shift. Behavioral medicine, in turn, was built on the achievements of the 1960s, but went far beyond. The 1970s witnessed dramatic theoretical progress in our understanding of psychological processes in medical disorders, but perhaps more importantly, there occurred a professional/political revolution that elevated the role of psychology in medical settings and spurred the acceptance of cognitive and behavioral interventions by our medical colleagues.

From the perspective of the 2000s, the significance and durability of changes in the 1960s and 1970s are beyond question. But what of the future of current changes? There are similarities between behavior modification, behavioral medicine, and behavioral sleep medicine that foster optimism. All three claim the following:

1. Though the emergence of the disciplines appeared sudden, it was not. All three draw on many years of basic research, successful clinical experience, and broad but poorly organized professional activity.

2. There is excitement, optimism, and professional ownership characterizing all three, and tangible evidence of this sense that something special is happening is mirroring the past. Expanded National Institutes of Health recognition and support, the emergence of organizational structures, and the creation of certification programs readily come to mind.

3. A burgeoning formal literature has appeared in all three time periods: books, both professional and lay, journals, and articles and chapters.

Will the success and impact of behavioral sleep medicine rival its preceding movements? It probably will not. Behavioral medicine as an offshoot of behavior modification was the beneficiary of the truly innovative, pioneering achievement of its predecessor, and though remarkable, we do not believe behavioral medicine had the breadth of societal impact attained by behavior modification. Similarly, behavioral sleep medicine can be viewed as a more narrow offshoot of behavioral medicine. Thus, by definition, the scope of impact will have to be more limited. We shall have to be content to witness and appreciate the emergence of behavioral sleep medicine as a more modest, but still meaningful, outgrowth of behavioral medicine and sleep medicine. Such a humble beginning, however, we hope, will be the progenitor of a time when there will be health providers board certified in behavioral sleep medicine in every sleep disorders center, the majority of clinical psychologists will have had exposure to behavioral sleep medicine in their graduate programs or internships, and patients will not stare blankly when you mention behavioral sleep medicine to them. Further, we hope that this book can contribute to forging this future and serve as an impetus for new research and the development of a broad range of cognitive, behavioral, and psychophysiologic interventions for each and all of the sleep disorders.

KENNETH L. LICHSTEIN
MICHAEL L. PERLIS

Acknowledgments

First and foremost, we would like to acknowledge the care, concern, and work efforts of the contributing authors, especially the senior authors: Rosalind Cartwright, PhD; Jack Edinger, PhD; Brett Kuhn, PhD; Tracy Kuo, PhD; Leon Lacks, PhD; Daniel Lewin, PhD; Charles Morin, PhD; Anne Rogers, PhD; Gerald Rosen, PhD; Avi Sadeh, PhD; Michael Smith, PhD; Arthur Spielman, PhD; and Edward Stepanski, PhD.

In an age where book chapters have less academic currency than they should, please know that we, and the nascent field of behavioral sleep medicine, are indebted to you.

We would also like to acknowledge the stalwart support of the American Academy of Sleep Medicine and, in particular, Daniel Buysse. Please know that all of us who are working to establish the subdiscipline are indebted to your vision, sense of collegiality, and unflagging support.

M.L.P.
K.L.L.

Contributors

Célyne Bastien
Universite Laval
Ecole de Psychologie
Sainte-Foy, Quebec, Canada

Richard R. Bootzin
Department of Psychology
University of Arizona
Tucson, Arizona

Rosalind D. Cartwright
Sleep Disorder Service
Rush-Presbyterian-St. Luke's
Medical Center
Chicago, Illinois

Deirdre Conroy
Sleep Disorders Center, City College of
New York
Sleep Disorders Center, New York
Methodist Hospital
Sleep-Wake Disorders Center, New York
Presbyterian, Cornell Medical Center
New York, New York

Jack D. Edinger
VA Medical Center
Durham, North Carolina

Amy J. Elliott
Munroe-Meyer Institute
University of Nebraska Medical Center
Omaha, Nebraska

Paul B. Glovinsky
Sleep Disorders Center, City College of
New York
Capital Region Sleep-Wake Disorders
Center
New York, New York

Daniel P. Kohen
Department of Pediatrics
University of Minnesota
Minneapolis, Minnesota

Brett R. Kuhn
Munroe-Meyer Institute
University of Nebraska Medical Center
Omaha, Nebraska

Tracy F. Kuo
Center for Excellence for Sleep
Disorders
Stanford University
Stanford, California

Clete A. Kushida
Center for Excellence for Sleep
Disorders
Stanford University
Stanford, California

Leon C. Lack
School of Psychology
Flinders University
Adelaide, South Australia

Daniel S. Lewin
School of Medicine
University of Pittsburgh
Pittsburgh, Pennsylvania

Kenneth L. Lichstein
Sleep Research Project
Department of Psychology
University of Memphis
Memphis, Tennessee

Mark W. Mahowald
Department of Neurology, University
of Minnesota
Minnesota Regional Sleep Disorders
Center, Hennepin County Medical Center
Minneapolis, Minnesota

Christina S. McCrae
Department of Psychology
University of Florida
Gainsville, Florida

Charles M. Morin
Universite Laval
Ecole de Psychologie
Sainte-Foy, Quebec, Canada

Janet Mullington
Department of Neurology
Beth Israel Deaconess Medical Center
Harvard University School of Medicine
Cambridge, Massachusetts

Sidney D. Nau
Sleep Research Project
Department of Psychology
University of Memphis
Memphis, Tennessee

Sara Nowakowski
University of Rochester Sleep Research
Laboratory
Department of Psychiatry
University of Rochester
Rochester, New York

Henry J. Orff
University of Rochester Sleep Research
Laboratory
Department of Psychiatry
University of Rochester
Rochester, New York

Michael L. Perlis
Department of Psychiatry
Department of Clinical and Social
Psychology, University of Rochester
University of Rochester Sleep Research
Laboratory
Rochester, New York

Ann E. Rogers
University of Pennsylvania School of
Nursing
Center for Sleep and Respiratory
Neurobiology
University of Pennsylvania School of
Medicine
Philadelphia, Pennsylvania

Gerald M. Rosen
Department of Pediatrics, University
of Minnesota
Minnesota Regional Sleep Disorders
Center, Hennepin County Medical Center
Minneapolis, Minnesota

Avi Sadeh
Department of Psychology
Tel Aviv University
Tel Aviv, Israel

Josée Savard
Universite Laval
Ecole de Psychologie
Sainte-Foy, Quebec, Canada

Leisha J. Smith
University of Rochester Sleep Research
Laboratory
Department of Psychiatry
University of Rochester
Rochester, New York

Michael T. Smith
Department of Psychiatry and Behavioral
Sciences
Johns Hopkins University School of
Medicine
Baltimore, Maryland

James P. Soeffing
University of Rochester Sleep Research
Laboratory
Department of Psychiatry
University of Rochester
Rochester, New York

Arthur J. Spielman
Sleep Disorders Center, City College of
New York
Sleep Disorders Center, New York
Methodist Hospital
Sleep-Wake Disorders Center, New York
Presbyterian, Cornell Medical Center
New York, New York

Edward J. Stcpanski
Sleep Disorder Service and Research
Center
Rush-Presbyterian-St. Luke's Medical
Center
Chicago, Illinois

Nancy M. Wilson
Sleep Research Project
Department of Psychology
University of Memphis
Memphis, Tennessee

SECTION I

Introduction to Behavioral Sleep Medicine

Chapter 1

A HISTORICAL PERSPECTIVE AND COMMENTARY ON PRACTICE ISSUES

EDWARD J. STEPANSKI AND MICHAEL L. PERLIS

Formally, *behavioral sleep medicine* (BSM) refers to the branch of clinical sleep medicine and health psychology that:

1. Focuses on the identification of the psychological (e.g., cognitive and/or behavioral) factors that contribute to the development and/or maintenance of sleep disorders
2. Specializes in developing and providing empirically validated cognitive, behavioral, and/or other nonpharmacologic interventions for the entire spectrum of sleep disorders

Behavioral sleep medicine is about to become a recognized subspecialty of sleep medicine, one with its own guidelines for training, board exam, journal, and now, with this book, its own principles and practice text. Thus, it seems appropriate to ask: "Where have we come from?" and "Where are we going?" A historical retrospective serves to help us address the former and acknowledges the work on which our field has been founded. The proposed commentary allows us to proactively consider the challenges that lie ahead.

TREATMENT DEVELOPMENT AND THE FOUNDATIONS FOR BEHAVIORAL SLEEP MEDICINE

Behavioral sleep medicine owes its existence as a subspecialty to the efforts to define and treat insomnia as a cognitive and behavioral disorder. Our field has two other, less well-recognized, sources:

1. The effort to define and treat pediatric sleep disorders behaviorally
2. The effort to apply cognitive and behavioral principles and practices to the full spectrum of sleep disorders

Accordingly, any attempt to provide a historical perspective on our field requires a review of how the various treatment modalities came into existence.

Treatment of Insomnia

Jacobson's well-known work on insomnia can arguably be cited as the beginning of BSM (1). Jacobson developed the tenets of progressive muscle relaxation (PMR) based on his work with patients he felt to have stress-related somatic problems. He theorized that heightened arousal contributed to a number of common medical complaints. PMR was a central treatment, but other stress management techniques were included in his treatment programs. The foundation for Jacobson's work can be traced to his training at Northwestern, Harvard, and the University of Chicago, where he trained with notable figures such as William James and Walter Cannon.

Relaxation Therapy

Jacobson provides a precise description of what would eventually be called *psychophysiological insomnia* in his 1938 book *You Can Sleep Well* (2). Although Jacobson is remembered for developing PMR as his major contribution, his writing also demonstrates a profound understanding of insomnia. In particular, his description of the behavioral and cognitive factors associated with insomnia is similar to our current understanding of these dimensions. He describes how the stresses of a modern society can lead to heightened arousal at night and then, in turn, to insomnia:

> What with electric lighting, automobiles, motion pictures, radios and other innovations, life after dark has become so attractive that most of the evening hours up to midnight are commonly occupied by some form of amusement—if only talking things over with friends and neighbors. (2, p. 182)

Every age has challenges that are in some ways unique but in a broader sense similar to those faced in every era. Reading Jacobson's case description of a patient with insomnia 70 years ago gives substance to the adage from psychotherapy that "the actors change, but the roles remain the same." In today's era, we would cite the Internet, satellite television, and 24-hour supermarkets as threats to a normal sleep-wake pattern in our version of modern society.

It is also interesting to note that concerns about pharmacological treatment for insomnia have not changed much over the years. Practitioners from the earlier era also expressed concerns about pharmacologic options for the treatment of insomnia (bromides and barbiturates):

> Today in most states sleeping medicines can be obtained only on a doctor's prescription, and this regulation has some merit because there are a few undisciplined persons who, if left to their own devices, would take large doses of these drugs every night without waiting to see if they were necessary for the obtaining of sleep. Many would rather take a drug than to make an effort to control emotions and calm down in the evenings. (3, p. 25)

Research aimed at understanding mechanisms underlying insomnia made further advances in the late 1960s. Much of this research took place at the University of Chicago under the direction of Rechtshaffen. Monroe (4), Hauri (5), Robinson (6), and Zimmerman (7) studied how physiological and cognitive arousal contributed to poor sleep. This research showed increased physiological arousal in poor sleepers compared to good sleepers, both before sleep onset and during the night (4). The role of physiological hyperarousal as a contributing factor in chronic insomnia continues to receive empirical support (8–9), and there is now evidence that central nervous system (CNS) arousal may also play a role in the disorder (10).

Despite the work of Jacobson and others, through the 1950s, insomnia was viewed as a consequence of a primary psychiatric or medical disorder. There was a struggle during the 1960s and 1970s about whether insomnia was always related to a psychiatric or medical disorder or could be "learned." The view that a primary psychiatric disorder was always to blame may be found in the writing of Kales (11). Acceptance of insomnia as a learned behavior was signified in the original nosological system published by the American Sleep Disorders Association (12). The term *psychophysiological insomnia* was used to denote an association between increased arousal and poor sleep, similar to the prevailing view that arousal might lead to hypertension or ulcers.

Aside from more basic research, many treatment outcome studies were conducted during the 1970s and early 1980s on relaxation-based treatment approaches to the treatment of insomnia. Progressive muscle relaxation was the approach most often studied. Studies using self-report measures of sleep tended to find a greater magnitude of change (13–15) than did those studies obtaining EEG measures of sleep (16–18). In general, it has been found that relaxation treatments generally did not show large effect sizes and were not better than placebo in some trials (19–20). The American Academy of Sleep Medicine (AASM) practice parameter paper for chronic insomnia rated PMR as empirically validated and well established (21).

One variant on "exercise"-oriented relaxation techniques (PMR, autogenics, and diaphragmatic breathing) is the use of biofeedback to diminish the hyperarousal that is thought to be associated with insomnia. Hauri published the best studies on the efficacy of biofeedback in the early 1980s (22–23). This research was particularly notable because he was able to show that increased arousal, measured by electromyography (EMG) levels, predicted successful treatment with EMG biofeedback but not sensory-motor rhythm (SMR) biofeedback. SMR biofeedback trains the individual to increase the 12 to 14 Hz type brain activity that tends to be associated with cortical synchronization and deeper sleep. This remains the only study to successfully show that treatment can be tailored based on patient characteristics. Other attempts to tailor treatment have not been successful and even showed that the nonpreferred treatment modality provided greater benefit than the predicted treatment (24). The AASM practice parameter paper rated biofeedback as empirically validated and probably efficacious as a treatment for chronic insomnia (21).

Over the past 15 years, relaxation therapies have gradually been replaced by other behavioral approaches and multicomponent cognitive-behavioral therapy (CBT) programs as described later. Biofeedback in particular appears to have fallen into disuse as a treatment for insomnia—probably because of the time-intensive nature of this treatment, with 15 to 62 one-hour sessions of training required for successful treatment (22).

Stimulus Control Therapy

Systematic intervention research investigating treatments for chronic insomnia had a renaissance in the 1970s. Principles of behavioral theory were applied to the problem of insomnia, and many new treatment approaches were formulated at this time. Bootzin used learning theory to create stimulus control therapy (SCT) for insomnia (25). Many investigators included SCT in their outcome research on treatment efficacy and showed significant improvement using self-report measures of sleep initiation and maintenance (15, 26). SCT continues to be one of the most commonly used behavioral treatments for insomnia and is included in multicomponent treatment programs for the treatment of insomnia. The AASM practice parameter recommendations for behavioral treatment of insomnia found that SCT had strong empirical evidence to support its efficacy and rated it as empirically validated and well established (21).

Sleep Hygiene

A list of rules to follow to promote better sleep in patients with insomnia was published and called *sleep hygiene* by Hauri in 1977 (27). This approach is extremely popular, and sleep hygiene education is almost universally recommended for the treatment of insomnia (28). The rules considered to constitute sleep hygiene have evolved over the years. There are few studies of sleep hygiene as a stand-alone treatment, and, instead, it appears to be considered a necessary, but not sufficient, approach in the treatment of insomnia (29).

Paradoxical Intention

The principles of paradoxical intention (PI) were used to formulate a treatment approach to insomnia (30). With PI, patients are instructed to stay awake for as long as possible after going to bed at night. Several studies reported positive results with PI using subjective outcome measures (30–32). In fact, the standards of practice statement rate this treatment as an empirically validated treatment based on an analysis of the literature, according to guidelines of the American Psychological Association (APA; 33). While overall effective, the research on PI as a treatment for insomnia suggests a highly variable treatment response across patients.

Sleep Restriction Therapy

In the 1980s, sleep restriction therapy (SRT) was developed by Spielman and colleagues (34). This behavioral treatment systematically reduces time in bed to increase homeostatic drive for sleep and then increases time in bed once sleep efficiency is increased. SRT has become a widely used treatment and is routinely included as part of CBT treatment programs for insomnia.

An important theoretical model for understanding the formation of chronic insomnia and its evolution over time was proposed in 1986 (35). This model classifies factors contributing to chronic insomnia as predisposing, precipitating, or perpetuating. Each of these types of factors plays a role in the formation and maintenance of insomnia, and the relative importance of these factors changes over the course of the insomnia. The least understood factors are predisposing factors although, as discussed previously, physiological hyperarousal appears to be a strong candidate as a predisposing factor for the development of chronic insomnia. Precipitating factors might be medical factors (e.g., pain), psychological factors (e.g., increased job stress), environmental factors (e.g., noise in the bedroom), or anything else (e.g., shift work) that would reasonably disrupt sleep acutely. These are the factors typically focused on in the nosological system for diagnosing sleep disorders (36). Perpetuating factors are behavioral and cognitive features of insomnia that typically develop when an individual has been struggling with insomnia for days or weeks. Examples include increasing time in bed to achieve more sleep, increasing use of caffeine to counteract daytime fatigue, self-medicating with alcohol, and ruminating throughout the day about the need to obtain additional sleep. This model is important because it provides a framework for understanding what is otherwise a disparate set of findings about the causes and consequences of insomnia. Additionally, it can serve to organize clinical interventions by targeting the appropriate set of factors based on the status of an individual patient.

Cognitive Therapy

Although the cognitive component of insomnia has been noted for decades, formalized cognitive therapy for insomnia is an innovation from the 1990s. A book on insomnia written by an editorial board of physicians for laypeople, notes that:

> Relaxation is more likely to come if the would-be sleeper hasn't any fear of insomnia; hence the physician does well when he keeps reminding a patient that nothing terrible need happen to him if he does not sleep. There are thousands of persons working hard and enjoying fair health who haven't had a good night's sleep for years. They do not go insane or come to any bad end. (3, p. 16)

In addition to the fear of insomnia, Jacobson notes that "many fear incapacity through fatigue" (37, p. 182). Indeed, the fear of being awake itself and the fear of daytime impairment are common among patients with insomnia. The interaction between cognitive and behavioral factors was also acknowledged in a 1938 book on insomnia:

> Nostrums, then, in insomnia are those pet schemes or remedies by whose aid the insomniac thinks to outwit his enemy, without realizing that often through his devoted attention to them he is setting up a ritual for himself which is fully calculated to keep the enemy in power. For these nostrums represent an attempt to defeat wakefulness or to avoid the anxiety incidental to lying awake, and as such signify that the individual is attempting to escape his anxiety through the use of some semi-magical device, thus turning his back on the need for understanding the problem and working out its solution along informed and intelligent lines. (38, pp. 134–135)

Patients themselves are also more likely to attribute their sleep difficulty to heightened cognitive arousal, rather than somatic arousal (39). A formal description of programmatic cognitive therapy designed for patients with insomnia is best described by Morin (40). Morin describes how misattributions, unrealistic expectations, and various cognitive errors contribute to emotional arousal and, ultimately, to insomnia. He then applies cognitive restructuring techniques that have been effective in the treatment of anxiety disorders and depression to changing these maladaptive cognitions that accompany insomnia. Cognitive restructuring teaches patients to evaluate their response to sleeplessness with a more realistic perspective. Integrating cognitive therapy with the behavioral therapies described previously is essential because many of the cognitive features inherent to insomnia lead to the behavioral changes that exacerbate the insomnia. For example, a fear of achieving fewer than eight hours of total sleep time may lead a patient to spend excessive time in bed.

The AASM practice parameter paper found insufficient evidence to establish the efficacy of cognitive therapy for the treatment of chronic insomnia as a single treatment (21). Cognitive therapy has most often been studied as part of a multicomponent therapy program.

Multicomponent Cognitive-Behavioral Therapy Programs

The current state-of-the-art program in the cognitive-behavioral treatment of insomnia combines sleep hygiene, stimulus control therapy, sleep restriction therapy, and cognitive therapy (40–41). These studies provide evidence that pre- to posttreatment changes exceed those that occur with time or placebo controls. These investigations have, in addition to being controlled clinical trials, the added advantage of both prospective self-report and polysomnographic measures of sleep continuity. It has been shown that CBT interventions have significantly greater durability than pharmacotherapy in older adults with primary insomnia (41). That is, while acute effects may be comparable, only CBT yields stable and long-term gains. These data challenge the conventional wisdom that in the short term, pharmacotherapy produces quicker and larger effects. This perspective is further challenged by the results of a recent comparative meta-analytic study that showed that CBT and pharmacotherapy produce comparable effects during acute treatment and that CBT may more profoundly reduce sleep initiation problems (43).

The multicomponent treatment program approach recognizes the failure of predicting which treatment will benefit a particular patient and avoids this problem by providing all treatment components to each patient. With improved understanding of the mechanisms that contribute to insomnia, it is expected that, eventually, clinicians will be able to match specific cognitive-behavioral therapies to a given patient based on individual patient characteristics. A recent study used the multicomponent program in general practice and found that two-thirds of those patients had sleep in the normal range at the end of treatment (44). The AASM practice parameter paper rates multicomponent treatment packages as empirically validated and probably efficacious for chronic insomnia (21).

As discussed previously, the success of CBT with primary insomnia is well established. Use of CBT for insomnia is also demonstrated by two meta-analytic studies conducted in the middle 1990s (45–46). This fact gives rise to the obvious question: How effective is CBT in patients with secondary insomnia, especially in subjects with medical and/or psychiatric conditions? Preliminary research shows that CBT is effective in such patients, and the magnitude of the treatment effects appears comparable (47–50).

Withdrawing Patients from Use of Hypnotic Medication

Assisting patients who are withdrawing from hypnotic medication is another area of interest for BSM specialists. It has been shown that introducing relaxation training, in conjunction with medication withdrawal, leads to less reliance on the medication (i.e., greater reduction in amount of medication used) as well as improved sleep (51). More research is needed to further refine treatment regimens to assist with tapering and discontinuing use of hypnotic medication.

Sleep and Sleep Disorders in Children

Enuresis

The behavioral treatment of enuresis was also initially developed during the 1930s. O. Hobart Mowrer presented his findings using the bell and pad treatment for enuresis at the American Orthopsychiatric Meeting in 1937 (52). This technique used the principles of classical conditioning to train children to awaken when they needed to urinate during the night. Bladder distention was the conditioned stimulus for the response of awakening. Mowrer provides a fascinating description of this work and its significance to practitioners at the time in his 1976 address to the APA (53). The immediate need to develop an effective treatment arose when he joined the staff of a residential institution for children with various emotional disorders. Half of the children at the institution suffered from enuresis; thus, development of an effective treatment approach was urgently needed. The technique proved to be effective, and estimates find that the bell and pad approach is over 70% effective (54). More than 60 years after its initial development, the bell and pad treatment is still the single most effective treatment for long-term control of enuresis.

Bedtime Refusal

It is fitting that the originator of behaviorism wrote about behavioral treatment for pediatric sleep disorders. John Watson wrote about the proper approach to establishing a regular sleep-wake schedule in young children (55). He recommended establishing a consistent set of nighttime rituals, including a bath, quiet play, followed by bedtime. Some obsolete advice includes a recommendation that the parent take a final look around the room to make sure the chamber pot is under the bed and that there is a flashlight on the nightstand for a child to use on awakening during the night. After this ritual, the parent leaves the room for the night.

  If he howls, let him howl. A week of this regime will give you an orderly bedtime. (55, p. 120)

Sixty years after this terse description by Watson, several empirical studies have shown that extinction procedures are efficacious as a treatment for bedtime refusal (56–57). According to standard criteria for judging the adequacy of empirical data, extinction is rated as a well-established treatment approach (58). Note that there is a less well-validated graded alternative to this implosive style procedure (see Chapters 14 and 16).

Nighttime Awakenings/Sleep Onset Association Disorder

The contemporary understanding of pediatric sleep disorders in behavioral terms made a giant leap forward with the publication of Richard Ferber's book in 1985 (59). He provided a model that discriminated among causes of sleep disturbance in children and also matched treatment regimens according to the specific disorder. His subtypes of disorders that can lead to difficulty initiating or maintaining sleep in infants and children include sleep onset association disorder and limit-setting disorder. Ferber describes how the most common pediatric sleep disorders are established through classical conditioning (sleep onset association disorder) or are maintained because of reinforcement from the parents (limit-setting disorder). Sleep onset association disorder occurs because the infant is conditioned to fall asleep in conjunction with certain circumstances that it cannot recreate during the night on awakening (e.g., being rocked by a parent). Therefore, the parent must again rock the child with each awakening to get the infant to return to sleep. Once understood in these terms, the treatment is intuitive: The infant must learn to fall asleep on his or her own to start the night.

Nighttime awakenings have also been successfully treated with extinction and graduated extinction procedures. Another approach to eliminate nighttime awakenings is use of scheduled awakenings (60). With this treatment approach, the child is awakened by the parent slightly before the usual time of the problematic awakening. The child is reassured and allowed to return to sleep. The scheduled awakenings are subsequently reduced in frequency and faded out. The empirical data to support this approach is rated as probably efficacious (61).

Parasomnias

A systematic approach to understanding and treating parasomnias has recently been proposed by the group at the Minnesota Regional Sleep Disorders Center, headed by Mark Mahowald. Categorization of parasomnias according to sleep state (NREM versus REM), as well as on the basis of whether they are primary or occur as secondary to other precipitants, has greatly improved clinical evaluation and treatment.

Non-REM parasomnias in children, such as sleepwalking and confusional arousals, may be managed with behavioral treatment (62). General behavioral changes include establishing a regular sleep-wake schedule and maintaining sufficient time in bed to avoid sleep deprivation. Sleep deprivation increases the likelihood of a NREM parasomnia because of the increased slow wave sleep observed with recovery sleep. Scheduled awakenings or scheduled nap interventions may also be useful because they precipitate lighter sleep. Measures to ensure the safety of the patient by removing obstacles from the bedroom and taking steps to keep the patient away from windows and stairs must also be a routine component of any behavioral treatment program for sleepwalking.

Nightmares can also be treated behaviorally. Use of imagery rehearsal therapy has been shown to be effective in the treatment of nightmares in patients with posttraumatic stress disorder (63).

Biological Rhythms and Circadian Rhythm Disorders

Circadian rhythm disorders occur when there is desynchrony between the biological and environmental clocks in the timing of the sleep-wake schedule. The most common of these disorders encountered in clinical practice is delayed sleep phase syndrome (DSPS). This disorder is marked by a biological sleep rhythm that is not prepared for sleep at the desired bedtime and promotes sleep during a time period later than the desired schedule.

Chronotherapy was the first behavioral therapy developed to treat DSPS (64). In brief, the treatment requires that the patient delay bedtime by one to two hours each night until the desired schedule is reached. The approach was based on the belief at the time that the intrinsic rhythm was a little more than 25 hours; therefore, it would be much easier for an individual to delay, rather than advance, the sleep phase. Discoveries since the initial description of chronotherapy suggest that this treatment, as initially conceived, might not be very effective. First, we now know that the intrinsic rhythm is about 24.18 hours, so the daily tendency to delay is slight (65). Second, and more importantly, the impact of exposure to bright light can be profound depending on its placement according to the phase response curve (66). Treatment with standard chronotherapy instructions, without regulating an individual's exposure to sunlight, would not be expected to produce a predictable shift in phase given the robustness of bright light in regulating circadian phase. An individual could potentially be exposed to sunlight on arising, which would precipitate a slight phase advance instead of a delay. Chronotherapy is being replaced with bright light therapy to accomplish the same goals for patients with DSPS.

Research aimed at determining if DSPS results from purely behavioral factors or is caused by an intrinsic deficit in circadian rhythm physiology is needed. Landmark research in this area suggests that adolescents have developmental changes in their circadian regulation that predisposes them to become phase delayed (67). It is also possible that decreasing homeostatic sleep drive contributes to the tendency to phase delay in adolescent individuals (68). Understanding this issue has great public health implications because adolescents start school earlier than they did 20 years ago and display evidence of chronic sleep deprivation (69).

Another circadian rhythm disorder encountered in clinical practice is shift work disorder. This disorder can also be treated behaviorally or with bright light therapy to achieve better regulation of the sleep-wake pattern (70). This disorder also has significant public health implications given the large number of workers performing shift work and the expectation that the proportion of workers engaged in shift work will continue to increase.

Adherence to Use of Nasal Continuous Positive Airway Pressure

An emerging area related to behavioral sleep medicine services is that of improving adherence to use of nasal continuous positive airway pressure (CPAP) in patients with obstructive sleep apnea (OSA). A landmark study from 1994 used covert sensors to objectively monitor the time of CPAP use and found that treatment adherence was significantly lower than what patients self-reported (71). Although the level of adherence to CPAP regimens appears similar to that found for other chronic medical treatments, the need to increase rates of adherence has been targeted as a critical goal in the field of sleep disorders medicine. Psychological factors were found to predict poor compliance (71), and further work to address improving adherence is warranted. Patients with OSA who are unable to comply with medical treatment often benefit from CBT-type interventions that range from additional clinician support and education (72) to desensitization procedures that target patients' phobic reactions to the use of CPAP (73). Formulation of other psychological interventions to target patients with poor compliance is needed (74).

CLINICAL PRACTICE ISSUES IN BEHAVIORAL SLEEP MEDICINE

Training in Behavioral Sleep Medicine

As the description of our clinical domain implies, BSM training requires that specialists acquire a broad-based knowledge of sleep medicine and behavioral medicine. The optimal course for such training is via clinical psychology curriculum with sleep medicine and sleep research components. Alternative courses may include other forms of clinical training with postdoctoral clinical experiences through fellowship programs and/or mentored apprenticeships.

Unfortunately, there are few formal training programs in BSM. At the predoctoral level, a handful of graduate school programs in psychology and/or internship programs offer clinical and/or clinical research training in sleep. For a list of BSM programs, see Table 1.1. Note that the curricula of the various programs and the extent to which they provide dedicated time to BSM are variable. Currently, there are no formal requirements for BSM training at either the graduate or internship levels, but one of the missions of the American Academy of Sleep Medicine's Presidential Committee on Behavioral Sleep Medicine is to develop such requirements, as well as a certification process for BSM specialists.

At the postdoctoral level, the American Academy of Sleep Medicine (AASM) has been accrediting fellowship training programs in sleep disorders medicine for physicians for about 20 years. As of 1999, there is a mechanism to accredit fellowship training programs for PhD candidates through the AASM.

Table 1.1   Behavioral Sleep Medicine Programs

Graduate Programs	Internship Programs
University of Arizona (Bootzin)	Brown University (Posner/Carskadon)
Bowling Green State University (Badia)*	Columbia University (Zammit)
Hahnemann University (Mindel)	Duke University (Edinger/ Wohlgemuth)
Laval University (Morin)	Harvard University (Dorsey)
Technion Israel Institute of Technology (Lavie)	Rush-Presbyterian-St. Luke's (Stepanski/Wyatt)
City College of New York (Speilman)	University of Arizona (Bootzin)
University of Memphis (Lichstein)	University of Ottawa (De Koninck)
University of Ottawa (De Koninck)	University of Pittsburgh (Buysse)*
University of Pittsburgh (Buysse) *	University of Rochester (Perlis/Giles)*
University of Rochester (Perlis/Giles)*	UCSD/SDSU Joint Program (Ancoli-Israel)
UCSD/SDSU Joint Program (Ancoli-Israel)	University of Washington (Vitiello)
University of Montreal (Montplaisir)	Eastern Virginia Medical School (Ware)*
University of Toronto (Moldofsky/Shapiro)*	
University of Washington (Vitiello)*	
Eastern Virginia Medical School (Ware)*	
Wright State University (Bonnet)	

*Denotes programs that offer clinical training opportunities but require special arrangements. This is necessary when the mentor does not have a primary faculty appointment in a degree-granting department and/or a primary affiliation with a clinical program or because there are limited slots available.

An advantage of an accredited training program is that graduates are automatically eligible for the American Board of Sleep Medicine exam. Guidelines to establish accredited fellowship programs for BSM are being formulated to prepare candidates for a new BSM board exam, administered by the American Academy of Sleep Medicine. As with the general sleep medicine fellowships, graduating from an accredited training program will allow candidates to be automatically eligible for the subspecialty board exam.

Barriers to the Clinical Practice of Behavioral Sleep Medicine

Taking a proactive stance in fostering growth within BSM requires that we address the question "What factors represent barriers to the widespread application of BSM treatment modalities?" One factor for all the treatment methods, apart from those for insomnia, is that they have limited empirical support and, as a result, are not reimbursed by third-party payers. It is hoped that, with an increase in clinical trial research, such therapies will gain credibility and become routinely remunerated with sleep disorders diagnostic codes and behavioral medicine procedure codes. This hope, however, is diminished by the fact that such a scenario has not yet played out with CBT of insomnia. Reimbursement has not been forthcoming despite having an empirically validated therapy that is effective and produces acute results comparable to, and long-term results superior to, medical therapy. A preponderance of data suggests that CBT should be the treatment of choice for chronic insomnia, yet this is not the case.

There are four interrelated reasons that CBT is not yet the standard of practice. First, behavioral interventions appear to be more costly. Second, there is a lack of awareness among health care professionals about the procedures and effectiveness of behavioral medicine in general and about BSM in particular. Third, there are only a few hundred clinicians in North America who are trained in, who are experienced with, and who specialize in the provision of BSM services. Fourth, most insurance companies and health plans, at least in the United States, do not provide coverage for the behavioral treatment of insomnia; and those that do, do so under mental health codes and benefits. We consider each of these in the following sections.

The Cost of Behavioral Sleep Medicine Treatment

Even the most expensive hypnotic medications do not, in the short run, rival the costs of behavior therapy. For example, a five-week trial of zolpidem or zaleplon costs approximately $166 compared to $350 for five weeks of behavioral treatment. This difference in short-term cost, however, needs to be placed in the broader context. What is the cost differential if the physician is willing to prescribe hypnotics for long-term use in a manner that is analogous to maintenance therapy with antidepressants? What happens when medical treatment is discontinued, regardless of treatment duration? In the case of the former, the initial consultation, follow-up visits, and prescription costs for one year alone easily exceed the cost of the five-week behavioral intervention. Maintenance of hypnotic medication therapy would be expected to cost at least $500 per year given intermittent dosing and more than $1,000 per year given nightly (qhs) use. In the latter, it can be expected (based on the data available) that the insomnia symptoms will recur following the discontinuation of pharmacologic treatment. As a result, the recurrent episode of insomnia, like the episode before treatment, will also have substantial indirect costs stemming from lost work productivity, absenteeism, fatigue-related injuries, and/or increased health care costs related to secondary medical and/or psychiatric morbidity.

One caveat, however, to this perspective is that relative costs of medical and behavioral treatment, as we have detailed them, depend on two assumptions—only one of which appears tenable. First, short-term behavioral therapy has long-lasting effects. This assumption appears viable. There is good empirical evidence showing that the clinical gains obtained with CBT interventions are durable for follow-up periods of up to a year. The second assumption is that when medical therapy is discontinued, the clinical gains are lost. This assumption has not, to our knowledge, ever been properly tested. That is, it is entirely possible that the long-term use of hypnotic medication may result in long-term gains, but such gains are evident only *after the withdrawal period*. To test this interesting possibility, a long-term trial needs to be undertaken (where time on the drug is evaluated in a dose response fashion), which includes a careful approach to medication withdrawal and longitudinal monitoring during and after the withdrawal period. If such studies found positive outcomes, a more accurate assessment of the relative costs of both pharmacologic and behavioral interventions would be possible.

In summary, long-term treatment with sedative hypnotics is undoubtedly more expensive. Short-term treatment, while more cost efficient in terms of direct dollars, is probably also more expensive given the indirect costs associated with recurrent episodes of insomnia (assuming that pharmacologic treatments are only palliative). Thus, the data to date suggest that behavioral sleep medicine interventions for insomnia are, in the long run, likely to be more economical.

Poor Understanding of Behavioral Medicine Treatment among Health Care Professionals

Despite the now-prevalent biopsychosocial approach to health care, many medical and mental health professionals have only a limited understanding of what constitutes behavioral medicine treatment—possibly for many reasons. Perhaps the most fundamental reason is that the biopsychosocial approach means a team approach to patient care as opposed to the application of psychological or behavioral approaches to medical disease. The latter, which is precisely the domain of behavioral medicine, is still controversial. Can we really affect medical illnesses with applications such as relaxation training, biofeedback, thought stopping, or stimulus control procedures? Can the course or intensity of a medical illness be changed by antidepressant effects of psychotherapy? These questions, which represent a direct challenge to the lingering dualistic perspective that there is a mind-body split, have yet to be answered in a way that suggests whether they are globally true. In the absence of such data, it is understandable that many medical and mental health professionals have only a limited appreciation of what constitutes behavioral medicine.

However, there is now sufficient data to justify the widespread education of medical and mental health professionals concerning our particular brand of behavioral medicine. That is, given the efficacy of the behavioral interventions for insomnia, there is no reason to suspend judgment. What is needed now is to educate the health care community so that it is commonly understood that BSM interventions for insomnia represent first-line treatment.

In summary, there is an understandable lack of awareness among the health care community as to the "power and potency" of behavioral treatment for insomnia. Ultimately, this will require a substantial publicity effort—one akin to that launched for sleep apnea. Ideally, such an effort would fall within the mission of the AASM and/or the National Institutes of Health (NIH) Center for Sleep Disorders Research. Such a campaign, however, will need to consider the supply side of the equation. While the tools for the job may exist, there is a lack of skilled personnel to wield them.

Shortage of Behavioral Sleep Medicine Specialists

There are simply not enough BSM specialists in this country. At best, there are 100 to 200 experienced providers (across a handful of states) to provide treatment for a community of patients that, by all estimates, is likely to be composed of more than 28 million individuals (given a conservative 10% prevalence estimate for just insomnia). The lack of available specialists in this arena results, at least in part, because only a handful of training opportunities in BSM are available across the entire educational spectrum for PhD clinicians. By our most recent estimates, there are 10 graduate programs, 8 clinical internships, and an undetermined (but likely smaller) number of sites that provide clinical fellowship training.

Graduate Training

The most direct solution to the very few graduate programs in BSM is to simply increase the number of programs and/or number of trainees in each program. While ideal, this is exceptionally difficult to implement. Assuming an adequate number of junior faculty available to develop new programs, starting new sleep research and sleep medicine programs is sufficiently costly that most universities are not inclined to risk the large investments required with less experienced individuals at the helm. Increasing the number of trainees in established programs, while not as complicated, is also difficult to implement. Funds must be secured to support new students at a time when funding for graduate training is less available. Moreover, establishing an increased number of trainee slots in existing programs often requires a substantial time burden for the would-be mentor, a burden that is usually unremunerated in the academic setting. The combination of these factors makes it unlikely that there can or will be a proliferation of programs or program slots dedicated to BSM based on intramural funding sources.

One possible solution to these problems is related to a new program established by the Sleep Research Society (SRS). This program offers salary support for junior faculty to be recruited to established programs and/or for mid-level faculty who wish to develop new sleep programs (for further information, see www.srs.grants). This societal-based program represents a welcome form of assistance. Our hope is that this program will make it possible for some training programs to be developed and/or additional junior faculty to be recruited to help grow extant programs. Unfortunately, the outcome from the SRS program is likely a limited one, given this society's emphasis on basic versus clinical research training.

Training opportunities at the internship and fellowship levels might represent another possible way to increase the number of clinicians who practice BSM. In fact, increasing the availability of training at this level would in some ways be more ideal because it would be open to a broader spectrum of candidates and allow for more focused and less time-intensive training.

Internship Training

While the number of internships that offer BSM training is on the rise, the growth rate is limited. Even when qualified personnel are available to lead such programs and to mentor students, establishing new rotations is often a complicated matter. A variety of issues must be considered, including how the new rotation will:

1. Compete with existing rotations for intern time
2. Obtain partial salary support monies
3. Inspire the extant training committees to undertake the administrative work of amending internship charters and so on

While there are no easy solutions to these problems and the burden of establishing more internship opportunities must inevitably be a grass roots labor, perhaps some progress could be made by dealing with this aspect of training at the highest level. That is, the leaders of the BSM section of the AASM could work with the internship accreditation component of APA to identify new regulations or incentives that inspire established programs to embrace BSM training. Such an effort might be based on APA's continuing efforts to enhance the training of predoctoral students in the provision of empirically validated therapies.

Postdoctoral Training

Establishing fellowship opportunities is generally less complicated than creating new graduate or internship programs, probably because it is accomplished based on the efforts of the individual. How do we ensure that such fellowships meet some minimum standard for training and that the trainees themselves emerge from these programs as qualified BSM specialists? The AASM's Presidential Committee on BSM has:

1. Formulated criteria for the certification of fellowship programs
2. Begun the process of establishing a board exam so that individuals may be credentialed in the area of BSM

No Third-Party Reimbursement or Only Partial Reimbursement under Mental Health

At one time, the most concrete reasons for third-party payers to refuse coverage for the behavioral treatment of insomnia were that:

1. It was not clear whether the disorder represented a substantial health problem.
2. There was not sufficient empirical evidence as to treatment efficacy (absolute or relative efficacy).

Both of these concerns have been addressed. A great deal of data shows that chronic insomnia is a highly prevalent problem, that it is associated with substantial medical and psychiatric morbidity, and that the costs to society are significant. There is also now clear evidence that CBT for insomnia is effective. The combination of these data has led some third-party payers to provide reimbursement for the nonpharmacologic treatment of insomnia, but as a mental health benefit.

The reimbursement of insomnia treatment under mental health raises some essential issues. One is: "Is insomnia a mental health condition?" Even if the answer to this question is no, the question "Is reimbursement based on the nature of the condition or by the mode of treatment?" must be answered. Most third-party payers have answered this by affirming the latter. Thus, we find ourselves in a situation where not only are there very few providers, but the impetus to become a provider is constrained by the unwholesome prospects that:

1. BSM services are not universally reimbursed.
2. When reimbursed, BSM specialists are required to have their patients carry a mental health diagnosis (one that is often at odds with how the patients conceive their disorder) and substantial copayments.

The combination of no payment, payment according to mental health fee schedules, and the loss of revenues associated with substantial patient copays has inevitably challenged the financial viability of delivering BSM services.

What is to be done about the reimbursement situation? At least two productive avenues could be pursued. First, the assumption behind nonparity, the assumption that nonpharmacologic interventions are less effective, must be challenged. The data from the Morin study (33, 41) and meta-analysis by Smith et al. (43) provide the basis on which such a challenge can be made to third-party payers and health care professionals. Second, BSM specialists need to capitalize on the movement to distinguish between, and provide separate Current Procedural Terminology (CPT) codes for, behavioral medicine services and mental health services. This movement, jointly sponsored by the APA and American Medical Association, will ostensibly allow for the cognitive and behavioral treatment of medical disorders to be reimbursed under medical benefits. The existence of special codes for behavioral medicine will be helpful and is likely to positively impact on the reimbursement of the behavioral treatment of insomnia. For further information about these new policies and CPT codes, see:

- www.apa.org/practice/cpt_faq.html
- www.apa.org/practice/pu/oct00/newcpt.html
- www.apa.org/monitor/nov00/codes.html

The issues that surround third-party reimbursement are complex and daunting although there is reason to be optimistic. The availability of new codes, in combination with strong empirical support for the efficacy of CBT for insomnia, will likely smooth the way for both routine reimbursement and the establishment of better reimbursement rates. Better reimbursement, along with enhanced training opportunities and a credentialing process, will in turn ensure that more qualified providers are available.

FUTURE DIRECTIONS

The past 30 years have seen a vast improvement in the understanding of the cognitive and behavioral factors that contribute to adult and pediatric sleep disorders. Additionally, the efficacy of CBT for insomnia has been established. However, a great deal of work remains in the application of CBT approaches to sleep disorders. Every area described here still has many challenges before treatment regimens are optimal. Behavioral sleep medicine is in a period of exceptional growth, with a marked expansion of interest beyond insomnia to include pediatric sleep disorders and circadian rhythm disorders.

Establishing the efficacy of CBT in younger patients with insomnia and in patients with secondary insomnia is needed. Both of the major outcome studies of CBT for insomnia were conducted in older adults with primary insomnia. Also, effectiveness studies that establish the portability of these treatments to various health care settings will be essential if these treatments are to be delivered to large numbers of patients in a cost-effective manner. An improved understanding of the mechanisms of insomnia across patient subtypes may yet lead to effective strategies for tailoring treatment recommendations to further enhance treatment effectiveness and reduce the time required for treatment. Research that assesses whether CBT can be combined effectively with pharmacological treatment is needed. The indications and limitations of combined treatment approaches may yield improved outcomes over current strategies that rely on either CBT or pharmacological treatments alone.

More empirical work to establish the effectiveness of behavioral treatments for pediatric sleep disorders is needed. Many of the commonly used behavioral treatments have few empirical studies on which to base clinical guidelines to optimize treatment efficacy. The need for effective treatments is enormous given the prevalence of parent reports of sleep-related disorders in their children (61).

The body of science underlying our understanding of biological rhythms is steadily growing, and regimens to treat the related sleep disorders continue to develop. However, a consensus on optimal treatments for common disorders such as delayed sleep phase syndrome or shift work disorder is still needed.

Finally, an intriguing area for research is identifying behavioral or psychological strategies that improve adherence to nasal CPAP treatment for patients with

OSA. This disorder is commonly encountered in sleep disorder centers and is associated with well-established behavioral and cardiopulmonary morbidity.

REFERENCES

1. Jacobson, E. *You Must Relax*. Chicago, IL: University of Chicago Press. 1934.
2. Jacobson, E. *You Can Sleep Well*. New York, NY: McGraw-Hill Book Company, Inc. 1938.
3. Alvarez, W. C., G. Blumer, L. Clendening, I. Cutter, H. W. Haggard, R. Matas, et al. Editorial Board. *Insomnia*. New York, NY: Harper & Brothers Publishers. 1942.
4. Monroe, L. J. Psychological and physiological differences between good and poor sleepers. *Journal of Abnormal Psychology* 72: 255–264, 1967.
5. Hauri, P. Effects of evening activity on early night sleep. *Psychophysiology* 4: 266–277, 1968.
6. Robinson, T. Presleep activity and sleep quality of good and poor sleepers. Unpublished doctoral dissertation, University of Chicago. 1969.
7. Zimmerman, W. B. Psychological and physiological differences between "light" and "deep" sleepers. Unpublished doctoral dissertation, University of Chicago. 1967.
8. Stepanski, E., F. Zorick, T. Roehrs, D. Young, and T. Roth. Daytime alertness in patients with chronic insomnia compared with asymptomatic control subjects. *Sleep* 11: 54–60, 1988.
9. Bonnet, M. H. and D. Arand. Hyperarousal and insomnia. *Sleep Medicine Reviews* 1: 97–108, 1997.
10. Perlis, M. L., H. Merica, M. T. Smith, and D. E. Giles. Beta EEG in Insomnia. *Sleep Medicine Reviews* 5: 364–375, 2001.
11. Kales, A. and J. Kales. *Evaluation and Treatment of Insomnia*. New York, NY: Oxford University Press. 1984.
12. Association of Sleep Disorders Centers. Diagnostic Classification of Sleep and Arousal Disorders; prepared by the Sleep Disorders Classification Committee, H. P. Roffwarg, Chairman. *Sleep* 2: 1–137, 1979.
13. Nicassio, P. and R. Bootzin. A comparison of progressive relaxation and autogenic training as treatments for insomnia. *Journal of Abnormal Psychology* 83: 253–260, 1974.
14. Haynes, S., H. Sides, and G. Lockwood. Relaxation instructions and frontalis electromyographic feedback intervention with sleep onset insomnia. *Behavior Therapy* 8: 644–652, 1977.
15. Lacks, P., A. Bertelson, L. Gans, and J. Kunkel. The effectiveness of three behavioral treatments for different degrees of sleep onset insomnia. *Behavior Therapy* 14: 593–605, 1983.

16. Borkovec, T. and T. Weerts. Effects of progressive relaxation on sleep disturbance: An electroencephalographic evaluation. *Psychosomatic Medicine* 38:
173–180, 1976.

17. Borkovec, T., J. Grayson, G. O'Brien, and T. Weerts. Relaxation treatment of
pseudoinsomnia and idiopathic insomnia: An electroencephalographic evaluation.
Journal of Applied Behavior Analysis 12: 37–54, 1979.

18. Coursey, R., B. Frankel, K. Gaarder, and D. Mott. A comparison of relaxation
techniques with electrosleep therapy for chronic, sleep-onset insomnia. A sleep
EEG study. *Biofeedback Self Regulation* 5: 57–73, 1980.

19. Borkovec, T. D. and D. C. Fowles. Controlled investigation of the effects of progressive and hypnotic relaxation on insomnia. *Journal of Abnormal Psychology* 82:
153–158, 1973.

20. Nicassio, P., M. Boylan, and T. McCabe. Progressive relaxation, EMG biofeedback
and biofeedback placebo in the treatment of sleep-onset insomnia. *British Journal
of Medical Psychology* 55: 159–166, 1982.

21. Chesson, A. L., W. M. Anderson, M. Littner, D. Davila, K. Hartse, S. Johnson,
et al. Practice parameters for the nonpharmacologic treatment of chronic insomnia. *Sleep* 22: 1128–1133, 1999.

22. Hauri, P. Treating psychophysiologic insomnia with biofeedback. *Archives of General Psychiatry* 38: 752–758, 1981.

23. Hauri, P., L. Percy, C. Hellekson, E. Hartmann, and D. Russ. The treatment of psychophysiologic insomnia with biofeedback: A replication study. *Biofeedback Self
Regulation* 7: 223–234, 1982.

24. Espie, C., W. Lindsay, N. Brooks, E. M. Hood, and T. Turvey. A controlled comparative investigation of psychological treatments for chronic sleep-onset insomnia. *Behavioural Research and Therapy* 27: 79–88, 1989.

25. Bootzin, R. R. Stimulus control treatment for insomnia. *Proceedings, 80th Annual
Convention* American Psychological Association: 395–396, 1972.

26. Lacks, P., A. Bertelson, J. Sugerman, and J. Kunkel. The treatment of sleep-
maintenance insomnia with stimulus-control techniques. *Behavioural Research
and Therapy* 21: 291–295, 1983.

27. Hauri P. *Current Concepts: The Sleep Disorders.* Kalamazoo, MI: The Upjohn
Company. 1977.

28. Buysse, D., C. Reynolds, D. Kupfer, M. Thorpy, E. Bixler, A. Kales, et al. Effects
of diagnosis on treatment recommendations in chronic insomnia—a report from
the APA/NIMH *DSM-IV* field trial. *Sleep* 20: 542–552, 1997.

29. Stepanski, E. J. and J. K. Wyatt. Use of sleep hygiene in the treatment of insomnia.
Sleep Medicine Reviews in press.

30. Ascher, L. M. and R. M. Turner. Paradoxical intention and insomnia: An experimental investigation. *Behavioural Research and Therapy* 17: 408–411, 1979.

31. Turner, R. M. and L. M. Ascher. Controlled comparison of progressive relaxation,
stimulus control, and paradoxical intention therapies for insomnia. *Journal of Consulting and Clinical Psychology* 47: 500–508, 1979.

32. Ladouceur, R. and Y. Gros-Louis. Paradoxical intention vs stimulus control in the treatment of severe insomnia. *Journal of Behavior Therapy and Experimental Psychiatry* 17: 267–269, 1986.

33. Morin, C. M., P. J. Hauri, C. A. Espie, A. J. Spielman, D. J. Buysse, and R. R. Bootzin. Nonpharmacological treatment of chronic insomnia. *Sleep* 22: 1134–1156, 1999.

34. Spielman, A. J., P. Saskin, and M. J. Thorpy. Treatment of chronic insomnia by restriction of time in bed. *Sleep* 10: 45–56, 1987.

35. Spielman, A. Assessment of insomnia. *Clinical Psychology Review* 6: 11–26, 1986.

36. American Sleep Disorders Association. *The International Classification of Sleep Disorders, Revised: Diagnostic and Coding Manual.* Rochester, MN: American Sleep Disorders Association. 1997.

37. Jacobson, E. *You Must Relax* (4th Edition). New York, NY: McGraw-Hill Book Company, Inc. 1962.

38. Millet, J. A. P. *Insomnia: Its Cause and Treatment.* New York, NY: Greenberg Publisher, Inc. 1938.

39. Lichstein, K. and T. Rosenthal. Insomniacs' perceptions of cognitive vs. somatic determinants of sleep disturbance. *Journal of Abnormal Psychology* 89: 105–107, 1980.

40. Morin, C. M. *Insomnia: Psychological Assessment and Management.* New York, NY: Guilford Press. 1993.

41. Morin, C. M., C. Colecchi, J. Stone, R. Sood, and D. Brink. Behavioral and pharmacological therapies for late-life insomnia: A randomized controlled trial. *Journal of the American Medical Association* 281: 991–999, 1999.

42. Edinger J. D., W. K. Wohlgemuth, R. A. Radtke, G. R. Marsh, and R. E. Quillian. Cognitive behavioral therapy for treatment of chronic primary insomnia: A randomized controlled trial. *Journal of the American Medical Association* 285: 1856–1864, 2001.

43. Smith, M. T., M. L. Perlis, A. Park, M. S. Smith, J. Pennington, D. E. Giles, et al. Comparative meta-analysis of pharmacotherapy and behavior therapy for persistent insomnia. *American Journal of Psychiatry* 159: 5–11, 2002.

44. Espie, C. A., S. J. Inglis, and L. Harvey. Predicting clinically significant response to cognitive behavior therapy for chronic insomnia in general medical practice: Analysis of outcome data at 12 months posttreatment. *Journal of Consulting and Clinical Psychology* 69: 58–66, 2001.

45. Morin, C. M., J. P. Culvert, and S. M. Schwartz. Nonpharmacological interventions for insomnia: A meta-analysis of treatment efficacy. *American Journal of Psychiatry* 151: 1172–1180, 1994.

46. Murtagh, D. R. and K. M. Greenwood. Identifying effective psychological treatments for insomnia: A meta-analysis. *Journal of Consulting and Clinical Psychology* 63: 79–89, 1995.

47. Dashevsky, B. A. and M. Kramer. Behavioral treatment of chronic insomnia in psychiatrically ill patients. *Journal of Clinical Psychiatry* 59: 693–699, 1998.

48. Lichstein, K. L., N. M. Wilson, and C. T. Johnson. Psychological treatment of secondary insomnia. *Psychology of Aging* 15: 232–240, 2000.

49. Perlis, M. L., M. C. Sharpe, M. T. Smith, D. W. Greenblatt, and D. E. Giles. Behavioral treatment of insomnia: Treatment outcome and the relevance of medical and psychiatric morbidity. *Journal of Behavioral Medicine* 24: 281–296, 2001.

50. Rybarczyk, B., M. Lopez, R. Benson, C. Alsten, and E. Stepanski. The efficacy of two behavioral treatment programs for comorbid geriatric insomnia. *Psychology and Aging* 17: 288–298, 2002.

51. Lichstein, K. L., B. A. Peterson, B. W. Riedel, M. K. Means, M. I. Epperson, and R. N. Aguillard. Relaxation to assist sleep medication withdrawal. *Behavior Modification* 23: 379–402, 1999.

52. Mowrer, O. H. Apparatus for the study and treatment of enuresis. *American Journal of Psychology* 51: 163–166, 1938.

53. Mowrer, O. H. Enuresis: The beginning work—what really happened. *Journal of the History of the Behavioral Sciences* 16: 25–30, 1980.

54. Rushton, H. G. Nocturnal enuresis: Epidemiology, evaluation, and currently available treatment options. *Journal of Pediatrics* 114: 691–696, 1989.

55. Watson, J. B. *Psychological Care of Infant and Child.* New York, NY: W.W. Norton and Company, Inc. 1928.

56. France, K. and S. Hudson. Behavior management of infant sleep disturbance. *Journal of Applied Behavior Analysis* 23: 91–98, 1990.

57. Adams, L. and V. Rickert. Reducing bedtime tantrums: Comparisons between positive routines and graduated extinction. *Pediatrics* 84: 756–759, 1989.

58. Mindell, J. Sleep disorders in children. *Health Psychology* 12: 151–162, 1993.

59. Ferber, R. *Solving Your Child's Sleep Problems.* New York, NY: Simon & Schuster. 1985.

60. Rickert, V. and C. Johnson. Reducing nocturnal awakening and crying episodes in infants and young children: A comparison between scheduled awakenings and systematic ignoring. *Pediatrics* 81: 203–212, 1988.

61. Mindell, J. Empirically supported treatments in pediatric psychology: Bedtime refusal and night wakings in young children. *Journal of Pediatric Psychology* 24: 465–481, 1999.

62. Mahowald, M. W. and G. M. Rosen. Parasomnias in children. *Pediatrician* 17: 21–31, 1990.

63. Krakow, B., M. Hollifield, L. Johnston, M. Koss, R. Schrader, T. D. Warner, et al. Imagery rehearsal therapy for chronic nightmares in sexual assault survivors with posttraumatic stress disorder: A randomized controlled trial. *Journal of the American Medical Association* 286: 537–545, 2001.

64. Weitzman, E. D., C. Czeisler, R. Coleman, A. J. Spielman, J. Zimmerman, W. C. Dement, et al. Delayed sleep phase syndrome: A chronobiological disorder with sleep onset insomnia. *Archives of General Psychiatry* 38: 737–746, 1981.

65. Czeisler, C. A., J. F. Duffy, T. L. Shanahan, E. N. Brown, J. F. Mitchell, D. W. Rimmer, et al. Stability, precision, and near-24-hour period of the human circadian pacemaker. *Science* 284: 2177–2181, 1999.

66. Czeisler, C. A. and S. B. Khalsa. The human circadian timing system and sleep-wake regulation. In M. Kryger, T. Roth, and W. C. Dement, eds. *Principles and Practice of Sleep Medicine* (3rd Edition). Philadelphia, PA: W.B. Saunders Company. 2000: 353–375.

67. Carskadon, M., S. Labyak, C. Acebo, and R. Seifer. Intrinsic circadian period of adolescent humans measured in conditions of forced desynchrony. *Neuroscience Letter* 260: 129–132, 1999.

68. Carskadon, M. A., C. Acebo, and R. Seifer. Extended nights, sleep loss, and recovery sleep in adolescents. *Archives Italiennes de Biologie* 139: 301–312, 2001.

69. Carskadon, M., A. Wolfson, C. Acebo, O. Tzischinsky, and R. Seifer. Adolescent sleep patterns, circadian timing, and sleepiness at a transition to early school days. *Sleep* 21: 871–881, 1998.

70. Eastman, C. and S. Martin. How to use light and dark to produce circadian adaptation to shift work. *Annals of Medicine* 31: 87–98, 1999.

71. Kribbs, N., A. Pack, L. Kline, P. Smith, A. Schwartz, N. Schubert, et al. Objective measurement of patterns of nasal CPAP use by patients with obstructive sleep apnea. *American Review of Respiratory Diseases* 147: 887–895, 1994.

72. Aloia, M., M. Perlis, D. Giles, L. DiDio, N. Illniczky, and D. Greenblatt. Improving compliance with CPAP in elderly patients with OSA. *Sleep* 22: S228–S229, 1999.

73. Speer, T. and R. Fayle. The effect of systematic desensitization and sensory awareness training on adherence to CPAP treatment. *Sleep Research* 26: 216, 1997.

74. Zozula, R. and R. Rosen. Compliance with continuous positive airway pressure therapy: Assessing and improving treatment outcomes. *Current Opinion in Pulmonary Medicine* 7: 391–398, 2001.

SECTION II

Assessment

Chapter 2

THE MEASUREMENT OF SLEEP

LEISHA J. SMITH, SARA NOWAKOWSKI, JAMES P. SOEFFING,
HENRY J. ORFF, AND MICHAEL L. PERLIS

The goal of this chapter is to provide clinicians unfamiliar with the measurement of sleep a comprehensive overview of this subject. In addition, we provide specific information about the characteristic sleep continuity and architectural abnormalities that occur in the five major intrinsic sleep disorders (obstructive sleep apnea, periodic leg movements of sleep, narcolepsy, primary insomnia, and delayed sleep phase syndrome). Clinicians who already have a substantial expertise in the area of sleep medicine and/or behavioral sleep medicine may also benefit from the information provided, given the detailed coverage of the technical aspects of polysomnography (PSG).

This chapter is divided into four sections:

1. Ways of measuring sleep
2. Principles of PSG
3. Polysomnographic evaluation of sleep disorders
4. Future directions concerning the measurement of sleep

WAYS OF MEASURING SLEEP

The four primary methods for measuring sleep are direct observation (e.g., nurse observations), self-report instruments (both questionnaires and sleep diaries), actigraphy, and PSG. While PSG represents the gold standard for both clinical and research applications, each of the assessment strategies has distinct advantages and disadvantages. Following, each form of assessment is described and critiqued.

Direct Observation

Apart from its ubiquitous use by bed partners and family members, direct observation is often used in a formal way in medical settings. For example, a nurse on an inpatient unit may observe and record whether patients are asleep or awake on some interval basis (e.g., every 30 or 60 minutes). For this measure, the observer necessarily relies on a variety of cues and on the context for those cues. As one might guess, the judgment that someone is asleep is made based on the following cues: recumbent body position, an absence of movement, slow and regular breathing pattern, blank facial expression, and closed eyes. These cues are not, in and of themselves or even in combination, likely to be sensitive and specific for sleep or wakefulness. The observer must also take context into account. For example, recumbent body position, absence of movement, slow and regular breathing pattern, blank facial expression, and closed eyes are suggestive of sleep *only if the subject is in bed.* The same cues observed while someone is lying on a sidewalk would not so much suggest sleep as they would suggest unconsciousness. Thus, both *cues* and *context* are important for the direct observation approach to assessing sleep.

Given the correct context, each of the major cues (along with repeated sampling) may be used to reasonably measure the occurrence of sleep and to derive estimates of:

1. How long it takes the patient to fall asleep (formally referred to as *sleep latency* [SL]).
2. How frequently the patient wakes up during the night (sometimes referred to as *frequency of nocturnal awakenings* [FNA]).
3. How much time the patient spends awake during the night (formally referred to as *wake after sleep onset* [WASO]).
4. How much total time the patient spends asleep throughout the night (formally referred to as *total sleep time* [TST]).

Collectively, these variables are referred to as *sleep continuity measures.*

The temporal resolution of direct observation is obviously limited to the sampling rate that is used. If bed checks occur at an hourly interval (q60), the resolution of the method is no better than plus or minus 60 minutes. Thus, estimates of sleep latency, wake after sleep onset, and total sleep time could be off by as much as an hour. Most would agree that this is too poor a resolution for research purposes, and many would argue that the q60 interval has little clinical value as well. A 15- or 30-minute interval is likely to be adequate, but such a high sampling rate is problematic for at least two reasons. First, even during third shift work, such a task would be unduly time consuming. Second, the monotony of such work would likely yield unreliable estimates. If these considerations were not important (i.e., a frequent sampling rate was used and the arbiter was completely vigilant about the task), there is still reason to question the absolute validity of the method. After all, the observer may simply be incorrect, even given all the right cues and context. That is, someone may be awake despite being in the right time and place for sleep and showing the telltale signs of sleep.

One way to enhance the validity of this approach is to determine if the patient is responsive and how much stimulation is required to elicit a response, the assumption being that a slow latency to response and/or the need for greater than usual levels of stimulation is indicative of sleep. Such an effort to enhance the validity of this method, however, runs the risk of having the measurement strategy alter the very thing one seeks to measure. That is, it is possible (if not likely) that any attempt to actively probe whether someone is asleep will result in an awakening and lead to underestimates of sleep quantity. Alternatively, refraining from actively probing the state of consciousness may lead to overestimates of sleep quantity.

Summary

The direct observation technique, given a high sampling rate (q15 or q30 minutes), may have some general utility within the hospital setting. The method, it seems to us, is not ideal for routine clinical or research use in studies which seek to specifically study sleep disorders.

Self-Report Measures

Retrospective Self-Report

This kind of measurement is commonly used socially to inquire about the quality and quantity of bed partner's and family members' sleep, hence, the ubiquitous "How did you sleep last night?" In the more formal application, retrospective self-report data are usually gathered using multi-item paper and pencil measures. Examples of the more established instruments include the Brock Sleep and Insomnia Questionnaire (BSIQ; 1), Pittsburgh Sleep Quality Index (PSQI; 2–3), and the Insomnia Severity Index (ISI; 4). More recently, our group has developed a computer-based multifactorial insomnia scale—the Rochester Sleep Continuity Inventory (RSCI). While, at the time of this writing, the instrument is still being validated, a copy of the program output is included as an appendix to illustrate the kind of information that such questionnaires typically gather (see Appendix 2.1 on p. 65).

Retrospective self-report instruments are usually administered on one occasion (at intake) but are often also used as pre- and postmeasures (e.g., the PSQI and ISI were expressly designed for this application). As with direct observation, this method allows for the acquisition of the standard sleep continuity parameters inclusive of SL, FNA, WASO, and TST. In addition, these measures may be used to gather a wide array of biopsychosocial information ranging from standard demographic information to medical and psychological profile information to family and relationship data. This is especially true of the longer survey instruments, which are often constructed as in-house measures.

The temporal resolution of retrospective reporting is obviously less of an issue for this assessment method. However, the issue is still relevant in two ways. First, when providing estimates of SL, WASO, and TST, patients are asked to do so in minutes, which leads to the question "Can patients make such estimates to this level of precision?" One way to address this issue is to consider what people are naturally inclined to do when asked to make such judgments. With the exception of total sleep time, most individuals appear comfortable with estimating the various parameters on a scale with minute or fractions of an hour units. Perhaps this is true because most subjects, for at least the first third of their lives, take less than an hour to fall asleep and are awake for less than an hour over the course of the night. Thus, the natural unit for such estimates is minutes.

It is also important to consider, irrespective of whether subjects are naturally inclined to estimate sleep continuity in terms of minutes, whether subjects can:

1. Actually make such fine discriminations
2. Log them into and recall them from long-term memory when asked to for the purposes of completing questionnaires

Second, when providing estimates of SL, WASO, and TST, subjects are asked to assess what is typical for them. Thus, retrospective self-report measures require that subjects understand the concept of "an average" or that they have some valid means of estimating what is typical for them. While it is hoped that such estimates are made based on true personal averages, it is more likely that retrospectively reported sleep continuity estimates are derived using heuristics. That is, subjects may estimate how they have been sleeping based not on their personal average, but rather on the worst case scenario (saliency), how they slept last night (recency), or how they slept on the first night of the time increment in question (primacy).

Summary

The value of questionnaires is primarily that they:

1. Are easy to administer
2. Allow for a comprehensive assessment
3. Usually require minimal explanation

4. Are inexpensive

5. Are likely to have sufficient sensitivity to resolve changes in sleep patterns over time

Perhaps the most serious limitation of the retrospective self-report measure in terms of validity is, as mentioned previously, that it is a single sample method, which requires subjects to provide estimates in terms of averages. The single sample method prevents the calculation of averages by the investigators and requires the subjects to, in the absence of veridical memory for the events in question, guesstimate using heuristics such as saliency, recency, and primacy. These issues withstanding, there is no question that retrospective estimates are clinically important; they (1) provide the means by which one may simply and comprehensively characterize the patient's chief complaint and (2) represent the appropriate starting point for treatment. Whether such instruments are ideal for research is open to debate. Retrospective measures are probably most useful when applied within simple between-subject design experiments, where groups are being compared at one time point for their natural sleep disturbance profiles. In contrast, retrospective measures are probably the least useful when used in pre- and post-study designs. In this context, the measurement strategy is challenged because it is open to experimental demand.

Prospective Self-Report (Sleep-Wake Diaries)

This form of measurement is the standard of practice for behavioral sleep medicine. The measurement strategy requires that subjects keep a daily log or diary for an extended time interval so that the behaviors of interest can be sampled across time. Like retrospective sleep continuity assessments, sleep diaries also require subjects to make estimates of how long it takes them to fall asleep, how many times they awaken across the night, and so on. All of the traditional sleep continuity variables may be obtained via this strategy, including SL, FNA, WASO, and TST. In addition, most clinicians and investigators use sampled data to derive one additional measure referred to as *sleep efficiency* (SE%). This variable is a ratio of *total sleep time* to *time in bed* (TST/TIB). This measure may be obtained using retrospective measures but is usually calculated when sleep diary data are available. While there are no industry standard sleep-wake sleep diaries, two are included in the appendixes as examples. Both are single-page instruments (one of which is double sided) that allow for daily information to be recorded for a seven-day time frame (see Appendixes 2.2 on pp. 66–67 and 2.3 on pp. 68–69).

The primary difference between the retrospective and prospective methods is that the estimate provided by the subject applies to only one time point (last night) and, therefore, does not require subjects to understand the concept of an average or use heuristics to form and relay impressions about their sleep quantity and quality.

The primary value with obtaining nightly estimates via the use of sleep diaries is that it allows the clinician/investigator:

1. To collect a reasonable sample on which to calculate measures of central tendency and night-to-night variability
2. The ability to conduct contingency analyses

With respect to the latter point, behavioral sleep medicine specialists often sample a standard repertoire of behaviors so that they can determine whether certain traditional factors are related to the incidence and severity of insomnia symptoms. For example, does the patient nap? Does sleep latency reliably get longer on the days that the patient naps? A covariation between these would suggest to the therapist that napping behavior needs to be modified or eliminated. Because many of the behavioral contingencies vis-à-vis insomnia have been well delineated (e.g., the maladaptive behaviors of napping, extending sleep opportunity, caffeine use, the use of alcohol as a sedative), these are often not included on, or measured with, sleep diaries. Prospective measurement, nonetheless, allows for the engagement of broad-based contingency analysis when the need arises.

The temporal resolution of prospective reporting, as with retrospective reports, is scaled in minutes. As noted previously, whether subjects can accurately accomplish this is open to question. Also open to question is whether the two forms of self-report actually yield significantly different data. That is, while it stands to reason that different methods will yield different parameter estimates, this need not be the case. To our knowledge, there are no published studies comparing prospective and retrospective estimates of sleep continuity. A preliminary study by our group suggests that the two methods do indeed provide different parameter estimates, but the direction of bias is not uniform (5). Our data show that when asked to make retrospective estimates on single survey instruments, patients report longer sleep latencies (+21.9 ±6.9 min) and less total sleep (−44.0 ±11.5 min) compared to diary data. This tendency toward more extreme estimates, however, was not reflected in retrospective estimates of number and duration of awakenings. When completing questionnaires, subjects report fewer awakenings (−0.72 ±0.28) and that awakenings are of shorter duration (−54.2 ±7.9 min) than those reported via sleep diaries. Because the direction of the bias is not constant, this suggests that retrospective assessments are not simply biased toward the exaggeration of symptoms. One alternative interpretation is that patients with insomnia, on interview (i.e., when assessed using retrospective instruments), may be more sensitive to sleep initiation difficulties and may not appreciate the extent to which sleep maintenance problems contribute to their insomnia. What factors mediate these discrepancies remain to be determined.

One final issue with respect to use of self-report measures to assess sleep continuity is whether such measures are truly useful because they are not objective measures, that is, forms of measurement that are made using instruments that do not require human judgment (observer or self report). At first blush, it seems obvious that the far superior strategy is to use objective measures like actigraphy or polysomnography. Since, however, the patient's perception of disability and/or disease cannot be irrelevant or inconsequential, it seems that in a one or the other scenario, self report measures of sleep continuity disturbance are actually more useful than the two widely used objective measures. While such a claim may seem to verge on the ridiculous, imagine the development of a miracle drug that yields perfect sleep when assessed by polysomnography but at the same time leaves the patient's initial presenting complaint unchanged. Given these circumstances, it is unlikely that the miracle drug would be a *big seller*. In short, self report cannot be irrelevant for clinical practice or clinical research. Such measures are required so that we can assess the patient's sense of disorder and recovery given treatment. Ultimately, the issue is not a matter of which measure is best, but rather which combination of approaches best allows us to be able to appreciate both the subjective and objective components of the disease in question.

Summary

The value of prospective measures is related to, in a word, *sampling*. Acquiring serial data allows for:

1. Stronger inferences about the frequency and severity of sleep continuity disturbance
2. The pursuit of proper contingency analysis, should the need arise

The primary problem with prospective self-report is, perhaps, the matter of getting good compliance. People may not remember, or may choose not, to fill out their diaries when they get up in the morning and thus may find themselves completing the diary at some later time. Needless to say, this practice undermines the inherent value of the method. As disturbing, the investigator/clinician is not in the position to determine whether the forms were completed each day on waking or minutes before the session. Thus, gaining and monitoring compliance represent a significant drawback of this approach. One final methodologic limitation is that there are no universally accepted forms of this measure; thus, it remains possible that different versions of sleep diaries may yield different characterizations of sleep continuity. A solution to both problems may be, however, at hand; diaries administered via the internet or via PDA devices will allow compliance to be assessed and thereby not only allow for adherence to be a measured variable but also may promote compliance given that patients/subjects know that this aspect of their behavior is being monitored.

Actigraphy

Actigraphy has its roots in a basic science methodology. In the basic application, the detection of movement and the absence of movement are used to infer when an animal is awake or asleep; the inference is that during wakefulness, there is a substantial amount of movement and that during sleep, movement occurs only sporadically.

When acquired from animals, movement is usually detected in one of two ways. In animals that use running wheels, the motion of the wheel itself is used to obtain activity counts (e.g., one turn = one count). In animals that do not use running wheels, motion detection grids or implanted telemetric devices may be used to obtain movement counts. In both cases, such data (when obtained along with some measure of temporal phase, e.g., nocturnal versus diurnal phase, clock time, and/or circadian time) allow for the calculation of total sleep, total wakefulness, frequency of nocturnal awakenings, wake after sleep onset, and amount of diurnal activity.

All of these strategies require that the movement data be sampled and summated for prespecified time intervals. These intervals are then assigned wake or sleep based on the activity counts that occur for the prespecified time intervals within the designated sleep phase. Diurnal activity, in turn, can be quantified by summing the activity counts for the designated wake phase. Finally, if the device also has a photo sensor or is capable of recording the moments of *lights-off* and *lights-on,* these measures can be used to determine the experimental equivalent of sleep opportunity or time in bed and allow inferences about sleep latency and sleep efficiency.

When movement recordings are made over successive 24-hour periods and are plotted in series (it is also helpful to double-plot such data), phase shifts in the sleep-wake cycle also can be detected (see Figure 2.1 and legend). Such data were and are extremely useful for chronobiologic research.

Similar principles are used with actigraphy. In this case, movement in the extremities is detected by placing a small motion detector on the wrist. The detector is housed in a wristwatch-like case and contains not only the detector but also an A-to-D converter, memory chips, a microprocessor, a clock, and a power source (see Figure 2.2).

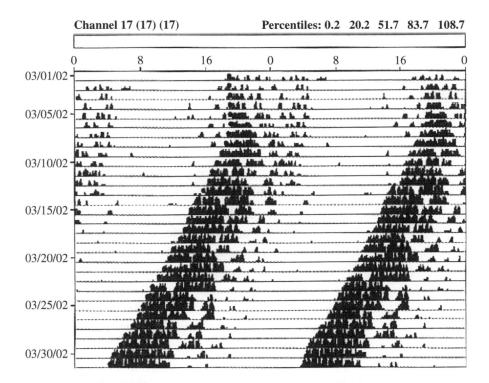

Channel 17 (17) (17)   Percentiles: 0.2   20.2   51.7   83.7   108.7

Figure 2.1   A Double Plotted Actogram of a Mouse Following Release into Constant Dark. Each line represents 48 hours. The initial rhythm remains close to the 24 h light/dark cycle; then the mouse free runs for a period of less than 24 hours. The plot is supplied by Susan Benloucif, PhD, Department of Neurology, Northwestern University Medical School.

The detector is typically a small piezoelectric accelerometer that generates voltages when there is movement across the radius-to-ulna axis or a wrist flexion-extension. In other words, most actigraphs are sensitive to movement in two planes (*x*, if you were moving your wrist as in waving, or *y*, as in dribbling a basketball). The sensors also detect movement in the *z* plane (such as throwing a punch) but are less sensitive to this form of movement. The resultant voltages

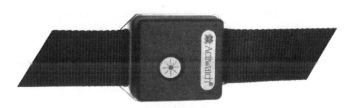

Figure 2.2   Picture of an Actigraph. Supplied by Mini-Mitter Co., Inc.

are then converted from analog signals to digital values, typically at a rate of about 30 times per second (range 10 to 32+ Hz). The values, which are scaled to a *byte* metric (0 to 255 counts), are summated online over fixed time increments (1 to 20 seconds) and are stored in memory in *bins*. The data in these bins may be further compressed by storing the summated counts as the sum total of multiple bins for a user-specified *epoch*. Epoch lengths range from 15 seconds to 15 minutes. Data may be acquired for periods of up to 30 days or more.

The epoch data for the entire measurement interval are transferred to a computer that has the setup and reader interface, visual displays for the data, and scoring algorhythms. The scoring algorhythms are applied to the epoch data, which are consecutively arrayed and are usually locked to clock time. Each epoch, usually of no longer duration than two minutes for the purposes of sleep scoring, is evaluated for whether it represents sleep or wakefulness. This determination is made according to one of several procedures, each of which uses a threshold approach. The threshold method may be assessed for either the amplitude or time domains. An example of an amplitude assessment is an epoch judged to be wake when the sum voltage for the epoch has a value of greater than some predetermined amount. An example of a time domain assessment (for instruments that retain the individual bin data) is an epoch judged to be wake when some percent of the total epoch time has voltages greater than some predetermined amount. The threshold for the three most well known commercial systems (Mini-Mitter Company, Inc., Ambulatory Monitoring Inc., IM Systems, Inc.) may also be adjusted by the investigator or clinician to suit the needs of an individual case (e.g., the sensitivity of the actigraph would have to be decreased for a patient with a persistent tremor).

Figure 2.3 shows an example of the data output from a subject studied with actigraphy. Note the clear differentiation between the wake and sleep periods, the ability to zoom in on the sleep window, the variable amplitude option (see upper right hand corner [scaling factor]), the event marks along the upper portion of the actogram, and the data summary at the bottom of the figure.

Unlike the basic science activity monitors, which require that the animal be kept in a defined space (in a grid or near telemetry receivers), actigraphic devices are fully portable and allow for unrestricted ambulatory studies. In addition to being able to obtain data on total wake time, total sleep time, frequency of nocturnal awakenings, wake after sleep onset, and sleep phase, actigraphs may also allow for the acquisition of a true sleep latency measure—one that allows the intent to fall asleep to be taken into account. This is simply done by fitting the actigraph with an event marker. When such a marker is available (a standard commercial offering), a button press indicates the subject's desire to fall asleep. The time elapsed from the event mark to when activity falls below the threshold

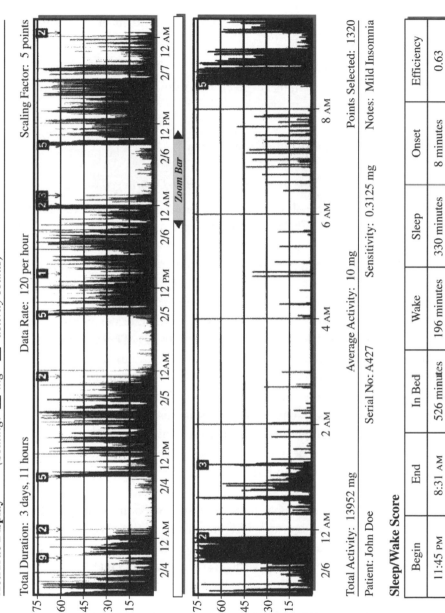

Figure 2.3 An Example of an Actogram

for wakefulness (for some predetermined number of consecutive epochs) equals sleep latency.

The three primary limitations of this technology are:

1. Very little work has been done to validate this form of measurement in sleep-disordered subjects.
2. The relative expense of the equipment as compared to self-report instruments.
3. The inability of the equipment, given its expense, to obtain more than just sleep continuity data.

Two of these issues are not substantial problems.

Few Validation Studies of This Technology in Sleep-Disordered Subjects

The application of this technology to sleep research and clinical sleep medicine, and particularly to the study of insomnia, is fairly recent. As of 2003, less than a dozen studies have been conducted to evaluate the validity of this method. Traditionally, these studies examine the association between actigraphically and polysomnographically assessed sleep continuity (6). Of these studies, most are in healthy good sleeper subjects. In general, the normative studies show epoch-to-epoch agreement rates of up to 97% and sleep parameter correlations for total time awake and/or total sleep time of up to $r = 0.94$ (7). These statistics correspond to an average discrepancy (in real time) of less than 10 minutes, where PSG measures tend to detect more sleep time (6, 8). Interestingly, none of the investigations to date evaluate the extent to which there is good convergence between actigraphic and polysomnographic measures of sleep latency. This is likely because both actigraph and PSG measures of sleep latency are variably defined and only the newer devices have the event markers required to measure the latency between the intent to fall asleep and the onset of sleep as measured by sustained inactivity.

As applied in clinical samples of patients with insomnia, actigraphy has been found to be less well correlated with PSG measures. While early studies suggest that the rate of disagreement between the measures is four times that observed in good sleepers, the most recent of the various studies suggests that these error rates are inflated. The most recent study suggests that the average correlation between the measures (for both patients with primary insomnia and sleep state misperception) is about $r = 0.77$ (9). While this degree of correlation is clearly of a smaller magnitude, the average discrepancy tends to be less than 25 minutes, where PSG measures once again tend to detect more sleep time. (Interestingly, this "offset" tends to be comparable to the subjective-objective discrepancy for total sleep time evident when PSG is compared to prospective self-report measures; 10.)

The reason that actigraphy, as compared to PSG measures, tends to underestimate total sleep time is unknown. Jean-Louis and colleagues suggest that this may be due to increased motor activity in the sleep of patients with insomnia (9). If true, this implies that more liberal threshold definitions may be used to reduce the error rate. An alternative explanation for the reduced accuracy of actigraphic measures, given that patients with insomnia do not exhibit more motor activity during sleep (10), may be related to the enhanced sensitivity of PSG measures. That is, if actigraphy requires 60 to 300 seconds time to make an accurate assessment of sleep (a time increment comparable to what humans take to distinguish sleep from wakefulness [11]) and given that PSG measures require only 30 seconds to reliably detect the occurrence of sleep, actigraphic measures might be up to 10 times less precise, especially for short duration bouts of sleep or for the initial sleep onset intervals following intermittent awakenings. In this case, the resolution of actigraphy might be enhanced by using algorhythms, which take context into account (not unlike human scoring of PSGs). One way this might be done is to increase the thresholds for the assessment of wakefulness when one or more contiguous epochs (before and/or after the epoch in question) are scored as sleep.

Regardless of whether the method has the same sensitivity and specificity as it does when applied to good sleepers, actigraphy may still be very useful for clinical work and clinical research. This is potentially true for essentially two reasons. First, actigraphy may be particularly useful for the assessment of treatment outcome because the measure (like PSG measures) is not confounded by expectancy effects and does not require much subject compliance to obtain data. Second, actigraphy may be exceptionally useful for the quantification of so-called "sleep state misperception." That is, actigraphy, in combination with prospective self-report measures, may allow for the resolution of the subjective-objective discrepancies that normally can be detected only with PSG. Both avenues should be explored in the future.

The Relative Expense of the Strategy

While the cost of this kind of instrumentation has substantially decreased over recent years, the average cost for a single system is approximately $2,500: The wrist actigraph costs between $850 and $2,000, the acquisition device or reader costs approximately $650, and the software that scores the actigraphic data starts at about $500 and may exceed $2,000. This kind of expense is far in excess of the costs of sleep diaries, even professionally printed versions. Thus, the upfront costs are higher, and the per diem costs are clearly greater. The upfront costs will continue to be a problem until such time that the purchase of actigraphs can be done in some other way than as a capital expense. Perhaps this could be resolved by having the manufacturers offer clinicians a way of distributing the expense over time (i.e., an extended payment plan). As for the per diem costs, this expense can be estimated as follows: If the use life of an actigraphic system is five years, 300 days per year, the cost per day of the least expensive system would be about $1.65 per day. The traditional week-long assessment, therefore, would cost approximately $12, and the typical eight-week course of treatment would cost approximately $100. While this expense is not exorbitant, it is still substantially more expensive than *paper-n'-pencil* measures. One way for these expenses to be offset, and to incentivize clinicians to use the method, is to have actigraphic assessments count as billable procedures which have, in turn, the standard CPT codes that allow for third-party reimbursement. Needless to say, being able to bill for the procedure will allow for the amortization of the capital expense and offer a potential avenue for a profit margin.

In the final analysis, the question of whether to use actigraphy cannot be only an economic one. The other important issue is, and must be, "How is patient care enhanced by the application of actigraphy?" There are several possibilities:

- When actigraphy is used as the primary means to assess sleep continuity:
    —Its objective nature allows for greater confidence in the validity of the data as compared to sleep diary data.
    —The probability of obtaining daily samples is enhanced by diminishing the need for patients to comply with the work of completing sleep diaries.
- When used in combination with sleep diaries, actigraphy may provide an inexpensive means to identify and quantify sleep state misperception.
- When actigraphy is used with on-board supplementary measures (e.g., event markers, photo, skin, and/or core body temperature sensors, respiratory effort data, and/or subjective event marking via on-board scoring keypads), the expanded assessment ability may allow for inexpensive screens for sleep-related circadian or respiratory disorders.

In addition to these considerations, actigraphy may greatly expand the clinician's ability to conduct interesting case series-type research. Two examples are:

1. The actigraph's ability to quantify diurnal activity may provide a means to evaluate the association of daily activity with sleep continuity.
2. The actigraph's ability to measure exposure to natural light may provide a means to evaluate the association of daily light exposure with sleep continuity.

Summary

The primary strengths of this measurement strategy are that it:

1. Allows for an assessment of sleep continuity that is free from either self-report or observer bias
2. Requires minimal subject compliance
3. Has excellent temporal resolution (allows for the detection of periods of wakefulness as brief as 60 seconds in duration)
4. Allows for the continuous assessment for periods of up to 60 days

As indicated previously, the primary concern about this technology is that very little work has been done to validate it in sleep-disordered subjects. We believe that actigraphy will be particularly valuable for the assessment and treatment of insomnia. To secure this promise, it will be necessary to establish that:

1. There is a stable, if not good, concordance between actigraphy and sleep diary and/or PSG assessed sleep continuity.
2. Sleep state misperception is adequately measured with actigraphy.
3. Actigraphy is sensitive enough (especially to sleep efficiency) to be used as a serial measure for treatment and treatment studies. Once these are demonstrated, it is entirely plausible that actigraphy will be to insomnia what the PSG is to OSA: the standard for clinical assessment.

Polysomnography

Direct observation, self report, and actigraphy, while useful for the measurement of sleep continuity, all suggest that sleep is a unitary state. That is, something that one is either in or not in, and once in, the state itself is a single thing. Introspection, however, would lead us to think otherwise. Certainly, it feels true that there is shallow and deep sleep and dream and "not-dream" sleep. This alone suggests that there are 2 to 4 stages or states of sleep. With the advent of PSG, it was found that such impressions are indeed rooted in something that can be objectively measured.

PSG, as it is used to define states of consciousness, is composed of three measures: electroencephalography (EEG), electromyography (EMG), and electrooccculography (EOG). Each of these measures, while based on different source potentials, capitalizes on naturally occurring electrical currents that are radiated from the scalp, muscles, and eyes. These currents can be represented continuously and plotted over time. Such graphs provide a moment-by-moment view of brain, motor, and eye movement activity. The combination of these plots allows for the detection and categorization of no less than five stages of sleep.

The measurement of sleep by PSG allows for objective measurement, excellent temporal (moment-by-moment) resolution, direct and quantitative measures of brain and somatic activity during sleep, and the ability to resolve substates that are not apparent with other measures. Coupled with other electrophysiological measures (e.g., electrocardiograms, nasal/oral air flow, etc.), this methodology paved the way for the first observations about the medical disorders that occur during sleep. Accordingly, the PSG mode of assessment is the gold standard for sleep research and neurologic and pulmonary sleep medicine. While PSG is not considered integral to the direct practice of behavioral sleep medicine, knowledge about the measure is required so that behavioral specialists can excel in our multi-disciplinary field.

PRINCIPLES OF POLYSOMNOGRAPHY

The Electroencephalographic Measure of Sleep: The Source Potential of the Electroencephalographic Signal

At the heart of PSG is the measure of the brain's electrical output. The formal term, *electroencephalography* (EEG), roughly translated, means "tracings or graphs of the electrical currents that are radiated from the scalp." A more formal definition is as follows: EEG is a continuous variance in voltage over time where the source potential for the voltage is derived from slow potential activity of the dendrites and somas residing within the first three layers of the cortex. This radiating activity, which is temporally and spatially summated, has characteristic voltages of between ~ 5 and ~ 200 microvolts (μV) and appears as an oscillating frequency with characteristic periodicities of between 0.5 and 45 Hz.

The voltage range may strike some as odd, given that the intracellular voltages of neuronal tissue is an order of magnitude larger (millivolt range). This difference in voltage results from the fact that the source signal obtained at the surface of the scalp is radiated through a variety of impeding media such as the arachnoid, dura and pia mater, periosteom, cerebral spinal fluid, bone, adipose, and epidural tissue. Thus, it can be said that the source voltage is attenuated as it is transmitted across the relatively large distance and through relatively nonconductive media to the electrode-sensor affixed to the scalp. This attenuation phenomena is schematically represented in Figure 2.4.

The voltage source may also seem curious. Slow potential activity, the graded potentials (IPSP and EPSPs) that continuously occur within somatic and dendritic

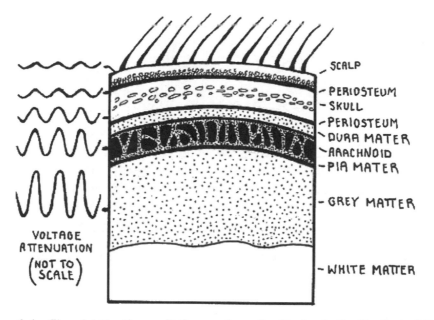

Figure 2.4   Signal Attention as It Occurs from the Cortex to the Surface of the Scalp. Note that the loss of signal is represented by the series of sine waves, which schematically represent the attenuation of signal as it passes through (and is impeded by) multiple layers of nonconductive media.

tissue, is the primary constituent of the EEG signal for two reasons. First, the most dorsal layer of the cortex (most proximal to the surface electrode [layer 1]) is composed largely of the apical dendrites from the pyramidal cells of the second and third layers of the cortex. This is schematically represented in Figure 2.5. Thus, the electrode picks up the radiating currents from that which is most close by. Second, because axonal tissue is wrapped in myelin, it is sufficiently insulated as to not leak much current.

The frequency range of the EEG concomitants of sleep is largely restricted to the lower portion of the EEG spectrum (0.5 to 14 Hz), while the EEG activity that is characteristic of wakefulness is largely restricted to the upper portion of the EEG spectrum (14 to 45 Hz). What actually constitutes the uppermost portion of the EEG spectrum during both wakefulness and sleep is somewhat controversial. Many investigators believe that pure EEG activity is limited to about 20 cycles per second (Hz) and that activity between 14 and 20 Hz (Beta) is unique to wakefulness and/or consciousness. Activity faster than 20 Hz, according to this point of view, is not thought to originate from the cortex but rather from the facial and scalp musculature. There is now, however, a growing body of evidence to suggest that activity from 20 to about 45 Hz does occur in the central nervous system and that such activity may represent sensory and information

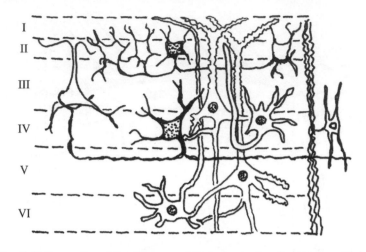

Figure 2.5   A Schematic of the Neuronal Substrate for the Source Potential for the EEG Signal

processing (12–17). This form of EEG is variably referred to as either *Gamma* or *40 Hz* activity. Interestingly, Beta and Gamma frequencies may co-occur with the traditional sleep EEG frequencies (0.5 to 14 Hz) and may be increased in the EEG sleep of patients with primary insomnia (18–19).

While the number of EEG measures that can be gathered from across the scalp has varied with time and the precision of this technology (the original standard system developed by Jasper [20] allowed for 21 measures of EEG activity), only one EEG is required to observe and differentiate four out of the five stages of sleep. As construed continuously, these stages appear to move from a kind of activity that is fast frequency and low voltage (formally referred to as *desynchronized EEG*) to a kind of activity that is slow frequency and high voltage (formally referred to as *synchronized EEG*). This progressive pattern of EEG slowing has been classified in terms of four stages. Characteristic tracings for each of these stages are illustrated in Figure 2.6.

The Purpose of Electroocculographic (EOG) and Electromyograpic (EMG) Measures in Polysomnography

With a single EEG measure (usually obtained from over the central region of the cortex in between the motor and sensory cortices [EEG designations C3, CZ, or C4]), the fifth stage of sleep or the so-called *third state of consciousness* cannot be reliably detected. This form of sleep has two unique characteristics (rapid eye movements and the absence of muscle tone), which require that two additional measures be used to characterize the state: EOG and EMG. Without

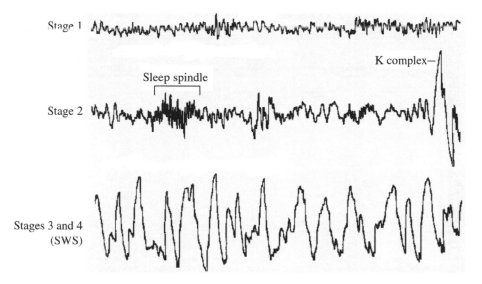

Figure 2.6   EEG of Stages 1, 2, and Slow Wave Sleep (Stages 3 and 4)

these measures, it is nearly impossible to distinguish between Stage 1 sleep and REM sleep (see Figure 2.7). Both have relatively desynchronous EEG patterns, but only REM sleep is accompanied by rapid eye movements and the sudden loss of muscle tone (atonia).

As a testament to how closely Stage 1 sleep resembles REM sleep, the first observations of REM sleep were misidentified and were referred to as *ascendant Stage 1* (21). Pictured in Figure 2.8 is a characteristic tracing of REM sleep.

While the functional correlate(s) of rapid eye movements are unknown, it is thought that the eye movements correspond to a variety of processes including scanning, emotional processing, and vestibulo-occular reflexes. The functional correlate of the loss of muscle tone appears to be more straightforward. Atonia is the electromyographic concomitant of the motor inhibition that occurs during REM sleep. This form of inhibition prevents the execution of coordinated voluntary movement during REM sleep and, presumably, prevents individuals from literally acting out their dreams (22).

Electrooculography is not only required for the reliable detection of REM sleep, it is also helpful in the effort to identify sleep onset. When a person begins

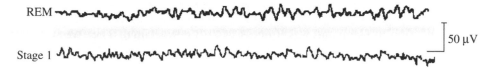

Figure 2.7   Example of the Similarity between the EEG of Stage 1 and REM Sleep

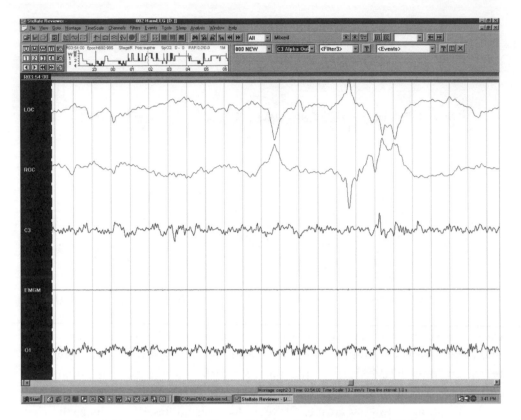

Figure 2.8   Stage REM Sleep, Stellate Harmonie-Luna™ Software

to fall asleep, the eyes will begin to slowly move back and forth. These movements are called *slow eye movements* (SEMs) and are usually observed within a few minutes of EEG-defined sleep onset (see Figure 2.9).

Regardless of whether one is seeking to measure SEMs or REMs, two channels of EOGs are generally required to represent eye movement. These channels are set up so that slow or fast eye movements are represented by (cross channel) out-of-phase oscillations. This strategy allows for the more precise differentiation between the slow EEG activity that occurs as an artifact in the EOG channels and frank eye movements. Examples of eye movement activity and how they are represented by EOG are shown in Figure 2.10.

One EEG, even in combination with EOG and EMG measures, while sufficient for the detection of sleep and wakefulness, is still not optimal. The five stages of sleep can be reasonably well identified with such a montage (collection of signals), but wakefulness within the context of sleep is best identified by a form of cortical activity that occurs predominately in the posterior regions of the cerebrum

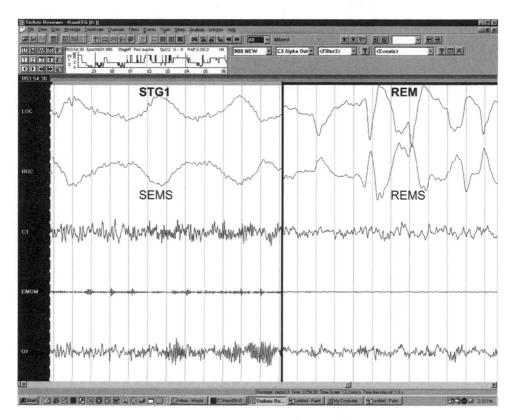

Figure 2.9   An Example of Slow (SEMs) and Rapid (REMs) Eye Movements

(mainly the parietal and occipital regions [P3, Pz, P4 and O1, Oz, O2]). This activity, which occurs when subjects are awake, relaxed, and have their eyes shut, is called *Alpha activity* (8.0 to 12.0 Hz). Alpha represents the disengagement of the visual system but sometimes occurs when subjects are inattentive or drowsy, regardless of whether their eyes are open or shut (see Figure 2.11).

The Multiple Measures Required for Clinical Polysomnography

Collectively, the use of two EOGs, two EEGs, and one EMG is referred to as *somnography* or *polysomnography.* This five-channel montage represents the gold standard for EEG sleep staging. Clinical PSG, however, requires even more measures. To assess for cardiac, respiratory, and/or peripheral neurologic disturbances, additional electrophysiologic measures are needed—measures that can be observed concomitantly (literally run alongside of) the traditional five-channel montage. Cardiac function is evaluated with an electrocardiogram (EKG). While

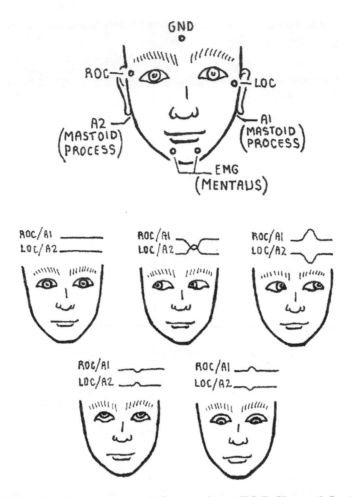

Figure 2.10   Eye Movements and Concomitant EOG Channel Oscillations

clinical EKGs (12-lead-type systems) are not generally acquired during sleep, a simple two-electrode configuration is used to monitor for the gross abnormalities that may occur during sleep.

The measure of respiratory activity during sleep is more complicated for two reasons. First, the assessment of respiratory function requires that all of the dimensions that come into play be evaluated, including air flow, respiratory effort,

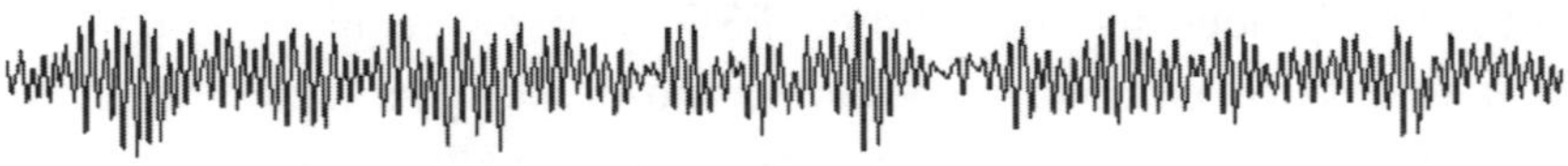

8–12 Hz Occipital Alpha Activity (Oz)

Figure 2.11   Waking EEG, Alpha Rhythm

and degree of arterial blood oxygenation. Thus, several measures are required. Second, none of the respiratory signals have natural source potentials and, therefore, cannot be directly measured with electrophysiologic techniques.

As for the various measures required, typically one or two channels (tracings) are dedicated to oral and/or nasal air flow, two channels are allocated to the measure of respiratory effort, and one channel is dedicated to the measure of blood oxygen content. The flow channels represent inhalation and exhalation. The effort channels usually depict thoracic and abdominal movement (the mechanical component of respiration). There are alternative ways to measure respiratory effort, such as those based on intercostal muscle activity or intraesophogeal pressure differentials.

As indicated previously, none of these measures are derived from naturally occurring signals (such as EEG, EMG, or EOG) but rather represent the various respiratory phenomena as varying voltages in time based on a principle known as *transduction*. This principle, as applied to sleep medicine, is simply this: Find a way to represent physiologic phenomena and how they change over time in terms of varying voltages.

In the case of oral/nasal airflow, the temperature of inhaled and exhaled air is used to modulate the conductivity of an exogenous voltage, which is generated by simply crossing dissimilar metals within a small sensor. Transduction occurs, in this case, because of changes in the conductivity of the metal as it is warmed and cooled. With cooling, more signal passes. With heating, less signal passes. Thus, an oscillating voltage is produced. In the case of respiratory effort, the expansion and contraction of the chest and/or abdomen modulate the conductivity of an exogenous voltage (usually supplied by a battery). The transducer in this case is an elastic material with metal particulate embedded in it. When the chest and/or abdomen expand, the metal particulate is spread apart and less signal passes. When the chest and/or abdomen contract, the metal particulate moves closer together and more signal passes. Thus, an oscillating voltage is produced. Finally, in the case of oximetry, there is a multistep process. A light beam is applied on one side of a heavily vascularized area (digital extremity or ear lobe). A photosensitive sensor is placed on the other side, which allows the amount of light that passes through the tissue to be measured. The light signal is then converted to a voltage. The result is that the more oxygenated the blood, the more light passes. The less oxygenated the blood, the less light passes. Thus, an oscillating voltage is produced.

The combination of these three transduced signals allows for the resolution of abnormal breathing patterns, including central sleep apnea (cessation of air flow in the absence of respiratory effort), obstructive sleep apnea (cessation of air flow in the presence of continued respiratory effort), hypopnea (reduction of air flow along with respiratory effort), and unusual respiratory patterns such as the Cheyne-Stokes respiration (crescendo-decresendo pattern) that occurs in, for example, patients with congestive heart failure.

The measure of abnormal limb movement or tone is accomplished, more often than not, by placing electromyographic leads on each of the legs over the tibial muscles. Two channels of EMG data are acquired, which can be used to detect the motor activity that occurs in association with restless leg syndrome or period leg movements of sleep. Additional EMGs on the extremities may be acquired and used to detect the motor activity that occurs with REM behavior disorder. Additional facial EMGs may be acquired and used to detect the motor activity that comes with nocturnal bruxism. Like EEG or EOG, the source potentials for EMG activity are endogenous currents that, in this case, radiate from neuronal motor end plates and/or from the muscle tissue itself.

While the number and arrangement of signals vary from lab to lab, most sleep disorders centers have a minimum montage of 12 channels, which includes two EOGs, two EEGs, one facial EMG (usually the mentalis muscle, measured because of all skeletal muscles, it remains the most active during sleep and thus is best suited to allow for the resolution of motor inhibition-produced atonia), one oral/nasal sensor, one EKG, two effort sensors, two tibial EMGs, and one measure of blood oxygenation. Most laboratories also include a broader EEG or EMG montage (e.g., in our lab, we acquire 10 EEGs and a minimum of two additional facial EMGs [corrugator muscles]). Other useful measures include a snore microphone, intercostal EMG, body position detectors, esophageal pH monitors (for the measurement of sleep-related acid reflux), measures of esophageal pressure, and so on.

POLYSOMNOGRAPHIC EVALUATION OF SLEEP DISORDERS

Polysomnographic Evaluation of Disorders of Excessive Daytime Sleepiness

In this section, we briefly profile the clinical and PSG concomitants of the five primary intrinsic sleep disorders: obstructive sleep apnea (OSA), period leg movements of sleep (PLMS), narcolepsy, primary insomnia (PI), and delayed sleep phase syndrome (DSPS). OSA, PLMS, and narcolepsy are reviewed as disorders of excessive daytime sleepiness, and PI and DSPS are reviewed as sleep initiation and maintenance disorders. Prior to explicating these disorders in text, Table 2.1 is provided for an at a glance perspective on how each of the disorders appears when assessed with PSG. Please note that the values in the table represent our best estimates as they are derived from literature. At present there are

Table 2.1 Average Sleep Variables for Healthy Good Sleepers (Normal) and Patients with Obstructive Sleep Apnea (OSA), Period Leg Movements of Sleep (PLMS), Narcolepsy, Primary Insomnia (PI), and Delayed Sleep Phase Syndrome (DSPS)

(Averages)	Disorder	Normal	OSA	PLMS	Narcolepsy	PI	DSPS
Sleep continuity measures	SL (minutes)	10	12[1]	20[7,8]	4[2,3]	56[4,5]	36[9]
	WASO (minutes)	10	??	54[7,8]	70[3]	45[5,6]	42[9]
	Number of awakenings (FNA)*	6?	10?	13[7,8]	13[3]	10?	8?
	TST (minutes)	420	346[1]	364[7,8]	416[2,3]	352[6]	446[9]
	SE %	>90%	81%[1]	81%[7,8]	85%[2,3]	79%[4,5,6]	90%[9]
Sleep architecture measures	Wake %	5%	1% ?	1% ?	1% ?	11%[4,5]	10%
	Stage 1 %	5%	11%[1]	15%[7,8]	19%[2,3]	10%[4,5]	3%[9]
	Stage 2 %	60%	71%[1]	46%[7,8]	48%[2,3]	56%[4,5]	52%[9]
	SWS %	15%	3%[1]	19%[7,8]	11%[2,3]	12%[4,5]	15%[9]
	REM %	15%	14%[1]	20%[7,8]	21%[2,3]	22%[4,5]	20%[9]
	SWS Latency	??	??	71[7,8]	??	Reduced?	
	REM Latency	90	134.0 ±6.5[1]	112[7,8]	43[2,3]	?	83.4[9]
Macro EEG findings	Frequent microarousals?	?	Yes	Yes	Yes	No	No ?
	Alpha intrusions	?	Yes	Yes	Yes	No	No ?
	Alpha sleep	?	??	No	??	No	No ?
Micro EEG Findings	Delta (δ)	?	Reduced?	Normal?	Normal?	High?	?
	Alpha (α) tonic-alpha sleep	?	Increased?	Increased?	Increased?	Normal?	?
	Sigma (σ)	?	?	?	?	High?	?
	Beta/Gamma (β/γ)	?	?	?	?	High	?

(continued)

Table 2.1 *Continued*

(Averages)	Disorder	Normal	OSA	PLMS	Narcolepsy	PI	DSPS
EMG findings	PLMs?	N	Variable	Yes	Variable	No	No
Respiratory findings	O/N respiratory pause?	N	Yes	No	No	No	No
	Respiratory effort pauses?	N	Yes	No	No	No	No
	50% reduction in O/N flow?	N	Yes	No	No	No	No
	5% or more O_2 desat.?	N	Yes	No	No	No	No
	Unusual respiratory findings? (e.g., Cheyne-Stokes)	N	Variable	No	No	No	No
EKG Findings	Brady/Tach Formation	N	Yes	?	No?	No	No?

*Most sources define "an awakening" as an event that is 30 seconds or more in duration.

1. Mendelson, W. B. "Sleepiness and Hypertension in Obstructive Sleep Apnea." *Chest* 101(4): 903–909, 1992.
2. Anonymous. "Randomized trial of modafinil as a treatment for the excessive daytime somnolence of narcolepsy." *Neurology* 54: 1166–1174, 2000.
3. Rosenthal, L. D., L. Merlotti, D. K. Young, F. J. Zorick, R. M. Wittig, T. A. Roehrs, et al. "Subjective and Polysomnographic Characteristics of Patients Diagnosed with Narcolepsy." *General Hospital Psychiatry* 12: 191–197, 1990.
4. Scharf, M. B., T. Roth, G. W. Vogel, and J. K. Walsh. "A Multicenter, Placebo-Controlled Study Evaluating Zolpidem in the Treatment of Chronic Insomnia." *Journal of Clinical Psychiatry* 55: 192–199, 1994 May.
5. Ware, J. C., J. K. Walsh, M. B. Scharf, T. Roehrs, T. Roth, and G. W. Vogel. "Minimal rebound insomnia after treatment with 10-mg zolpidem." *Clinical Neuropharmacology* 20(2): 116–125, 1997 April.
6. Edinger, J. D., et al. "Cognitive Behavioral Therapy for Treatment of Chronic Primary Insomnia, A Randomized Controlled Trial." *Journal of the American Medical Association* 285(14): 1856–1864, 2001 April.
7. Saletu, M., P. Anderer, B. Saletu, C. Hauer, M. Mandl, B. Semler, et al. "Sleep laboratory studies in periodic limb movement disorder (PLMD) patients as compared with normals and acute effects of ropinirole." *Human Psychopharmacology* 16: 177–187, 2001.
8. Saletu, M., P. Anderer, G. Saletu-Zyhlarz, W. Prause, B. Semler, A. Zoghlami, et al. "Restless legs syndrome (RLS) and periodic limb movement disorder (PLMD): Acute placebo-controlled sleep laboratory studies with clonazepam." *European Neuropsychopharmacology* 11: 153–161, 2001.
9. Kayumov, L., G. Brown, R. Jindal, K. Buttoo, and C. M. Shapiro. "A Randomized, Double-Blind, Placebo-Controlled Crossover Study of the Effect of Exogenous Melatonin on Delayed Sleep Phase Syndrome." *Psychosomatic Medicine* 63: 40–48, 2001.

no universally agreed upon standards for how each of the intrinsic sleep disorders appear on PSG measures.

Excessive Daytime Sleepiness (EDS) is defined as the inclination to fall asleep at inappropriate times and places. Disorders classified as *EDS disorders* all have sleepiness (as opposed to fatigue) as a prominent and defining symptom. The three primary disorders that fall within this class (primarily by prevalence) are obstructive sleep apnea, periodic limb movements of sleep, and narcolepsy.

Obstructive Sleep Apnea

Obstructive Sleep Apnea (OSA) is the most prevalent of the EDS disorders and is most commonly found in middle-age and older adults and in overweight men. It is present in 1% to 2% of the population, and its male to female ratio is 8:1. Individuals with OSA have a characteristic snoring pattern of loud snores or brief gasps alternating with 20- to 30-second periods of silence. Other symptoms include disorientation, grogginess, mental dullness, incoordination on waking, morning headaches, and dryness of the mouth.

On PSG, patients with OSA show reasonably normal sleep continuity profiles and abnormal sleep architecture. Patients fall asleep quickly, tend to not awaken for prolonged periods (> five minutes), and have normal total sleep time and relatively normal sleep efficiencies (see Table 2.1). Patients with OSA, however, exhibit frequent microarousals (awakenings lasting less than 15 seconds at a rate of 10 to 60+ an hour). When evaluated with a full clinical montage, these arousals are clearly preceded and/or precipitated by apneic events. These respiratory disturbances are characterized by reduction or cessation of air flow, along with continued respiratory effort. In the PSG example of an apneic event (see Figure 2.12), the top two channels are EOGs, the third and fifth channels are EEGs (C3 and O1, respectively), the fourth channel is a mentalis EMG, and the sixth channel represents oral/nasal airflow.

As indicated previously, OSA patients show severely abnormal sleep architecture. In general, REM sleep is substantially suppressed and slow wave sleep is somewhat decreased. The percent of time spent in Stage 1 is increased, while Stage 2 remains normal. Little is known about the quantitative EEG (QEEG) abnormalities as they occur in OSA, but it stands to reason that the Alpha component of their EEG is increased given the frequent occurrence of microarousals.

Periodic Limb Movements of Sleep

The general prevalence of periodic limb movements of sleep (PLMS) is unknown; it is recognized as being rare in children and is increasingly prevalent with advancing age. PLMS are common in up to 34% of patients over 60 years old, and they occur in 1% to 15% of patients with insomnia. There are no sex

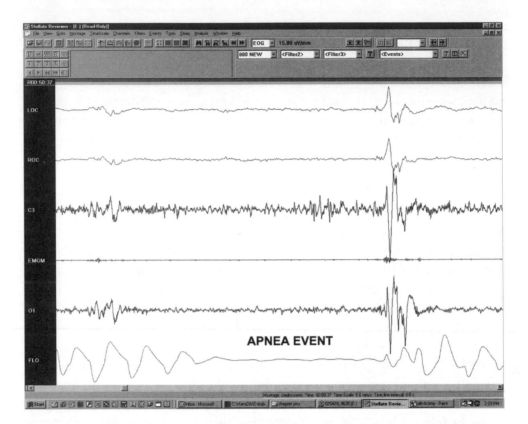

Figure 2.12   Example of an Apnic Event, Stellate Harmonie-Luna™ Software.
Note: **Only one respiratory trace is available because this was a screening study as opposed to a clinical assessment.**

differences in this disorder. The most prominent symptom of PLMS is repetitive movement of the great toe, which may also be accompanied by leg twitches. On occasion, the movements interfere with the ability to initiate or maintain sleep. The disorder is, however, more often characterized by the occurrence of frequent microarousals, which are thought to lead to excessive daytime sleepiness.

On PSG, the sleep continuity and architecture profiles are similar to those observed in OSA. Patients fall asleep quickly, tend to not awaken for prolonged periods, and have normal total sleep time and relatively normal sleep efficiencies (see Table 2.1). As with OSA, patients with PLMS exhibit frequent microarousals. When evaluated with a full clinical montage, the arousals are clearly preceded and/or precipitated by myoclonic events. These events appear as repetitive bursts of EMG activity in the channels dedicated to the monitoring of leg movement. Figure 2.13 is an example PSG of period leg movement activity. The montage for this figure is the same as the prior example except that the last two channels are tibial EMGs.

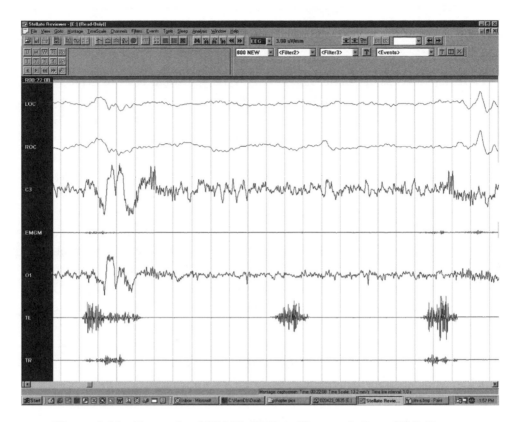

Figure 2.13   Example of PLMS, Stellate Harmonie-Luna™ Software

Unlike OSA, the sleep architecture of PLMS is relatively normal. There is little to no REM suppression, presumably because the motor inhibition of REM sleep blocks PLM events from occurring. If abnormalities are apparent, they are evident as modest reductions in the amount of slow wave sleep and increases in Stage 1 sleep.

Whether PLMS require clinical management is somewhat of a controversial issue because many patients have substantial PLMS but are asymptomatic (without sleep complaint). This may be true because PLMS can occur in the absence of the microarousals that are thought to be responsible for sleep disturbance and daytime sleepiness. Our position on this issue is that if the patient is symptomatic and PLMS are detected, treatment is indicated.

Narcolepsy

Narcolepsy is the least common of the intrinsic sleep disorders with a prevalence of between 0.03% and 0.16% in the general population. While the disorder does not occur preferentially in either of the sexes, the syndrome shows a strong familial pattern. There is also now clear evidence at the molecular level that the disease, or at least the predisposition for the disease, is genetically mediated (23–25).

Narcolepsy is a syndromic disorder. The four cardinal features (the Narcoleptic Tetrad) are excessive daytime sleepiness, sleep paralysis, hypnagogic and hypnopompic hallucinosis, and cataplexy. EDS, as defined previously, is the inclination to fall asleep at inappropriate times and places. Sleep attacks differ from EDS because they occur suddenly, without warning, and are often precipitated by the experience of strong emotion. *Sleep paralysis* refers to the inability to move or speak during the transition between sleep and wakefulness. Hypnagogic and hypnopompic hallucinosis, which also occurs at sleep-wake transitions, is characterized by florid visual, tactile, kinetic, and auditory perceptual experiences. Hypnagogic hallucinations occur just before sleep onset, and hypnopompic hallucinations occur on awakening. The former is the more common. In both cases, the hallucinations themselves are often centered on threat-related experiences and are accompanied by an overwhelming sense of dread or the feeling of impending death. Finally, cataplexy (muscle weakness or sudden loss of postural tone) occurs when the motor inhibitory systems of REM sleep are inappropriately engaged during wakefulness. This symptom, which is also brought on by strong emotion, may be experienced as a kind of weakness (e.g., that requires that the person lean against something for support) or may actually result in what appears outwardly as fainting.

On PSG, patients with narcolepsy show both sleep continuity and architecture abnormalities. The sleep continuity effects, although nonspecific, are pervasive and include both sleep initiation and maintenance problems. The initiation difficulties are characterized by multiple peri-sleep onset awakenings. That is, it is not so much that these patients have difficulty falling sleep as it is that they have problems with sustaining consolidated sleep following sleep onset. The maintenance difficulties are characterized by frequent awakenings, which span the range from microarousals to extended periods of wakefulness. The microarousals may be attributable to the co-occurrence of PLMS. The extended wake after sleep onset intervals may be related to a variety of factors ranging from the fundamental dysregulation of the neuronal apparatus that is responsible for the timing, onset, and offset of both NREM and REM sleep to the same behavioral factors that are thought to be responsible for PI (e.g., poor sleep hygiene, conditioned arousal, etc.). The combination of the various sleep continuity disturbances results in very low sleep efficiency.

The sleep architecture effects that occur with narcolepsy are more specific and are REM sleep related. Narcoleptics have, as a defining feature of their PSGs, very short REM latencies with an average of about 20 minutes, depending

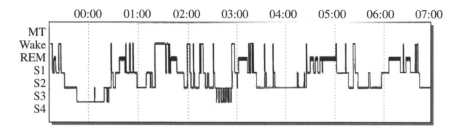

Figure 2.14   Sample Hypnogram for a Narcoleptic Patient. Supplied by the Strong Sleep Disorders Center.

on the time of day. For example, it is not uncommon to observe what are referred to as *SOREMPs* (Sleep Onset REM Periods) during the nocturnal phase, and it is commonplace to observe such phenomena during daytime naps. In these ontogenetically atavistic instances, patients may exhibit REM latencies in the 0 and 10 minutes range. We refer to SOREMPs as *ontogenetically atavistic* because infants normally enter sleep through REM and then later in life assume the more adult pattern where sleep is initiated by first cycling through Stages 1 through 4. Apart from reduced REM latency, narcoleptics also exhibit increased REM time and REM percent and larger proportions of Stage 1 sleep. Stage 2 and slow wave sleep remain normal. For a typical narcoleptic hypnogram, see Figure 2.14. A *hypnogram* is a standard graphic for portraying how the various sleep stages map in time over the course of the night, with time in epochs on the abscissa and sleep stage on the ordinate. Note the short sleep and REM latency and the frequent occurrence of wake after sleep onset awakenings.

POLYSOMNOGRAPHY EVALUATION OF INSOMNIA AND DELAYED SLEEP PHASE SYNDROME

Insomnia

The true prevalence of insomnia for the general population is unknown. Survey data, which often does not discriminate between primary and secondary insomnia (nor take into account severity or chronicity), indicate that a one-year prevalence of insomnia complaints is between 30% and 40%. Chronic insomnia is thought to occur in about half as many people. The complaint occurs with increasing prevalence beginning in young adulthood or in middle age and is rare in childhood. In adolescence, the complaint occurs with some substantial frequency when individuals cannot sleep within their preferred sleep phase, but this type of sleep initiation problem is thought to be developmental or (when persistent and severe) related to circadian dysrhythmia. In short, specific complaints of insomnia are more prevalent with increased age and among women. In general, it is thought that younger adults with PI tend to complain more of difficulty initiating sleep, while midlife and elderly adults usually complain of middle of the night or early morning awakenings. Recent work by Lichstein and colleagues, however, does not support this age-by-insomnia-type characterization (26–28).

As indicated previously, much of the population prevalence work is based on surveys that use single-item questions to assess for the presence or absence of insomnia. Such questions, more or less, assume "if they have it, and it is severe and chronic enough, they'll know." Interestingly, this situation is not substantially improved within the nosological structures. Most of the formal classification systems simply define insomnia in terms of problems initiating and/or maintaining sleep that are associated with daytime distress or impairment (29). The nosologies do not specify quantitative criteria for:

1. How much wakefulness (prior to desired sleep onset or during the night) is considered abnormal
2. How little total sleep must be obtained to fall outside the normal range
3. How frequently these difficulties must occur to be considered pathologic

With respect to how much wakefulness, most investigators consider 30 or more minutes to fall asleep and/or 30 or more minutes of wakefulness after sleep onset to represent the threshold between normal and abnormal sleep. With respect to how much sleep, most investigators are reluctant to fix a value for this parameter, in part because representing what is pathological with one number is too confounded by factors such as age, prior sleep, and the individual's basal level of sleep need, and in part because it is possible to have profound sleep initiation or maintenance problems in the absence of sleep loss. Of the investigators that are inclined to set minimums, most specify that the amount of sleep obtained on a regular basis be equal to, or less than, either 6.5 or 6.0 hours per night. Finally, there is also no fixed benchmark for frequency of complaint. Most investigators require that subjects experience problems on three or more nights per week, but this may have more to do with increasing the odds of studying the occurrence of the disorder in a laboratory than an inherent belief that less than three nights per week is normal.

The problems with definitions are not limited to the quantitative formulation of what constitutes PI. The lack of formal criteria also serves to cloud the distinction between primary and secondary insomnia. At present, PI is considered an independent diagnostic entity (distinguished from secondary insomnia or circadian rhythm disorders) when it appears that cognitive and behavioral factors maintain the disorder (as opposed to acute or unresolved medical and/or psychiatric conditions or phase delay or advance problems). The importance of behavioral factors for PI is explicitly acknowledged in the American Academy of Sleep Medicine's nosology (the International Classification of Sleep Disorders-Revised [ICSD-R]). In this disease classification system, PI is referred to as *psychophysiologic insomnia* (30). The change in terminology reflects that the disorder, to be deemed primary, must have both psychological and physical components. More specifically, *psychophysiologic insomnia* is defined as "a disorder of somatized tension and learned sleep-preventing associations that results in the complaint of insomnia and associated decreased functioning during wakefulness" (30).

As evident from this description, PSG evaluation is not required to establish the diagnosis of PI. On such measures, however, patients with PI reliably exhibit (relative to good sleeper controls) sleep continuity abnormalities including increased sleep latency, increased wake after sleep onset time, and decreased total sleep. The PSG findings, however, do not correspond in a one-to-one fashion to patient perceptions of sleep continuity. Patients with insomnia routinely report more severe sleep disturbance than is evident on traditional PSG measures (31–33). Some have argued that this discrepancy might be explained by the finding that patients with PI show a greater degree of psychopathology, including tendencies to somatize internal conflicts and exaggerate symptoms (e.g., 34–36). We have argued that the subjective-objective discrepancy findings are not psychologically based but rather reflect the persistence of sensory and information processing into NREM sleep. Persistent sensory and information processing, in turn, is thought to make it difficult for patients with insomnia to distinguish wakefulness from sleep states (37). The extent to which one or both of these factors contribute to the discrepancies between subjective and objective measures of sleep in insomnia continues to be a matter of ongoing debate.

Whether sleep architecture is normal in PI is also a matter of debate. Some investigators suggest that the sleep architecture of PI is similar to that which is evident in insomnia secondary to major depression. That is, patients with PI exhibit some or all of the "sleep stigmata" of depression, including reduced REM latency, reduced slow wave sleep, and increased REM time (33–36). Data from our laboratory suggest that the sleep architecture of patients with PI is largely normal, especially with respect to REM parameters. In our hands, we do not observe either reduced REM latency or increased REM time. Interestingly, we also do not observe slow wave sleep deficits. In fact, we have preliminary data that suggest that, at least in the first half of the night, patients with insomnia may exhibit more slow wave activity than is normal. Moreover, the latency to slow wave sleep (although rarely a calculated variable) may also be shorter than usual. These findings suggest that the mechanisms that govern the homeostatic component of sleep may be dysregulated in patients with PI. Such data, along with the quantitative EEG methods (power spectral analysis and/or digital period analysis), which show increased high frequency activity at sleep onset and during NREM sleep (17, 37–40), suggest that PSG may be more useful for the assessment of PI than has been previously thought.

Delayed Sleep Phase Syndrome

There are a variety of chronobiologically based sleep disorders (e.g., delayed and advanced sleep phase syndromes, non-24-hour sleep-wake disorder, time zone change syndrome [jet lag], shift work sleep disorder). For further information on delayed sleep phase syndrome (DSPS), see Chapter 12 and the Suggested Readings Appendix at the end of this book for general information on this whole class of sleep disorders.

We present information on DSPS, and only on DSPS, in this chapter for two reasons. First, patients with this disorder often have PSG evaluations and/or seek treatment at insomnia clinics or behavioral sleep medicine services. Second, patients with DSPS may exhibit on PSG semi unique sleep continuity and sleep architectural profiles.

The general prevalence of DSPS is estimated between 5% and 10%. These numbers are likely to be substantially lower than the real population prevalence for two reasons. First, because phase delay occurs developmentally and is often compatible with the social preferences of the individuals most likely to be affected, the occurrence of the phenomenon becomes "pathologized" only when the delay is extreme or interferes with daytime performance. Second, surveys are not likely to have the discriminatory power to distinguish between sleep onset problems as they occur in PI and as they occur in DSPS. Thus, some percentage of self-reported sleep onset problems, especially in individuals younger than 30, is likely reported or described as PI.

While there is a progressive phase delay over much of the first two decades of life, DSPS is thought to be rare in children and in the elderly. During adolescence, there is a 10:1 ratio with the disorder occurring more frequently in males. This sex ratio is thought to diminish to roughly a 1:1 occurrence rate in individuals in their third decade of life. The most prominent symptom of DSPS is, as the name suggests, a phase delay. Specifically, this refers to the notion that the individual's preferred sleep phase no longer falls in the normal 10 P.M. to 7 A.M. zone, but instead is delayed to some later time interval (e.g., 3 A.M. to 11 A.M.). When allowed to sleep ad libitum, many individuals with this disorder do not complain of sleep disturbance. If, however, the vocational or social dictates of individuals' lives require them to sleep according to a nonpreferred schedule, sleep initiation and/or maintenance problems occur. The magnitude of these problems is directly related to the degree to which the enforced and the preferred schedules are misaligned.

The two most common sleep continuity complaints that occur with DSPS are that the individual takes too long to fall asleep and/or does not get enough sleep. The sleep onset problem results when individuals, for social or work-related reasons, go to bed earlier than they would prefer (e.g., 11 P.M. versus 3 A.M.) and then find that they take several hours to fall asleep. The failure to get enough sleep most often occurs when they go to bed at the desired time but truncate their sleep period to meet the need to be awake and functioning at an early hour.

While it is possible, if not likely, that DSPS may evolve in such a way as to share features with PI (e.g., conditioned arousal, sleep-related worry, and the engagement of maladaptive behaviors that perpetuate and exacerbate the sleep problem), DSPS may also exist in the chemically pure form and, as such, is a fundamentally different disorder from PI, despite the shared symptom profiles.

On PSG, the sleep continuity profiles closely approximate the patient's complaints. Reports of taking hours to fall asleep are corroborated. Once asleep, the architecture is normal and the various sleep stage latencies (such as REM latency) are normal despite the late nocturnal phase (see Table 2.1).

FUTURE DIRECTIONS AND MEASUREMENT OF SLEEP

Throughout this chapter, we have endeavored to explicate what each of the available measurement strategies are and how each conveys useful information. We also hope that we have communicated that:

- Self-report information, especially when gathered prospectively, is of substantial value for the understanding of patients' experience of their sleep disorders and the effectiveness of the treatments they receive.

- Actigraphy is a valuable, but underused, methodology—one that may have a substantial role to play in the objective measure of sleep continuity abnormalities across all the sleep disorders, and perhaps a special application in patients with PI.

- PSG is the gold standard for pulmonary and neurologic sleep medicine. Its utility as a diagnostic procedure for behavioral sleep medicine has yet to be established. Our sense is that PSG has much more of a role to play in the assessment of PI than is, perhaps, currently appreciated. The value of this method is less related to the simple fact that "it is a more objective measure" and more related to its capacity to provide information on:

1. Homeostatic dysregulation (abnormalities in the amount and/or timing of slow wave sleep)
2. Assessment of central nervous system arousal in the form of QEEG measured high-frequency activity, as it occurs in subjects with insomnia

Apart from these issues, there is the question of "What value do the newer technologies (such as quantitative EEG [QEEG], evoked response potentials [ERPs], and functional imaging) have with respect to the assessment of sleep disorders?" The newness (if not the complexity, relative unavailability, and expense) of these approaches as applied to sleep disorders relegates their use primarily to the clinical research domain. The potential value of each and the value of "co-registration" studies cannot be underestimated.

QEEG has already been shown to be of use vis-à-vis the study of the CNS effects of GABAnergic agents (41–43), the slow wave sleep deficits in insomnia secondary to major depression (MDD; 44–46), and the occurrence of high-frequency EEG activity in patients with PI (17, 37–40).

ERPs, though surprisingly rarely applied to the study of sleep disorders, have been used to study sensory and information processing abnormalities in patients with insomnia (38) and motor abnormalities in patients with PLMS (39–41).

Functional imaging, in its various forms, has been productively applied to the study of OSA (42–44; for a review, see 45), PLMS (46–48), insomnia secondary to major depression, and PI. The OSA studies have been useful for the evaluation of dilator muscle activity and airway patency. The PLMS studies have been useful for assessing the CNS sources of the efferent activity that occurs before myoclonic activity. The functional imaging studies of insomnia secondary to MDD have allowed for the detection of hyperactivation of the limbic system during REM sleep. These data may greatly enhance our ability to understand why the REM sleep stigmata are so well correlated with clinical history and course. Finally, there is (to our knowledge) only one functional imaging study in patients with PI (49). This study showed that patients with insomnia, as compared to good sleepers, show substantial cerebral deactivation immediately following sleep onset. These data, along with the QEEG findings of increased slow wave sleep and shortened slow wave sleep latencies, support the point of view that the discharge of the homeostat occurs abnormally in patients with PI.

Each of these considerations supports the point of view that alternative measures used along with traditional methods will greatly enhance our ability to understand the pathophysiology of the various sleep disorders. Such information may greatly inform both the practice of behavioral sleep medicine and the development of alternative treatments.

APPENDIX 2.1: RSCI OUTPUT

The Rochester Sleep Continuity Inventory (RSCI)

Individual Report for _____, 41 year old Female

Name:
Age: **41**   Height: **5'3"**   Ethnicity: **Caucasian**   Occupation: **Attorney**
Sex: **Female**   Weight: **115**   BMI: **20.37**   Education: **JD**
Self-reporting   Self-reporting
medical conditions: psych conditions:

Prescription medication:	Type	Amount	Schedule	Time
	excedrine	500 mg	occasional	AM/PM
	multivitamin	unknown	daily	AM

Alcohol use: **No**   Nicotine use: **No**

Caffeine use: Coffee: Tea: Caffeinated Soda: Chocolate:
                 ½ cup   **1 can**   **1 candy bar**

Sleep Disturbance Severity: 39   **Insomnia Severity: 56**   **Overall Severity: 74**
     Sum: 1–3   Sum: 1–4   Sum: 1–5
     Max = 60   Max = 80   Max = 105

I: SUM OF SEVERITY & CONSEQUENCES & WORRY   Test Date: **24-Jan-02**

		5	10	15	20
1. Initiation Problems:	14				
2. Maintenance Problems:	13				
3. Early Morning Awakenings:	12				
4. Daytime Consequences:	17				
5. Sleep-Related Worry:	18				

II: CONTRIBUTING FACTORS

		5	10	15	20	25
6. Factor 1 - Conditioning Component:	11					
7. Factor 2 - Circadian Component:	7					
8. Factor 3 - Homeostatic Component:	10					
9. Factor 4 - Sleep Hygiene Factor:	14					

III: AROUSAL COMPONENTS

		5	10	15
10. Factor 1 - Cognitive Arousal:	13			
11. Factor 2 - Somatic Arousal:	5			
12. Factor 3 - Cortical Arousal:	8			

Sleep duration **390**   Needed **420**   Is this a problem? **Yes**   How long? **240 months**   Sleepy? **Once in the last 1 year**

The Rochester Sleep Continuity Inventory (RSCI): Individual Report for a 41-Year-Old Female

APPENDIX 2.2: ROCHESTER SLEEP DIARY

(See pp. 66–67.)

Name: _____   Date: _____

COMPLETE IMMEDIATELY BEFORE BED CONCERNING HOW YOU FELT TODAY:

	MON	TUES	WED	THUR	FRI	SAT	SUN	MEAN
Typical day? (yes/no)*								
Fatigue (none 0—1—2—3—4—5 a lot)								
Stress (none 0—1—2—3—4—5 a lot)								
Alert (not very 0—1—2—3—4—5 very)								
Concentration (good 0—1—2—3—4—5 bad)								
Mood (bad 0—1—2—3—4—5 good)								
Time spent exercising (min.)								
Time spent outside today (min.)								
Number of alcoholic beverages								
Prescriptions today (yes/no)								
OTC meds today (yes/no)								
Pain today (none 0—1—2—3—4—5 a lot)								
Health (felt fine 0—1—2—3—4—5 bad)								
Menstruate today (yes/no)								
Menstrual pain (none 0—1—2—3—4—5 bad)								

* Please indicate on the back of this sheet why any given day was not typical and/or what medications you took on any given day.

COMPLETE IMMEDIATELY ON AWAKENING:

	MON	TUES	WED	THUR	FRI	SAT	SUN	MEAN
Time to bed (clock time)								
Time out of bed (clock time)								
Time to bed (dev frm 11 time)								
Time out of bed (dev frm 7)								
Time to fall asleep (SL)								
Number times awakened (NUMA)								
Wake after sleep onset (WASO)								
Total amount time out of bed (TTOB)								
Total sleep time (TST) (min.)								
Sleep quality (good 0—1—2—3—4—5 poor)								
Fatigue (none 0—1—2—3—4—5 a lot)								
SE and TIP to be autocalculate.								

SE and TIB to Be Autocalculate

APPENDIX 2.3: PITTSBURGH SLEEP DIARY

WESTERN PSYCHIATRIC INSTITUTE AND CLINIC
SLEEP AND CHRONOBIOLOGY CENTER
PITTSBURGH SLEEP DIARY (PghSD)

Please keep this booklet by your bed and fill it out last thing at night and first thing in the morning. There are 14 sheets in the booklet, one sheet for each night of sleep. Please fill out the left half of the sheet last thing at night, the right half first thing the following morning. We realize that estimates of time to fall asleep and time awake during the night are not going to be exact, just do the best you can.

When answering questions about how well you slept, your alertness and mood on awakening, please consider the line to represent your own personal range. Place a mark somewhere along the line to represent your feelings at that time. We are using the line so that you are not required to give "yes" or "no" answers but can give one of a whole range of possible answers. Please try to use the whole scale, rather than simply putting your marks at one end or the other.

Name: _____   ID#: _____

SLEEP DIARY   **BEDTIME**   KEEP BY BED

Please fill out this part of the diary last thing at *night*.

Day: _____   Date: _____

Today, when did you have: Breakfast: _____   Lunch: _____

                          Dinner: _____
(if none, write "none")

How many of the following did you have in each time period? (if none, leave blank)

	Before or with Breakfast	After Breakfast before/with Lunch	After Lunch before/with Dinner	After Dinner
Caffeinated drinks	_____	_____	_____	_____
Alcoholic drinks	_____	_____	_____	_____
Cigarettes	_____	_____	_____	_____
Cigars/pipes/plugs (of chewing tobacco)	_____	_____	_____	_____

Which drugs and medications did you take today? (prescribed and over the counter)

Name	Time	Dose
_____	_____	_____
_____	_____	_____

What exercise did you take today? (if none, check here)

Start _____   End _____   Type _____

Start _____   End _____   Type _____

How many daytime naps did you take today? (if none, write 0) _____ give times for each:

Start _____   End _____   Start _____   End _____

Start _____   End _____   Start _____   End _____

SLEEP DIARY   **WAKETIME**   KEEP BY BED

Please fill out this part of the diary first thing in the *morning*.

Day: _____   Date: _____

Went to bed last night at   _____

Lights out at   _____

Minutes until fell asleep   _____

Finally woke at   _____

Awakened by (check one):   Alarm clock/radio   ☐
                            Someone whom I asked to wake me   ☐
                            Noises   ☐
                            Just woke   ☐

After falling asleep, woke up this many times during the night (circle)

   0   1   2   3   4   5   more

total number of minutes awake _____

Woke to use bathroom (circle # times)

   0   1   2   3   4   5   more

Awakened by noises/child/bedpartner (circle # times)

   0   1   2   3   4   5   more

Awakened due to discomfort or physical complaint (circle # times)

   0   1   2   3   4   5   more

Just woke (circle # times)

   0   1   2   3   4   5   more

Ratings (place a mark somewhere along the line):

   Sleep Quality:
      very bad · very good

   Mood on final wakening:
      very tense · very calm

   Alertness on final wakening:
      very sleepy · very alert

REFERENCES

1. Cote, K. A. and R. D. Ogilvie. The Brock Sleep and Insomnia Questionnaire: Phase 1. *Sleep Research* 22: 356, 1993.

2. Buysse, D. J., C. Reynolds, and T. Monk. Quantification of subjective sleep quality in healthy elderly men and women using the Pittsburgh Sleep Quality Index. *Sleep* 14: 331–338, 1991.

3. Buysse, D. J., C. F. Reynolds, T. H. Monk, S. R. Berman, and D. J. Kupfer. The Pittsburgh Sleep Quality Index: A new instrument for psychiatric practice and research. *Psychiatry Research* 28: 193–213, 1989.

4. Bastien, C., A. Vallières, and C. M. Morin. Validation of the Insomnia Severity Index as an outcome measure for insomnia research. *Sleep Medicine* 2: 297–307, 2001.

5. Cragg, K., M. Perlis, M. Aloia, J. Boehmler, A. Millikan, D. Greenblatt, et al. Questionnaire vs. diary assessments of sleep complaints. *Sleep* 22: 244, 1999.

6. Jean-Louis, G., D. F. Kripke, R. J. Cole, J. D. Assmus, and R. D. Langer. Sleep detection with an accelerometer actigraph: Comparisons with polysomnography. *Physiology Behavior* 72: 21–28, 2001.

7. Jean-Louis, G., D. F. Kripke, W. J. Mason, J. A. Elliott, and S. D. Youngstedt. Sleep estimation from wrist movement quantified by different actigraphic modalities. *Journal of Neuroscience Methods* 105: 185–191, 2001.

8. Jean-Louis, G., H. von Gizycki, F. Zizi, J. Fookson, A. Spielman, J. Nunes, et al. Determination of sleep and wakefulness with the actigraph data analysis software (ADAS). *Sleep* 19: 739–743, 1996.

9. Jean-Louis, G., F. Zizi, H. von Gizycki, and P. Hauri. Actigraphic assessment of sleep in insomnia: Application of the actigraph data analysis software (ADAS). *Physiology and Behavior* 65: 659–663, 1999.

10. Perlis, M. L., D. E. Giles, W. B. Mendelson, R. R. Bootzin, and J. K. Wyatt. Subjective—objective discrepancies in psychophysiologic insomnia: A neurocognitive perspective. *Journal of Sleep Research* 6: 179–188, 1997.

11. Lehmann, D., W. K. Strik, B. Henggeler, T. Koenig, and M. Koukkou. Brain electric microstates and momentary conscious mind states as building blocks of spontaneous thinking: I. Visual imagery and abstract thoughts. *International Journal of Psychophysiology* 29: 1–11, 1998.

12. Basar-Eroglu, C., D. Struber, M. Schurmann, M. Stadler, and E. Basar. Gamma-band responses in the brain: A short review of psychophysiological correlates and functional significance [Review] [69 refs]. *International Journal of Psychophysiology* 24: 101–112, 1996.

13. Desmedt, J. E. and C. Tomberg. Transient phase-locking of 40 Hz electrical oscillations in prefrontal and parietal human cortex reflects the process of conscious somatic perception. *Neuroscience Letter* 168: 126–129, 1994.

14. Galambos, R., S. Makeig, and P. J. Talmachoff. A 40-Hz auditory potential recorded from the human scalp. *Proceedings of the National Academy of Sciences of the United States of America* 78: 2643–2647, 1981.

15. Joliot, M., U. Ribary, and R. Llinas. Human oscillatory brain activity near 40 Hz coexists with cognitive temporal binding. *Proceedings of the National Academy of Sciences of the United States of America* 91: 11748–11751, 1994.

16. Loring, D. W., M. Ford, and D. Sheer. Laterality of 40 Hz EEG and EMG during cognitive performance. *Psychophysiology* 21: 34–38, 1984.

17. Sheer, D. Focused arousal and 40 Hz EEG. In R. Knight and D. Bakker, eds. *The Neuropsychology of Learning Disorders*. Baltimore, MD: University Press. 1976: 71–87.

18. Perlis, M. L., Merica, H., Smith, M. T., and D. E. Giles. Beta EEG in insomnia. *Sleep Medicine Reviews* 5: 364–375, 2001.

19. Perlis, M. L., M. T. Smith, H. J. Orff, P. J. Andrews, and D. E. Giles. Beta/Gamma EEG activity in patients with primary and secondary insomnia and good sleeper controls. *Sleep* 24: 110–117, 2001.

20. Jasper, H. H. The ten-twenty electrode system of the international federation. *Electroencephalography and Clinical Neurophysiology* 10: 371–375, 1958.

21. Aserinsky, E. and N. Kleitman. Regularly occurring periods of eye motility and concomitant phenomena during sleep. *Science* 118: 273–274, 1953.

22. Chase, M. H. and F. R. Morales. The atonia and myoclonia of active (REM) sleep. *Annual Review of Psychology* 41: 577–584, 1990.

23. Chemelli, R. M., J. T. Willie, C. M. Sinton, J. K. Elmquist, T. Scammell, C. Lee, et al. Narcolepsy in orexin knockout mice: Molecular genetics of sleep regulation. *Cell* 98: 437–451, 1999.

24. Lin, L., J. Faraco, R. Li, H. Kadotani, W. Rogers, X. Lin, et al. The sleep disorder canine narcolepsy is caused by a mutation in the hypocretin (orexin) receptor 2 gene. *Cell* 98: 365–376, 1999.

25. Mignot, E. Genetic and familial aspects of narcolepsy. *Neurology* 50: S16–S22, 1998.

26. Lichstein, K. L., H. H. Durrence, D. J. Taylor, A. J. Bush, and B. W. Riedel. Quantitative criteria for insomnia. *Behaviour Research and Therapy* 41: 427–445, 2003.

27. McCrae, C. S., N. W. Wilson, K. L. Lichstein, H. H. Durrence, D. J. Taylor, A. J. Bush, et al. 'Young old' and 'old old' poor sleepers with and without insomnia complaints. *Journal of Psychosomatic Research* 54:11–19, 2003.

28. Lichstein, K. L., H. H. Durrence, B. W. Riedel, D. J. Taylor, and A. J. Bush. *Epidemiology of Sleep: Age, Gender, and Ethnicity*. Mahwah, NJ: Erlbaum. Unpublished manuscript.

29. World Health Organization. *The ICD-10 Classification of Mental and Behavioral Disorders: Clinical Descriptions and Diagnostic Guidelines*. Geneva, Switzerland: World Health Organization. 1992.

30. American Sleep Disorders Association. *The International Classification of Sleep Disorders: Diagnostic and Coding Manual*. Rochester, MN: American Sleep Disorders Association. 1990.

31. Carskadon, M., W. Dement, M. Mitler, C. Guilleminault, V. P. Zarcone, and R. Spiegel. Self-reports versus sleep laboratory findings in 122 drug-free subjects with complaints of chronic insomnia. *American Journal of Psychiatry* 133: 1382–1388, 1976.

32. Coates, T. J., J. Killen, J. George, E. Marchini, S. Hamilton, and C. Thoresen. Estimating sleep parameters: A multitrait-multimethod analysis. *Journal of Consulting and Clinical Psychology* 50: 345–352, 1982.

33. Frankel, B. L., R. Coursey, R. Buchbinder, and F. Snyder. Recorded and reported sleep in primary chronic insomnia. *Archives of General Psychiatry* 33: 615–623, 1976.

34. Kales, A., A. Caldwell, and T. Preston. Personality patterns in insomnia. *Archives of General Psychiatry* 33: 1128–1134, 1976.

35. Kales, A., E. Bixler, A. Vela-Bueno, R. Cadieux, C. Soldatos, and J. Kales. Biopsychobehavioral correlates of insomnia. III: Polygraphic findings of sleep difficulty and their relationship to psychopathology. *International Journal of Neuroscience* 23: 43–56, 1984.

36. Bonnet, M. H. and D. L. Arand. Physiological activation in patients with sleep state misperception. *Psychosomatic Medicine* 59: 533–540, 1997.

37. Perlis, M. L., D. E. Giles, W. B. Mendelson, R. R. Bootzin, and J. K. Wyatt. Psychophysiological insomnia: The behavioral model and a neurocognitive perspective. *Journal of Sleep Research* 6: 179–188, 1997.

38. Wang, W., S. Z. Zhu, L. C. Pan, A. H. Hu, and Y. H. Wang. Mismatch negativity and personality traits in chronic primary insomnia. *Functional Neurology* 16: 3–10, 2001.

39. Trenkwalder, C., S. F. Bucher, W. H. Oertel, D. Proeckl, H. Plendl, and W. Paulus. Bereitschaftspotential in idiopathic and symptomatic restless legs syndrome. *Electroencephalography Clinical Neurophysiology* 89: 95–103, 1993.

40. Mosko, S. S. and K. L. Nudleman. Somatosensory and brainstem auditory evoked responses in sleep-related periodic leg movements. *Sleep* 9: 399–404, 1986.

41. Wechsler, L. R., J. W. Stakes, B. T. Shahani, and N. A. Busis. Periodic leg movements of sleep (nocturnal myoclonus): An electrophysiological study. *Annuals of Neurology* 19: 168–173, 1986.

42. Baik, U. B., M. Suzuki, K. Ikeda, J. Sugawara, and H. Mitani. Relationship between cephalometric characteristics and obstructive sites in obstructive sleep apnea syndrome. *Angle Orthodontist* 72: 124–134, 2002.

43. Arens, R., J. M. McDonough, A. T. Costarino, S. Mahboubi, C. E. Tayag-Kier, G. Maislin, et al. Magnetic resonance imaging of the upper airway structure of children with obstructive sleep apnea syndrome. *American Journal of Respiratory and Critical Care Medicine* 164: 698–703, 2001.

44. Kamba, M., Y. Inoue, S. Higami, Y. Suto, T. Ogawa, and W. Chen. Cerebral metabolic impairment in patients with obstructive sleep apnoea: An independent association of obstructive sleep apnoea with white matter change. *Journal of Neurology, Neurosurgery, and Psychiatry* 71: 334–339, 2001.

45. Schwab, R. J. Imaging for the snoring and sleep apnea patient. *Dental Clinics of North America* 45: 759–796, 2001.

46. Ruottinen, H. M., M. Partinen, C. Hublin, J. Bergman, M. Haaparanta, O. Solin, et al. An FDOPA PET study in patients with periodic limb movement disorder and restless legs syndrome. *Neurology* 54: 502–504, 2000.

47. Trenkwalder, C., A. S. Walters, W. A. Hening, S. Chokroverty, A. Antonini, V. Dhawan, et al. Positron emission tomographic studies in restless legs syndrome. *Movement Disorders* 14: 141–145, 1999.

48. San Pedro, E. C., J. M. Mountz, J. D. Mountz, H. G. Liu, C. R. Katholi, and G. Deutsch. Familial painful restless legs syndrome correlates with pain dependent variation of blood flow to the caudate, thalamus, and anterior cingulate gyrus. *Journal of Rheumatology* 25: 2270–2275, 1998.

49. Smith, M. T., M. L. Perlis, V. U. Chengazi, J. Pennington, J. Soeffing, J. M. Ryan, et al. Neuroimaging of NREM sleep in primary insomnia: A Tc-99-HMPAO single photon emission computed tomography study. *Sleep* 25: 325–335, 2002.

SECTION III

Sleep Medicine

Chapter 3

SLEEP APNEA: A CHALLENGE FOR BEHAVIORAL MEDICINE

ROSALIND D. CARTWRIGHT

Recently, sleep apnea, or more specifically, obstructive sleep apnea (OSA), has had a remarkable impact on public awareness as a new health problem. The close association of snoring and pauses in breathing during sleep with the presence of hypertension and increased vulnerability to stroke has been confirmed in sleep studies of large samples of persons who were followed for their health status over the next few years (1). No doubt it is this disorder that has brought the field of sleep medicine to the attention of health care professionals who might otherwise not have included a review of their patients' sleep as part of their routine care.

There are two major forms of sleep apnea: central sleep apnea and the obstructive type. In the central type, there are short pauses in respiration during sleep, each lasting 10 or more seconds, during which no effort is being made by the lungs and diaphragm to move air. In the obstructive type, the pauses are usually longer and occur in spite of continued effort by the muscles of the chest and abdominal wall to sustain breathing by their pumping action. In the central form, the breathing pause is due to failure of the brain's respiratory center to send a signal to the muscles to contract, while in OSA, the muscles do their work but cannot pass air freely because of some blockage in the upper airway. Central apnea affects fewer persons and is more likely to occur in infants under the age of one year because of some neurological immaturity or in elderly persons who have suffered a stroke or some other neurodegenerative disorder. The obstructive form is much more common, particularly in middle-age males who have some narrowing of the throat—perhaps because of their cranial-facial structure or because their neck size increased as they gained weight. Either restricts the oropharyngeal space (the opening behind the tongue). When a person with a narrow airway lies down to sleep, the muscles that hold the throat open during the day relax. The tongue also relaxes and may fall back, narrowing the breathing space further. This combination of a narrow structure plus changes in muscle tone with sleep can lead to a few short pauses in breathing during the transition from waking to sleep. These may be normal events. Sleep apnea is diagnosed only when the pauses are longer and more frequent and occur not just at the beginning but throughout sleep. These pauses lead to a reduced level of oxygen in the blood and to frequent arousals to restart breathing.

The diagnosis of OSA must be established in a sleep laboratory using monitoring devices that show the frequency of two types of episodes—the complete cessation of breathing for at least 10 seconds (apnea) and the partial reduction of the airflow by 30% or more, with a drop in the level of oxygen saturation of 4% or more from the sleep baseline. This second type is called *hypopnea*. Both of these interruptions of regular respiration are considered in making the diagnosis of this disorder (2).

Over the past 20 years, the recognition of OSA has spawned an industry for the manufacture and distribution of increasingly sophisticated recording equipment for its diagnosis and mechanical devices for its control. OSA is responsible for increased funding from the National Institutes of Health in support of research into its prevalence and health consequences, with an emphasis on the strong association of OSA and cardiovascular disorders. OSA has also been the impetus behind the development of new, specialized advanced training programs in sleep medicine to prepare physicians and clinical psychologists for the management of this and other disorders of sleep. Altogether, there has been more focus on the understanding and control of this sleep-related breathing disorder than on all the other disorders of sleep.

Among the risk factors for OSA are a number of lifestyle behaviors, including smoking, alcohol use, and the poor eating habits that contribute to obesity. These have received less attention and represent an opportunity for behaviorally trained clinicians to develop treatment programs that can be integrated into the care of these patients. This chapter focuses on the place of behavior change programs in the management of OSA, its prevention, and the role of the health psychologist in this endeavor. The new postdoctoral training program for psychologists in sleep medicine opens up this field for the collaborative treatment of OSA with medically trained persons. Psychologists have played a role in developing treatment strategies and in carrying out research. Now they have the opportunity to be important members of the treatment team as well.

CLINICAL INTERVIEW (SIGNS AND SYMPTOMS)

OSA was not unknown before it achieved its new name and fame. It was first called the *Pickwick syndrome* (3), named for Joe, the lazy fat boy character in

Charles Dickens' novel, *The Pickwick Papers* (1). Joe had three outstanding traits: He was obese, he was constantly falling asleep when he was supposed to be awake and attentive to his job, and when he slept, he snored very loudly. These are still the most easily recognized signs identifying those who are most likely to demonstrate a repetitive pattern of obstructed breathing during sleep. Before a patient is referred for an all-night sleep recording to confirm this diagnosis, both the patient and his or her bed partner should be interviewed by either a physician or clinical psychologist to explore whether the patient has Joe's three characteristics:

1. *Snoring:* Has there been an increase in the frequency and severity of the snoring recently? Is the snoring more continuous and louder after nights when the patient has used alcohol during the evening? Does the snoring worsen when the patient sleeps on his or her back? Are there periods of silence broken by snorting or gasping sounds? (The more positive answers to these questions, the more likely the diagnosis.)

2. *Body weight:* What is the patient's present weight in relation to norms for his or her age and sex? Has there been a weight gain that accompanied the increase in snoring severity? What is the neck size in inches? Has there been a recent increase in collar size? (A body mass index above 35 and collar size above 16.5 inches correlate positively with OSA diagnosis.)

3. *Daytime sleepiness:* Is the patient having trouble staying awake during the day? Has he or she fallen asleep while driving? At work? While watching TV? (The more severe the excessive daytime sleepiness [EDS], the more likely the patient will need a diagnostic sleep study.)

Patients are often not the best reporters on these key symptoms—partly because they are asleep at the time, but also these changes occur slowly and so may go unrecognized. It is better to get this information from someone who has observed their sleep. Patients can usually supply information about other associated symptoms: whether they have experienced changes in mood, a decrease in sex drive, a presence of sweating during the night particularly in the region of the neck and chest, an increase in the number of times they awaken to urinate, nocturnal heartburn, or awakening with a dry mouth. During this interview, it should also be noted whether the patient has a history of hypertension and whether the hypertension is being treated and controlled by medication. Does the patient have a short, thick neck, a short lower jaw, or receding chin (micrognathia or retrognathia), a large tongue, or difficulty breathing through one nostril at a time? Is the patient's tongue large, the uvula long or thick; is the space at the back of the throat crowded? All of these indicate that the patient is a good candidate for a sleep laboratory evaluation to rule out OSA.

POLYSOMNOGRAPHIC ASSESSMENT AND DIAGNOSIS

The diagnosis of OSA requires at least one night of polysomnographic recording of the patient's sleep carried out during his or her usual sleep hours. This must include continuous monitoring of respiration by nasal/oral airflow, the percent of oxygen in the blood usually measured by pulse oximetry, the effort exerted by the muscles in the chest and abdominal walls, as well as the usual monitors of the brain waves of waking and sleep, chin muscle tone, snoring, periodic movements of the legs, and the EKG. To meet the criteria for the diagnosis of OSA, the frequency of episodes of complete or partial obstruction of the airflow during sleep must be more than the number and length of these seen during normal sleep. It is normal for a few brief episodes of complete or partial respiratory pausing at the onset of sleep but also during the rapid eye movement (REM) sleep episodes when there is a natural and profound loss of tone in the muscle of the head and neck. This can also result in a few short apneic episodes. The diagnosis of OSA is made by calculating the total number of times the flow of air from the nose and/or mouth stops completely or is reduced for 10 or more seconds, divided by the number of hours of sleep. This value is called the *Apnea + Hypopnea Index* (A+HI). The severity of OSA is divided into three rough categories: mild, when the A+HI falls between 5 and 15 events per hour; moderate, with A+HI between 15 and 29; or severe, when this number is greater than 30. In addition to this number, the diagnosis considers number and severity of the episodes of oxygen desaturation, the number of awakenings, and the severity of the waking consequences of such sleep.

The typical pattern of respiration during sleep in an OSA patient is of loud snoring followed by periods of silence, when no air passes through the nose or mouth in spite of continued effort by the muscles of the chest and abdomen. This indicates a blockage in the upper airway, preventing the free flow of air. The silence of the apneic period is broken by a gasping noise as the effort to breath results in a breakthrough of the obstruction and a brief arousal when normal breathing resumes. In patients who are severely affected by OSA, this pattern of snoring, silence, and gasping may repeat as often as 100 times each hour of sleep. OSA is a progressive problem. In the first stage, there is only intermittent snoring and a mild interference with free breathing. Next, there is both snoring and a mild to moderate number of respiratory pauses. Finally, there is the full-blown disorder with long pauses accompanied by severe drops in the oxygen saturation measure and many arousals during the night. The consequent degree of daytime sleepiness is related to the degree of severity of the disordered breathing during the prior sleep and the number of arousals it causes.

The prevalence of OSA in the United States depends on where the cutoff point is set between normal and abnormal breathing. When the cutoff point is set at five or more episodes per hour, the expectation is that 9% of adult women and 24% of men will qualify for this diagnosis (5). This very high number is something of a surprise to those unfamiliar with sleep medicine. Only recently was it recommended that the diagnostic criterion be set at this level. Previously, the criterion was 10 events per hour. At that level, the prevalence figures for OSA most often quoted were 2% for women and 4% for men. The change was based on recent research showing that even those who exhibited a very mild degree of sleep-disordered breathing are at greatly increased risk for the development of hypertension and/or stroke when studied four years later (6).

In addition to the impact of OSA on physical health, this sleep problem takes a toll on the mental, social, and economic health of those afflicted. Like Dickens' character Joe, they often have difficulty maintaining daytime wakefulness, which has been implicated in their reduced work productivity and increased rate of motor vehicle accidents (7–8). Over time, those with untreated OSA show changes in personality, an irritable mood, memory problems, and often a loss of libido (9). All of these constitute a stress on the individual's partner as well. The profound sleepiness of these patients limits their ability to engage in social activities, and their loud snoring may preclude their sharing a bed (10).

A telephone survey of 1,154 adults, conducted by the National Sleep Foundation (11), asked about the frequency of the respondent's snoring. Thirty-two percent of men and 18.8% of women replied that they snored every night or almost every night, which would put them at least in the first stage of this disorder. Another question asked whether they had pauses in their breathing during sleep. Eight and a half percent of the men surveyed and 4.9% of women reported they had such pauses every, or almost every, night. This disproportionate rate between the sexes has been confirmed in sleep laboratory studies not only in the United States but also in many other countries (12). The typical picture of the OSA patient is of an overweight, middle-age male with a short, thick neck (13), but this disorder also occurs in women, although with less frequency until they have passed menopause, and in persons of all ages and even in those who are within normal weight for their age if they have a small airway because of some external structural feature or show a crowded internal space behind the tongue because of enlarged tonsils, a thick uvula, or tongue base. Given the high prevalence of OSA among adult males of working age, it is not surprising that much effort is being expended to develop treatments to restore unobstructed breathing in sleep.

MEDICAL TREATMENTS FOR OBSTRUCTIVE SLEEP APNEA

Surgery

Once OSA was recognized, it was logical to turn to surgery as the first method to create a more open airway. If the A+HI were in the severe range, a tracheostomy might be performed to bypass the upper airway obstruction. This allowed the patient to breath freely during sleep through a tube inserted in the neck. Although this was an effective treatment, it was a rather drastic solution, most appropriate for those who were morbidly obese, severely affected by hypoxemia, or when the patient needed temporary support while in emergency status. For patients whose breathing was less severely compromised, more traditional surgeries, such as a tonsillectomy, adenoidectomy, and correction of a deviated nasal septum were often performed in an effort to provide a more patent nasal/oral airway. These were helpful for some children who had very enlarged tonsils but were rarely of sufficient help in adult cases.

The first surgery designed specifically for OSA was the uvulopalatopharyngeoplasty (UPPP), developed by Fujita et al. in 1981 (14). This involved removing the uvula and trimming the soft palate, tonsils, and other redundant soft tissue in the upper airway. This surgery was popular for about 10 years even though the procedure was painful, expensive, and generally successful in reducing the rate of apneic pauses per hour of sleep by only half the preoperative level in 30% to 50% of the cases (15). Follow-up sleep recordings showed the A+HI in many patients to be as high after surgery as before, and some had unpleasant side effects as well. A modified version of this approach, called the *laser-assisted UPPP* (LAUPP), developed by Kamami (16), had the advantage of being an outpatient office procedure. This has largely replaced the traditional UPPP although it is no more successful than the original. It, too, is most helpful for those who are primarily at the early stages of this problem, bothered by snoring, or snoring with a mild degree of sleep apnea (17). The LAUPP is often done as a series of three or more treatments before reaching the desired level of success.

More aggressive surgeries have been developed to reshape the cranial-facial features of patients whose bony structure restricts their posterior airway space (18). Bringing both the upper and lower jaws forward an average of about 10 millimeters in a series of steps has proved successful in two large case series (19–20).

A more recent innovation addresses the problem of the crowded upper airway by injecting radio frequency waves into the soft palate by means of a curved needle. This technique, called *radio frequency ablation* (RFA), stiffens the tissue internally, which reduces the flutter of the uvula and soft palate associated with snoring (21–22). This is a short outpatient procedure no more painful than a dental appointment, which is most beneficial for those on the low end of the severity continuum, that is, with socially bothersome snoring or mild apnea. The RFA technique has also been used to reduce the thickness of a bulky tongue base (23) and to shrink the nasal turbinates if either appears to contribute to upper airway obstruction. A modification of this approach, called *injection snoreplasty,* has recently been reported. In this procedure, a chemical—Sotradecol—is injected instead of the radio frequency waves to reduce the palatal flutter. Little is known yet of the long-term effectiveness of these new methods.

For patients who are massively obese and whose sleep-disordered breathing is severe, surgery that reduces the size of the stomach capacity by gastric bypass (gastroplasty or bariatric surgery) is another surgical option. It is reported to be highly successful in controlling OSA in a recent study (24). Gastroplasty has not often been recommended in the past because it was seen as a risky procedure. It is now being performed as a minimally invasive surgery. A study of OSA patients who had traditional gastric bypass surgery to reduce their weight were found at follow-up to show a return of sleep apnea even when there had not been any associated gain in weight (25). Patients whose airways are prone to collapse during sleep appear likely to continue this episodic loss of tone after all of the so-called "corrective" surgeries.

Mechanical Treatments

Nasal Continuous Positive Airway Pressure

By far, the most common treatment prescribed for this disorder is also the one that brings the most rapid and complete reversal of the sleep-related episodes of obstruction. This method holds the upper airway open mechanically by delivering pressurized air through a nasal mask attached by flexible tubing to a bedside compressor. The level of pressure needed to control the snoring and sleep-disordered breathing must first be established in the sleep laboratory by gradually increasing the pressure until free breathing is restored. This technique, developed originally by Sullivan et al. in 1981 (26) is known as *nasal CPAP* (continuous positive airway pressure). This technique, introduced into the United States in 1985, has undergone many improvements. The noise of the air blowing into the mask has been reduced, the units have been made lighter for those who must travel with their equipment, and the masks now fit better with fewer problems of air leaks. Some patients who resist using the mask because they feel uncomfortable or even claustrophobic when being enclosed can use a system that delivers the air directly into the nostrils through nasal pillows. They can also be desensitized before the sleep test by learning to relax during short periods of using the system during the day. The air can now be heated and humidified before it is delivered to avoid nasal dryness, and chin straps can be added for those CPAP users who breathe through their mouths while sleeping, thereby bypassing the benefit of the pressurized air. Some units are equipped with "smart cards" the patient can swipe periodically and mail to their clinician. When downloaded, these cards show the number of hours the patient has used the CPAP device each night. This permits the clinician to monitor the patient's adherence to this treatment and allows any problems to be addressed directly.

Patient adherence is the major problem associated with CPAP treatment. It is, after all, a clumsy piece of equipment to be used all night, every night. Studies that have tracked the actual hours of use in the home report similar results: About half of the patients for whom this is prescribed actually use the CPAP machine for at least four hours of sleep on 70% of the monitored nights (27). If control of the respiratory events during sleep is necessary for the reversal of the symptoms of excessive daytime sleepiness, elevated morning blood pressure, cognitive difficulties, and irritable mood (28–29), the poor rate of adherence to this treatment is a worrisome problem.

Investigations of the variables associated with good and poor compliance with CPAP treatment suggest that it is those patients who experience immediate relief from excessive daytime sleepiness who are most likely to continue to wear their equipment most consistently (30). Some patients never accept this treatment option; others do initially, then simply discontinue using their device. Still others do not use it for enough hours to obtain the needed benefit. After a patient is diagnosed, equipment is typically ordered from a vendor of home health equipment for a trial period during which the machine is rented through the patient's medical insurance plan. After this period, the patient may be required to assist the insurance company in the purchase of the machine and may be reluctant to contribute to the purchase if the machine is not being used regularly. Dropout rates at this point have been estimated between 5% and 30% (31).

Establishing whether those who continue nightly use have adequate hours is more complicated because there must be some agreement about what constitutes a "therapeutic dose." A seminal study of adherence by Kribbs et al. (27) recommended two separate definitions. Minimally acceptable and optimal use was defined as using CPAP at least four and seven hours, respectively, on at least five of seven nights. While 46% of the participants in this study met criteria for minimal use, only 6% met criteria for optimal use. Average use for the entire group was 5.3 hours per night. These findings are consistent with other studies of adherence, reporting rates of 4.7 to 5.6 hours of use per night in patients receiving standard clinical care (32–35). It stands to reason that these less than optimal rates of CPAP use produce only partial improvements in day-time functioning (36).

Several studies have examined the effects of supportive or cognitive-behavioral techniques for improving adherence to CPAP in moderate to severe OSA patients (37–38). A support group and verbal reinforcement strategies have been only modestly effective. Likar et al. (39) found that patients attending an OSA support group used CPAP about one hour per night more than those who did not attend. Similarly, in a study of verbal reinforcement, Fletcher and Luckett reported that CPAP adherence was increased by about one hour per night compared to a control group (40). Three months later, treatments were switched across the groups. Both the size and direction of the initial effect in the experimental group remained, suggesting that the intervention worked best when it occurred early in treatment.

In keeping with the notion that there may be a "critical window" for improv-ing the time used, Hoy et al. tested an intensive CPAP setup protocol versus standard clinical care. The intensive setup consisted of home education of both the patient and his or her spouse, three nights of CPAP titration, and home visits by nurses at 7, 14, 28, and 120 days to troubleshoot any difficulties. This inten-sive intervention improved CPAP use by only 1.5 hours per night compared to a group receiving standard clinical care. At the six-month follow-up, the intensive group still used CPAP only an average of 5.4 hours per night (41).

In contrast to this expensive, intensive early intervention, Chervin et al. (39) found that the provision of literature on sleep apnea was sufficient to produce in-creased adherence. In this study, *bibliotherapy* was more effective than was a se-ries of supportive phone calls. Patients receiving the literature used their CPAP about 1.5 hours per night more (7 hours per night on average) than those receiv-ing supportive phone calls, who averaged 5.5 hours per night. This was about 2.5 hours per night more than a group who received no intervention (4.5 hours per night on average). The only statistically significant difference in this study was between the literature and no intervention control groups. While the results from this study seemed promising, the literature provided information similar to that already used in most sleep centers. Given that most centers report poor adher-ence despite using this type of literature, these results need to be replicated.

Aloia and colleagues (42) employed a motivational enhancement interven-tion designed to increase compliance. Before receiving their CPAP, two matched groups of six patients each received either a 45-minute face-to-face session of motivational enhancement intervention (MEI) or an attention control intervention. The MEI was designed to decrease ambivalence toward treatment. The control group received the same amount of face-to-face therapy time, but the content consisted solely of educational information on sleep architecture and the participant's evaluation of the clinic. A second session took place one week later. Machine nightly use was downloaded at 1, 4, and 12 weeks posttreatment initiation.

Participants in the two conditions did not differ at week 1. A trend was evident at week 4, however, with an overall mean increase of only 1.3 hours per night. The two groups significantly differed in terms of hours of CPAP use at week 12 with motivational treatment subjects using CPAP 3.2 hours more than the control subjects. Using a six-hour minimum of CPAP per night as the cutoff at the 12-week follow-up point, five of six experimental treatment subjects were classified as compliant compared to one of the six control subjects.

Finally, systematic desensitization and sensory awareness techniques have also been used to improve adherence. In a six-month follow-up study, CPAP was discontinued in only 13% of the group desensitized to CPAP as compared to a 47% discontinuation in the control group. While effective, this intervention is considered by some to be too time- and cost-intensive. Therefore, this form of intervention may be best for the subjects who have discontinued their treatment.

Overall, attempts to improve compliance through patient education programs, regular follow-up phone calls, support groups, motivational interviewing, and desensitization procedures have been only moderately successful. To date, systematic desensitization appears to be useful for preventing the discontinuation of CPAP therapy, and motivational interviewing looks to be a promising intervention for increasing nightly use time.

This leaves the problem of CPAP being the best treatment option available for normalizing sleep-disordered breathing but one that is accepted and used by only half of those for whom it is prescribed who receive only standard clinical care. Patients report that it is just too much bother, too large, too difficult to keep in place, and generally more nuisance than they can tolerate. The data from the downloads from the equipment typically show that those who are not using the CPAP all night start the night with it on but remove it when they get up to go the bathroom and do not replace the mask when they return to bed. This means that in the last two or three hours of sleep, when REM sleep is more prominent and when apneic events are longer and more severe, these patients are not being protected by the CPAP treatment. This is a point at which behaviorally trained clinical psychologists can make a contribution to the care. However, few clinical services have incorporated this into their usual care. Patients who refuse CPAP or drop out may switch to a different kind of device. When offered a trial of both CPAP and an oral appliance, patients more often choose to continue their treatment with the oral appliance even when it proves to be less effective in controlling their OSA than the CPAP (43). Further work on improving CPAP adherence is a priority area of research for health psychologists.

Oral Appliances

A large number of mouth pieces, designed to be worn during sleep for the control of snoring and OSA, have been approved by the FDA (44). Most of these must be fitted by a dentist. They work on one of two principles—either to hold the tongue forward during sleep to prevent it from retrolapsing against the posterior pharyngeal wall (45) or to move the lower jaw forward (46). Both will increase the posterior airway space and tighten the tongue (genioglossis) muscle that typically relaxes during sleep. These devices have also undergone design improvements since they were first introduced. Some are now adjustable even by the bed partner in the home, and some have built-in monitors to provide information on how often they are being used (47–48). They are about 80% effective in controlling snoring and mild to moderately severe OSA. However, when the A+HI is in the severe range, greater than 30 events per hour, the proportion of patients who achieve trouble-free breathing with an oral appliance drop to about 30%. As discussed later, severity of OSA is positively correlated with a differential rate of A+HI by sleep position. Those with a higher rate of apnea when they sleep on their backs than when in a side position are more likely to be successfully treated with an oral appliance (49–50).

Combined Surgical and Mechanical Treatments

Control of sleep-disordered breathing often needs more than one treatment. An oral appliance that does not permit mouth breathing is not useful for patients who have difficulty breathing through their nose. Once the nasal airway has been opened by treating congestion due to sinus infection or allergy or by performing surgery to correct a structurally narrowed nasal passage due to polyps, enlarged turbinates, or a deviated septum, some find they can use an oral appliance to control snoring and moderately severe apnea with good success (51). In general, combining treatments should proceed from less to more invasive. If an initial UPPP surgery has removed most of the soft tissue of the palate, the patient who does not get adequate control of symptoms (50% of patients) may no longer have the option of using a nasal CPAP with success.

Pharmacological Treatments

Many agents have been explored for their effectiveness in stimulating respiration during sleep in hopes of finding a medication treatment for the sleep apneic patient. Neither theophylline nor medroxyprogesterone has proved useful. For patients whose apnea is confined to REM sleep, nortriptyline or protriptyline, both of which have a REM sleep suppression effect, have been used on occasion with some effectiveness. The magic pill has yet to be developed that will be generally effective for this disorder.

BEHAVIORAL TREATMENTS

Sleep Position Training

Part of the evaluation of patients for OSA includes determining whether they have been observed to snore more often and more loudly and to have more frequent and longer breathing pauses when they sleep on their backs than when they turn and sleep in a side position. Despite the fact that Gastaut et al. (3) had noted this differential in the original paper on OSA, the early sleep laboratory evaluations did not always differentiate the rate of respiratory events by the time slept in various sleep positions and did not take this into account in making the treatment plan. This may well have resulted in the overdiagnosis and inflated reports of the severity of the OSA disorder. This was particularly likely to occur in patients who remained in the supine position while being tested because of fear of displacing the electrodes by any body movement, even though this was not their usual sleep posture when sleeping at home (52). Chart reviews of large unselected samples of patients ($N = 574$ and $N = 184$) who had been diagnosed with OSA showed that 56% to 60% sustained A+HI rates that were two or more times higher while they slept supine than when they slept in the lateral position (53–54). This ratio proved to be highly reliable from night to night and inversely related to the severity of the apnea and to the degree to which the patient was overweight. Recognizing that OSA severity varies by sleep position in a majority of patients, the guidelines for diagnosing this disorder were written to include the requirement that sleep posture be monitored.

If roughly half the patients who are referred for evaluation of a sleep-related breathing disorder have a dramatic improvement in their ability to breath freely when they spontaneously turn from back to side, this appears to be another opportunity to use a behavior change strategy as a treatment. There were some reports of homemade devices already being effective in controlling snoring by making the supine position uncomfortable. Sewing or pinning a tennis ball to the back of the pajama top was one that still finds its way into the popular press (55). Lloyd developed a position monitor for training OSA patients through the use of an auditory signal. The device consisted of a small position-sensitive monitor mounted on a Velcro strap worn around the chest. This produced a loud beep if a patient remained sleeping on his or her back for more than 15 seconds. Eight of

10 patients tested with this equipment for one laboratory night responded by reducing their supine sleep time to zero (56). For home use, a digital counter was attached to the monitor. This accumulated the number of times the signal was activated each night. The patient was instructed to log this number each morning and reset the counter to zero for the next night. When this display showed a consistent reading of zero for a week, the patient was assumed to be trained. In one experimental study testing this assumption, the results showed that not all positional OSA patients could be trained at home to a satisfactory level of control by using a monitor over an eight-week period (57). Fourteen of 20 patients averaged fewer than five signals on the last week of their home training period. The six who still needed more than five signals to avoid back sleep were those most severe on their diagnostic night (mean A+HI = 52). However, when retested in the laboratory without the help of the signal after their home training period, their average A+HI had dropped to 19.3. This was not significantly higher than the posttraining mean A+HI of the 14 patients who appeared to be trained at home (mean A+HI = 15.6). The difference between the groups is that half of the 14 who recorded few home signals were now within normal limits on their laboratory follow-up night (A+HI < 5), whereas none of those who still needed more auditory cues at home were within normal limits when retested without the signal. The question of whether and for how long this training can be maintained without some reinforcement has not been formally tested. Another finding from that study was that the mean number of signals for slow learners during home training (mean = 14.4 by the eighth week) was reduced to a mean of only two on the posttraining laboratory night when they were allowed to have the signal turned on. This is a warning that performance in the sleep laboratory may not always be a good representation of the patient's unmonitored sleep at home. When patients are aware that they are being watched and tested, they proved to be much more able to control their sleep position behavior in the laboratory setting.

Reporting the severity of respiratory disturbance by sleep position per hour of sleep is now more common. If the A+HI is at, or nearly, within normal limits in lateral sleep, wearing a nightshirt with a vertical pocket to hold three or four tennis balls in a line down the spine helps train the sleep apnea patients to avoid supine sleep. However, there are only a few laboratory studies testing the effectiveness of these T-shirts to control sleep-disordered breathing. One study showed that avoiding supine sleep over a one-month interval using such a T-shirt resulted in a lower mean blood pressure for all 13 of a group of positional OSA patients, even though they had no change in their body weight during this period. These patients wore ambulatory blood pressure monitoring equipment for a 24-hour period to compare their blood pressure (B/P) before and after being trained to avoid sleeping on their backs. Both those patients who were initially hypertensive and those who were not reduced their B/P by avoiding supine sleep (58).

Combined Position Training and Mechanical Devices

A few studies have looked into whether the CPAP pressure needed to control OSA is lower during lateral than supine sleep, for both patients who do and do not have more severe apnea during back sleep. These suggest a small but significantly lower pressure required during lateral sleep. It is difficult to have enough time in a usual single night of clinical evaluation to establish the effective pressure in each body position for both REM and NREM sleep stages and whether this difference is large enough to justify combining CPAP treatment with position training (59–60).

To examine the optional treatment for OSA patients who were positional on their diagnostic sleep test, 60 patients were assigned to eight weeks of home treatment of four different types (61). The patients were randomly assigned to:

1. Use an oral appliance.
2. Use the posture alarm for position training.
3. Use a combination of oral appliance and the posture alarm.
4. Learn to avoid supine sleep on their own.

They were then tested in the laboratory for two more nights, one with and one without their devices in place. Thirty-seven of the 60 (62%) had an A+HI within normal limits on the posttreatment night when they were allowed to use their various treatment strategies to avoid supine sleep. Twenty (33%) were normal also on the second night without the treatment instruments in place, indicating the breathing problem was now controlled. Group 3, who received the combined treatment, had the highest number who were successfully treated with 11 of the 15 patients (73%) having fewer than five respiration events per hour on the follow-up night. Those who were more obese and whose apnea was initially more severe were less successful with the treatments used in this study.

Weight Loss

Because many OSA patients are overweight, a change in eating habits is clearly one kind of behavioral program that should be of help in managing this disorder. How much weight must be lost to normalize sleep-related respiratory problems is unknown, which makes it difficult to set a target for any specific patient. Few studies of single cases report a logarithmic relation of apnea and body weight (62). Also in contrast to gastroplasty, weight loss accomplished by a change in eating habits is a slow process. This means some more immediately effective treatment is typically needed in the interim. Many patients use a CPAP until they have lost 20 to 40 pounds, sufficient to justify a new sleep laboratory evaluation. This new test starts without any pressure through the CPAP mask to establish the current level of the respiratory problem. If there are no episodes of apnea or snoring or if these appear to be fewer than five per hour, the CPAP will not be initiated. If during the first hour or two the patient is snoring and exhibiting respiratory events that lead to episodes of oxygen desaturation and arousals, the balance of the night is used to establish the CPAP pressure the patient now needs to control these events. If the sleep study demonstrates that the loss of weight has improved the patient's breathing problem from severe to a mild or moderate level, a substitute for the CPAP may then be appropriate. This might be an oral appliance or positional training or both.

Weight loss is difficult for the OSA patient to achieve and even harder to maintain. This difficulty is partly because of a problem common to many programs, which attempt to change behaviors that have a negative impact on health—the problem of patients' feeling of failure when they break the rules by yielding to temptation on one or more occasion. Often, they then feel justified in giving up all effort to change. At this point, the clinician needs to redefine this as a slip, rather than a total failure. When a weight reduction program is carried out as a group treatment, those who have shared the experience of an occasional slip are more effective in encouraging the patient's continued effort than is an individual therapist—especially one who is slender. For the same reason, if both members of a couple are overweight, programs for the two of them work better than when only one needs to change his or her eating behavior. The partner who does the shopping and meal preparation, even when not overweight, needs to be involved in the treatment planning for the apneic patient to ensure that treatment is not sabotaged. Many obese OSA patients do most of their eating outside the home. Sometimes a simple change in restaurant eating can make a significant difference in weight. One patient whose A+HI when he was first diagnosed was over 100 used a CPAP while trying to lose weight. On reevaluation eight months later, his A+HI was 0. He had lost weight by changing from taking his clients out to dinner to taking them to lunch, where he felt comfortable ordering only a salad for himself (52).

A formal dietary controlled weight loss program is not always affordable, nor is it reimbursable or even necessary when patients are encouraged by a behaviorally trained psychologist to make changes on their own in their eating behavior. Simple, easy to remember rules with periodic checkups often work better than calorie counting or complicated exchange programs.

Weight Loss Rules

1. Keep a daily record of when and what you eat. Review this food log to become more aware of your own intake of foods and drinks. Before buying, look at the labels for calorie and fat content.
2. Limit yourself to three meals a day with no between-meal snacks.
3. Drink a glass of water before each meal and avoid carbonated soft drinks.
4. Use a smaller plate to reduce portion size and no seconds.
5. Slow down your eating; pause between bites.
6. Become aware of when you feel full—and then stop.
7. Don't skip breakfast, eat a fast-food lunch, and load up at dinner. You have more chance of burning off calories by working than by sleeping on a full stomach.

All of these statements have a similar thrust: They put patients in charge of their eating behavior and give them the chance to make choices that will effect significant weight changes. This program works well with periodic clinic visits to weigh in, review the food log, and receive feedback and reinforcement from the behavioral clinician.

Part of any weight loss program should include attention to the patient's use of alcohol, not only because of its high caloric value but for the direct effect that alcohol has on relaxing the muscles of the upper airway (63–64). Late night alcohol increases snoring frequency and loudness and has also been demonstrated to markedly reduce the tone of the upper airway muscles, leading to an increase in the number and length of the respiratory pauses even in nonapneic persons (65) and especially in those who are in the severe range of this disorder.

Exercise

Physical exercise has often been abandoned by sleep apnea patients, especially those who are having a major problem with excessive daytime sleepiness. Many state they just do not have the energy to engage in any exercise. Here, too, the interim use of a nasal CPAP can tide a patient over and give the symptom relief needed to engage in a weight loss and exercise program. When they have reduced their weight and increased muscle tone sufficiently to bring the A+HI down to more moderate levels, alternate treatments can be introduced. Patients are often more willing to accept a CPAP as an adjunct treatment than if they feel it will be needed for a lifetime. Once patients experience a marked increase in energy from using the CPAP for at least six hours per night, they can more easily incorporate physical exercise into their daily routines. Here, too, some simple habit changes that fit into their usual daily schedule and are less expensive than a health club membership can be implemented and monitored by a health psychologist sleep clinic team member:

1. Take a walk at lunchtime or after dinner for 20 minutes, and gradually increase this time. Walking with the bed partner is a good plan if possible.
2. Use the stairs rather than the elevator at least for one floor, and gradually increase the number of flights you walk.
3. Park a block or more away from your destination and walk the rest.
4. Use a bicycle instead of a car whenever possible.
5. Stand up instead of sitting when talking on the telephone.

Smoking Cessation

A history of smoking is a risk factor for the development of sleep apnea. If the patient is still an active smoker, every effort should be made to help him or her to stop. Many programs have been successful in helping patients control this behavior. The most important ingredient in this success is the patient's own motivation to quit. Without this, no program has much chance of working. When the patient is motivated but having difficulty making this change, a program that combines pharmacologic and behavior change elements increases the probability of success. The pharmacologic agents that are used most often, the nicotine patch or Wellbutrin, which reduce nicotine craving, are coupled with a gradual programmed reduction in number of cigarettes smoked per day. Again, this can be administered by the psychologist team member of the sleep center.

Summary of Studies

The most useful summary of these studies using a combination of treatment strategies is that CPAP and a concurrent weight loss program is the best initial treatment for the severely apneic patient who is overweight and does not show any positional benefit from side sleep. If, following some weight loss, the patient then shows a marked positional difference in apnea severity, an oral appliance and position training can replace the CPAP. Patients should be encouraged to continue their weight loss program until they are within their ideal body weight for their height. This sequential management program requires more systematic follow-up and care than is usual for clinical patients to receive and insurance programs to support. Those who, on diagnostic testing, are positional are more likely to be more moderately affected by OSA and less overweight. If their A+HI is at, or close to, normal limits during lateral sleep, they may be treated by position training alone. However, most of these will still require treatment for some snoring and mild respiratory events that persist in lateral sleep. These may be controlled with the addition of an oral appliance.

Behavioral treatments aimed at controlling eating, smoking, and alcohol drinking behaviors should be part of the routine care offered to all OSA patients. All patients with this diagnosis need to understand their vulnerability to relapse even after successful treatment. Further, treatments can be phased in and out as needed and as appropriate to their stage of severity and willingness to adhere to them. This approach to a combination of mechanical and behavioral treatments appears to have the best likelihood of being effective in controlling OSA and is best delivered by a team trained in the management of sleep problems.

FUTURE DIRECTIONS FOR PRACTICE AND RESEARCH

Although this chapter has emphasized the role of behavior change in the treatment of OSA, some patients require more aggressive treatment. Some patients' cranial facial structure restricts the size of the upper airway, and others must have a patent nasal airway established before all else. Surgery may have to be the first step in these cases. In some families where the father has already been diagnosed, his sons may look like him and snore like he snores. For them, preventive measures may be in order to defeat further progression into frank OSA. Education of the public and changes in public policy can have an impact on the behaviors that contribute to the risk of developing overt OSA:

1. Some local school boards has initiated programs to help counteract the rising rates of obesity among adolescents by terminating long-term contracts that make high-calorie soft drinks available in the schools and by attention to school lunch menus to limit fast foods.
2. Smoking cessation campaigns are already targeting young people who smoke, and requiring proof of age before purchase of cigarettes is an added deterrent.
3. Proof of age is also being employed to help discourage early drinking (signs saying "We Card").
4. Education programs for primary care physicians are increasing their awareness of the connection among hypertension, body habitus, weight

gain, and snoring and between these and OSA. There is already evidence showing that short courses on sleep disorders for HMO physicians have increased their ability to identify patients at an early stage of the development of this disorder and greatly reduce the number of visits and health care costs (66).

5. The campaign to teach the mothers of newborns to put their infants to sleep on their backs ("Back To Sleep") has had a marked effect on reducing the prevalence of Sudden Infant Death Syndrome (SIDS). Pediatricians should now be educating mothers that, once their child is past the danger age for SIDS, they should train their children to become side sleepers for life.

If public education and continuing education programs for physicians and psychologists can help bring about changes in eating, smoking, exercise, alcohol drinking, and sleep position behaviors, the problems of Dickens' Joe with obesity, excessive sleepiness, and snoring would be less of a national problem and fewer adults would develop OSA with its consequent health problems. Toward achieving this goal, behaviorally trained psychologists are key players in developing the programs and testing their efficacy in well-designed research studies.

REFERENCES

1. Peppard, P., T. Young, M. Palta, and J. Skatrud. Prospective study of the association between sleep-disordered breathing and hypertension. *New England Journal of Medicine* 342: 1378–1384, 2000.

2. American Academy of Sleep Medicine Task Force. Sleep-related breathing disorders in adults: Recommendations for syndrome definition and measurement techniques in clinical research. *Sleep* 22: 667–689, 1999.

3. Gastaut, H., C. Tassinari, and B. Duran. Polygraphic study of the episodic nocturnal and diurnal manifestations of the Pickwick syndrome. *Brain Research* 2: 167–186, 1961.

4. Dickens, C. *Pickwick Papers*. New York, NY: Signet Classics. 1964.

5. Young, T., M. Palta, J. Dempsey, J. Skatrud, S. Weber, and S. Badr. The occurrence of sleep-disordered breathing among middle-aged adults. *New England Journal of Medicine* 328: 1230–1235, 1993.

6. Nieto, F. J., T. Young, B. Lind, E. Shahar, J. Samet, S. Redline, et al. Association of sleep-disordered breathing, sleep apnea, and hypertension in a large community-based study. *Journal of the American Medical Association* 283: 1829–1836, 2000.

7. Pack, A. I., A. M. Pack, and E. Rodgman. Characteristics of crashes attributed to the driver having fallen asleep. *Accident Analysis and Prevention* 27: 769–775, 1995.

8. Findley, L. J., M. E. Univerzaat, and R. Guchu. Vigilance and automobile accidents in patients with sleep apnea or narcolepsy. *Chest* 108: 619–624, 1995.

9. Bassiri, A. and C. Guilleminault. Clinical features and evaluation of obstructive sleep apnea-hypopnea syndrome In M. H. Kryger, T. Roth, and W. C. Dement, eds. *Principles and Practice of Sleep Medicine* (3rd Edition). Philadelphia, PA: W.B. Saunders Company. 2000: 869–878.

10. Cartwright, R. and S. Knight. Silent partners: The wives of sleep apneic patients. *Sleep* 10: 244–248, 1987.

11. Johnson, E. *Sleep in America: 2000.* Washington, DC: National Sleep Foundation. 2000.

12. Partinen, M. and C. Hublin. Epidemiology of sleep disorders In M. H. Kryger, T. Roth, and W. C. Dement, eds. *Principles and Practice of Sleep Medicine* (3rd Edition). Philadelphia, PA: W.B. Saunders Company. 2000: 558–579.

13. Davies, R. J. O. and R. J. Stradling. The relationship between neck circumference, radiographic pharyngeal anatomy and obstructive sleep apnea syndrome. *European Respiratory Journal* 3: 509–514, 1990.

14. Fujita, S., W. Conway, and F. Zorick. Surgical correction of anatomic abnormalities in obstructive sleep apnea: Uvulopalatopharyngeoplasty. *Otolaryngology: Head and Neck Surgery* 89: 923–934, 1981.

15. Sher, A., K. Schechtman, and J. Piccirillo. The efficacy of surgical modifications of the upper airway in adults with obstructive sleep apnea syndrome. *Sleep* 19: 156–177, 1996.

16. Kamami, Y. Laser CO2 for snoring: Preliminary results. *Acta Otorhinolaryngol Belgium* 44: 451–456, 1990.

17. Walker, R., M. Grigg-Damberger, and C. Gopalsami. Laser assisted uvulopalatoplasty for snoring and obstructive sleep apnea: Results in 1970 patients. *Largynoscope* 105: 938–943, 1995.

18. Jamieson, A., C. Guilleminault, and M. Partinen. Obstructive sleep apneic patients have craniomandibular abnormalities. *Sleep* 9: 469–477, 1986.

19. Riley, R., N. Powell, and C. Guilleminault. Maxillofacial surgery and obstructive sleep apnea: Review of 80 patients. *Otolaryngology: Head and Neck Surgery* 101: 353–361, 1989.

20. Prinsell, J. Maxillomandibular advancement surgery in a site-specific treatment approach for obstructive sleep apnea in 50 consecutive patients. *Chest* 116: 1519–1529, 1999.

21. Powell, N., R. Riley, and R. Troell. Radio frequency volumetric tissue reduction of the palate in subjects with sleep-disordered breathing. *Chest* 113: 1163–1174, 1998.

22. Cartwright, R., T. Venkatesan, D. Caldarelli, and F. Diaz. Treatments for snoring: A comparison of somnoplasty and an oral appliance. *Largynoscope* 110: 1680–1683, 2000.

23. Powell, N., R. Riley, and C. Guilleminault. Radio frequency tongue base reduction in sleep-disordered breathing: A pilot study. *Otolaryngology: Head and Neck Surgery* 120: 656–664, 1999.

24. Dixon, J., L. Schachter, and P. O'Brien. Sleep disturbance and obesity: Changes following surgically induced weight loss. *Archives of Internal Medicine* 161: 102–106, 2001.

25. Pillar, G., R. Peled, and P. Lavie. Recurrence of sleep apnea without concomitant weight increase 7.5 years after weight reduction surgery. *Chest* 106: 1702–1704, 1994.

26. Sullivan, C., F. Issa, and M. Berthon-Jones. Reversal of obstructive sleep apnea by continuous positive airway pressure applied through the nares. *Lancet* 1: 862–865, 1981.

27. Kribbs, N., A. Pack, L. Kline, P. Smith, A. Schwartz, N. Schubert, et al. Objective measurement of patterns of nasal CPAP use by patients with obstructive sleep apnea. *American Review of Respiratory Diseases* 147: 887–895, 1993.

28. Meslier, N., T. Lebrunt, and V. Grillier-Lanoir. French survey of 3,225 patients treated with CPAP for obstructive sleep apnea: Benefits, tolerance, compliance and quality of life. *European Respiratory Journal* 12: 185–192, 1998.

29. Faccenda, J. F., T. W. Mackay, N. Boon, and N. J. Douglas. Randomized placebo-controlled trial of continuous positive airway pressure on blood pressure in sleep apnea/hypopnea syndrome. *American Journal of Respiratory and Critical Care Medicine* 163: 344–348, 2001.

30. Meurice, J., P. Dore, and J. Paquereau. Predictive factors of long term compliance with nasal continuous positive airway pressure treatment in sleep apnea syndrome. *Chest* 105: 429–433, 1994.

31. Collard, P., T. Pieters, G. Aubert, P. Delguste, and D. O. Rodenstein. Compliance with nasal CPAP in obstructive sleep apnea patients. *Sleep Medicine Reviews* 1(1): 33–44, 1997.

32. Engleman, H. M., S. E. Martin, and N. J. Douglas. Compliance with CPAP therapy in patients with sleep apnea/hypopnea syndrome. *Thorax* 49: 263–266, 1994.

33. Krieger, J. and D. Krutz. Objective measurement of CPAP compliance with nasal CPAP treatment for obstructive sleep apnea syndrome. *European Respiratory Journal* 1: 436–438, 1988.

34. Rauscher, H., D. Formanck, W. Popp, and H. Zwick. Self-reported vs. measured compliance with nasal CPAP for obstructive sleep apnea. *Chest* 103: 1675–1680, 1993.

35. Reeves-Hoche, M. K., R. Meck, and C. W. Zwillich. Nasal CPAP: An objective evaluation of patient compliance. *American Journal of Respiratory and Critical Care Medicine* 149: 149–154, 1994.

36. Engleman, H. M., S. E. Martin, I. J. Deary, and N. J. Douglas. Effect of continuous positive airway pressure treatment on daytime function in sleep apnea/hypopnea syndrome. *Lancet* 343: 572–575, 1994.

37. Anstead, M., B. Phillips, and K. Bach. Tolerance and intolerance to continuous positive airway pressure. *Current Opinion in Pulmonary Medicine* 4: 351–354, 1998.

38. Chervin, R., S. Theut, C. Bassetti, and M. Aldrich. Compliance with nasal CPAP can be improved by simple interventions. *Sleep* 20: 284–289, 1997.

39. Likar, L., T. Panicera, A. Erickson, and S. Rounds. Group education sessions and compliance with nasal CPAP therapy. *Chest* 111: 1273–1277.

40. Fletcher, E. C. and R. A. Luckett. The effect of positive reinforcement on hourly compliance in nasal continuous positive airway pressure users with obstructive sleep apnea. *American Review of Respiratory Diseases* 143: 936–941, 1991.

41. Hoy, C. J., M. Vennelle, R. N. Kingshott, H. M. Engleman, and N. J. Douglas. Can intensive support improve continuous positive airway pressure use in patients with the sleep apnea/hypopnea syndrome? *American Journal of Respiratory and Critical Care Medicine* 159: 1096–1100, 1999.

42. Aloia, M. Maximizing patient's potential: Strategies to improve CPAP compliance in elderly apnea patients. *Advance for Managers of Respiratory Care* 9(6): 31–33, 2000.

43. Ferguson, K., T. Ono, and A. Lowe. A randomized cross-over study of an oral appliance vs. nasal continuous positive airway pressure in the treatment of mild-moderate obstructive sleep apnea. *Chest* 109: 1269–1275, 1996.

44. Lowe, A. Oral appliances for sleep breathing disorders. In M. H. Kryger, T. Roth, and W. C. Dement, eds. *Principles and Practice of Sleep Medicine* (3rd Edition). Philadelphia, PA: W.B. Saunders Company. 2000: 929–939.

45. Cartwright, R. and C. Samelson. The effects of a nonsurgical treatment for obstructive sleep apnea. *Journal of the American Medical Association* 248: 705–709, 1982.

46. Clark, G. Mandibular advancement devices and sleep disordered breathing. *Sleep Medicine Reviews* 2: 163–174, 1998.

47. Schmidt-Nowara, W., A. Lone, L. Wiegand, R. Cartwright, G. Perez-Guerra, and S. Mann. Oral appliances for the treatment of snoring and obstructive sleep apnea: A review. *Sleep* 18: 501–510, 1995.

48. Pancer, J., M. Al-Faifi, and V. Hoffstein. Evaluation of a variable mandibular advancement appliance for the treatment of snoring and sleep apnea. *Chest* 116: 1511–1518, 1999.

49. Cartwright, R. What's new in oral appliances for snoring and sleep apnea: An update. *Sleep Medicine Reviews* 5: 25–32, 2001.

50. Cartwright, R. Predicting response to the tongue retaining device for sleep apnea syndrome. *Archives of Otolaryngology* 111: 385–388, 1985.

51. Caldarelli, D., R. Cartwright, and J. Lilie. Obstructive sleep apnea: Variations in surgical management. *Largynoscope* 95: 1070–1073, 1985.

52. Cartwright, R. Obstructive sleep apnea: A sleep disorder with major effects on health. *Disease-A-Month* 47: 105–148, 2001.

53. Oksenberg, A., D. Silverberg, and E. Arons. Positional vs. nonpositional obstructive sleep apnea patients: Anthropometric, nocturnal polysomnographic and multiple sleep latency test data. *Chest* 112: 629–639, 1997.

54. Lloyd, S. and R. Cartwright. Physiologic basis of therapy for sleep apnea. *American Review of Respiratory Diseases* 136: 525–526, 1987.

55. Editorial Note: Patient's wife cures his snoring. *Chest* 84: 582, 1984.

56. Cartwright, R., S. Lloyd, J. Lilie, and H. Kravitz. Sleep position training as treatment for sleep apnea syndrome: A preliminary study. *Sleep* 8: 87–94, 1985.

57. Cartwright, R. Home modification of sleep position for sleep apnea control. In L. Miles and R. Broughton, eds. *Medical Monitoring in the Home and Work Environment.* New York, NY: Raven Press. 1990: 123–128.

58. Berger, M., A. Oksenberg, D. Silverberg, E. Arons, H. Radwan, and A. Iaina. Avoiding the supine position during sleep lowers 24h blood pressure in obstructive sleep apnea (OSA) patients. *Journal of Human Hypertension* 11: 647–664, 1997.

59. Pevernagie, D. and J. Shepard. Relations between sleep stage, posture and effective nasal CPAP levels in OSA. *Sleep* 15: 162–167, 1992.

60. Oksenberg, A. and D. Silverberg. The effect of body posture on sleep-related breathing disorders: Facts and therapeutic implications. *Sleep Medicine Reviews* 2: 139–162, 1998.

61. Cartwright, R., R. Ristanovic, F. Diaz, D. Caldarelli, and G. Alder. A comparative study of treatments for positional sleep apnea. *Sleep* 14: 546–552, 1991.

62. Browman, C., M. Sampson, and S. Yolles. Obstructive sleep apnea and body weight. *Chest* 85: 435–436, 1984.

63. Remmers, J. Obstructive sleep apnea: A common disorder exacerbated by alcohol. *American Review of Respiratory Diseases* 130: 153–155, 1984.

64. Scrima, L., M. Broady, and K. Nay. Increased severity of obstructive sleep apnea after bedtime alcohol ingestion: Diagnostic potential and proposed mechanism of action. *Sleep* 5: 318–328, 1982.

65. Berry, R., M. Bonnet, and R. Light. Effect of ethanol on the arousal response to airway occulsion during sleep in normals. *American Review of Respiratory Diseases* 145: 445–452, 1992.

66. Johnson, S. Sleep medicine as preventive medicine. In S. Poceta and M. Mitler, eds. *Sleep Disorders: Diagnosis and Treatment.* Totowa, NJ: Humana Press. 1998: 199–220.

Chapter 4 ————————————————————————

PERIODIC LIMB MOVEMENTS: ASSESSMENT AND MANAGEMENT STRATEGIES

JACK D. EDINGER

Periodic limb movements (PLMs) are curious phenomena characterized by repetitive, stereotyped movements of the lower and, sometimes, upper extremities during sleep. Typically, PLMs consist of dorsiflexions of the ankle and extension of the great toe lasting 0.5 to 4.0 seconds and occurring repetitively every 20 to 40 seconds (range = 5 to 90 sec.) with remarkable periodicity. The degree of movement may vary from subtle dorsiflexion of the ankle or toes to pronounced movement of the ankle along with partial flexion of the knee and hip. The latter is reminiscent of the triple flexion response or exaggerated Babinski sign that is elicited in some patients with upper motor neuron lesions (1). In some individuals, flexions of the arm or upper body jerks may be observed as part of the PLM complex. Usually PLMs are most prominent during stages 1 and 2 of NREM sleep, but they may also be seen during slow wave sleep, REM episodes, and periods of quiet wakefulness before sleep onset (2). Nocturnal sleep monitoring studies show some individuals manifest PLMs with little apparent sleep disturbance, whereas others display frequent EEG arousals associated with their occurrence (2).

At present, PLMs remain poorly understood and arguably controversial sleep-related motor events. Whether these sleep-related movements represent a discrete sleep disorder or are merely an incidental finding remains hotly debated by sleep experts. This chapter briefly reviews what is known about the etiology, prevalence, and potential clinical significance of PLMs. Subsequently, the diagnosis, periodic limb movement disorder (PLMD) is discussed, and assessment methods used in establishing this diagnosis are considered. The latter portions of the chapter provide a brief review of pharmacological approaches to PLMD and present a rationale for the incorporation of alternative behavioral treatments in the management of PLMD patients. In addition, the nature and efficacy of several behavioral treatments for PLMD are considered. The chapter concludes by posing a number of important questions designed to stimulate continued interest in research concerning behavioral treatments with PLMD.

ETIOLOGY

Originally called *nocturnal myoclonus,* PLMs were first described about 50 years ago by Symonds (3), who viewed these and several other sleep-related movements as epileptic variants. Although this view failed to gain wide acceptance, the exact etiology of PLMs remains an open question. However, electrophysiological studies conducted to determine the origins of PLMs primarily have implicated subcortical CNS areas in the production of these phenomena. Those studies conducted to explore cortical involvement have either failed to identify cortical prepotentials immediately preceding PLMs or found only nonspecific potentials that mimicked those seen just before voluntary limb movements (4–5). More recently, a neural imaging study employing functional MRI showed the occurrence of PLMs was associated specifically with activation of subcortical areas including the red nuclei and pontine sites (6). Observations of PLMs occurring during spinal and epidural anesthesia and in cases of complete spinal cord transection imply that spinal cord areas may also contribute significantly to PLM activity (7–9). Furthermore, all studies of PLMs have demonstrated their 20- to 40-second periodicity, which mirrors the periodicity seen during sleep and coma for functions such as blood pressure, respiration, intraventricular fluid pressure, and pulse frequency (10–11). This observation, in turn, suggests the likely involvement of an underlying CNS (brainstem or spinal cord) pacemaker in PLM events. Finally, the effectiveness of opioids and L-dopa for reducing PLM-related sleep complaints has suggested the neurochemical basis of these phenomena may reside in the dopaminergic and/or opiate systems (12).

Previous research has provided significant insights into the etiology of PLMs, but there are important questions about this phenomenon's origins that remain unanswered. For example, the unique CNS sites and processes involved in the manifestation of PLMs remain unclear because those previously cited studies implicating subcortical regions examined individuals who had PLMs as well as the related condition *restless legs syndrome* (RLS). Unlike PLMs, RLS is a waking phenomenon characterized by annoying paresthesias that occur most often in the lower limbs and encourage frequent voluntary, albeit sleep-delaying, limb movements to relieve them. Whether the same subcortical (i.e., red nuclei, pons) regions would be implicated in similar studies of individuals manifesting PLMs without RLS remains an open question. Further complicating current under-standing of PLMs is the fact that ingestion of various medications as well as the presence of a varied array of sleep, medical, neurologic, and psychiatric disor-ders all seem to enhance an individual's likelihood of manifesting sleep-related PLMs. However, what may be common to these conditions is that they all disrupt normal sleep-wake functioning. As suggested originally by Coleman, Pollak, and Weitzman (13), PLMs may arise from chronic disturbances "of the daily sleep-wake schedule and specific sleep stages [that] induce or disinhibit an underlying periodic process in the central nervous system." Thus, it remains possible that PLMs may imply no specific CNS pathology at all but rather an unmasking of normal CNS pacemaker activity that is typically suppressed in those with nor-mal, nondisturbed sleep-wake functioning.

PREVALENCE AND SIGNIFICANCE OF PERIODIC LIMB MOVEMENTS

Because PLMs occur primarily during sleep, it has been difficult to establish the prevalence of this phenomenon in the general population via usual epidemio-logical survey techniques. Approximately 70% to 80% of all patients with the related condition, RLS, also have PLMs, whereas it is estimated that about one-third of all individuals with PLMs have RLS (12, 14). It should, therefore, be possible to estimate the population prevalence of PLMs based on what is known about RLS's population prevalence. One North American population survey showed that 10% to 15% of the general population has complaints suggestive of RLS (15). Based on the coincidence of RLS and PLMs, it would be expected that between 7% and 12% of the general population would have both RLS and PLMs. Because PLMs are about three times more prevalent than RLS, PLMs should be present in 21% to 36% of the population at large. However, the preva-lence among older adults may be somewhat higher. One study (16), for example, showed that 45% of a randomly selected community sample composed of 427 senior adults (age > 65 years) had five or more PLMs per hour of sleep during home-based sleep recordings.

Clinic population studies suggest that PLMs are fairly common among those who present for evaluation and treatment of sleep complaints. Studies conducted at individual sleep disorders centers have shown that 5.7% to 13% of all patients presenting with sleep complaints meet minimal criteria for the diagnosis of PLMD by virtue of having five or more PLMs per hour of sleep (13, 17–18). More recently, a national cooperative study of 19 accredited sleep disorders centers showed that PLMD was a primary diagnosis in 2.6% and secondary diagnosis in

16.4% of all patient contacts across centers (19). Consistent with these speculations, clinic studies suggest advanced age may place individuals at increased risk for sleep-disruptive PLMs. Case series studies have shown that older individuals are more prone to receive a PLMD diagnosis and older PLMD patients are likely to have substantially more limb movement activity (i.e., greater numbers of PLMs and PLM-related arousals) during sleep than are their younger counterparts (17, 20). However, longitudinal studies conducted among older adults suggest that PLM frequency and associated sleep disruption may not worsen with additional aging (13, 21).

These prevalence data suggest PLMs are reasonably common among sleep clinic patients, but the unique and specific clinical significance of such phenomena remains controversial. Fueling this controversy are previous studies that have shown PLMs are common to a variety of other sleep disorders as well as to normal, noncomplaining older adults (13, 19, 22). Research designed to relate PLMs to daytime symptoms or other indexes of nocturnal sleep disturbance has found, at best, very weak associations that are of questionable clinical significance (13, 17, 23–24). Such findings have led to the view that PLMs are merely epiphenomena arising from sleep-wake disruptions caused by other sleep disorders or the normal aging process (2, 24–25). One renowned sleep expert has accordingly argued that PLMD should be dropped from the International Classification of Sleep Disorders (ICSD) until there is convincing evidence that PLMs cause sleep-wake complaints (26). However, somewhat more moderate opinions have prevailed over the years, and those who have studied PLMs rather extensively have suggested that such phenomena appear to play a significant role in the sleep-wake complaints of at least some patients (14, 25). Consequently, consideration of PLMD in the diagnostic work-up of sleep-disordered patients remains an acceptable practice and, indeed, falls within currently recommended practice parameters (27). Nonetheless, there is a sufficient basis for controversy concerning the PLMD diagnosis and, as discussed later, this controversy provides a reasonable rationale for considering varied treatment approaches in the management of those patients who manifest PLMs during their sleep.

CLINICAL ASSESSMENT AND DIAGNOSIS

Because PLMs during sleep are found in noncomplaining individuals, the mere presence of these movements does not necessarily warrant a sleep disorder diagnosis. As indicated in the ICSD (28), PLMD should not be assigned as a formal diagnosis unless the patient presents with a sleep-wake complaint and manifests a minimum of five PLMs per hour of recorded sleep. Patients meeting these criteria usually complain of difficulty maintaining sleep or excessive daytime sleepiness whereas those who suffer both from PLMD and RLS usually also complain about difficulties initiating sleep (14). PLMD sufferers often are unaware of their limb movements during sleep, but bed partners who are disturbed by these phenomena frequently provide impetus for such individuals to seek treatment. Indeed, it is not uncommon for bed partners to complain more about the PLMs than do the patients themselves (14).

Establishment of a PLMD diagnosis begins by carefully interviewing both the patient and bed partner. When the patient reports a history of RLS or the bed partner describes the patient's repetitive and stereotyped movements during sleep, a PLMD diagnosis becomes likely. Certain demographic and historic data also may raise clinical suspicion about PLMD. The presence of one of the comorbid medical conditions or use of one or more of the psychoactive substances listed in Table 4.1 may also make PLMD likely. The patient's age also should be a consideration. Although some young adults suffer from this condition, most often, PLMD is diagnosed in middle-age and older adults. One case series study (29) showed that PLMD with or without RLS was diagnosed in 12.8% of all sleep clinic patients under age 40 but in 32.8% of all patients who were 40 years old or

Table 4.1   Psychoactive Substances and Medical, Neurological, and Psychiatric Conditions Related to PLMs

Psychoactive Substances	Medical Disorders	Neurologic/ Psychiatric Disorders
Alcohol (ethanol)	Chronic fatigue syndrome	Attention deficit disorder
L-dopa	Congestive heart failure	Akathisia
Serotonin-reuptake blockers	Obstructive pulmonary disease	Amyotropic lateral sclerosis
Tricyclic antidepressants	Diabetes	Huntington's disease
	Fibrositis/fibromalgia	Issacs' syndrome
	Impotence	Multiple sclerosis
	Leukemia	Myelopathies
		Parkinson's disease
		Peripheral neuropathies
		Posttraumatic stress disorder
		Radiculopathies
		Seizure disorder
		Spinal cord lesions
		Startle disease
		Stiff-man syndrome

older. However, demographic and interview data do not always result in accurate clinical impressions about the presence/absence of PLMD. We (29) found that PLMD was predicted accurately in only 14 (56%) of 25 patients who eventually were determined to have this condition by overnight sleep monitoring. Our clinical prediction of PLMD was also incorrect in 9 (12%) of the 75 patients later found to have no evidence of this condition during their sleep recordings. Thus, when no clear clinical indexes (e.g., restless legs complaints) herald the presence of PLMs, additional objective testing is needed and generally recommended for the establishment of a PLMD diagnosis.

As with other primary sleep disorders, polysomnography (PSG) remains the gold standard for the diagnosis of PLMD. Typically, the PSG recording montage for assessment of PLMs includes bilateral anterior tibialis recording with separate channels devoted to each leg. When available channels are limited, tibialis activity from both legs can be summed and displayed on one channel. According to the standard PSG scoring criteria (28), limb movements are counted as PLMs if they consist of a series of four or more movements occurring at intervals of 5 to 90 seconds during any sleep stage. Furthermore, each discrete PLM event should have a 0.5- to 5-second duration. The raw count of PLMs throughout the entire night conveys some meaningful information, but usually the number of movements per hour of sleep (i.e., Movement Index [MI]) and the number of PLMs associated with EEG arousals (sleep stage changes, awakenings, etc.) per hour of sleep (PLM Arousal Index [AI]) are calculated to connote the level of PLM severity. According to the most recent edition of the ICSD (28), a complaint of insomnia or excessive daytime sleepiness accompanied by a PLM MI in the range of 5 to 24 would suggest *mild* PLMD, such complaints accompanied by a MI between 25 and 50 would be considered *moderate* PLMD, and similar complaints accompanied by a MI greater than 50 or an AI greater than 25 would be considered *severe* PLMD. Those patients having MIs less than 5 are not assigned a PLMD diagnosis.

Because PLM activity may vary considerably from night to night (12), the reliability of a single PSG for connoting usual PLMD severity might be questioned. However, one study conducted by Montplaisir and colleagues (30) showed that 76% of 49 patients undergoing two consecutive nights of sleep monitoring were found to have MIs of 5 or greater on each night. In another study, we (31) found considerable night-to-night variability in the PLM indexes shown by some patients across three consecutive nights of home sleep monitoring. Nonetheless, ICSD PLMD severity classifications were fairly similar across nights for most patients, particularly for those with severe PLMD. Given these findings, it can be expected that a single night of PSG recording should be sufficient to establish a PLMD diagnosis for most patients although some PLMD patients may require a second study to confirm this diagnosis.

Given the cost and inconvenience of PSG, there has been some interest in using alternate, less expensive, and more convenient forms of objective monitoring to assist in the diagnosis of limb movements. Some authors (32–33) have suggested monitoring leg activity by means of actigraphy. Early applications of actigraphy to detect leg movements suggested this technology has a relatively modest ability to predict PLM indexes during sleep (32). More recent work (34) has shown that a specially designed actigraph unit containing a computerized program to detect duration, intensity, and intervals between leg movements provides highly accurate estimates of the number of PSG-detected leg movements throughout the nocturnal recording period. Despite these latter findings, such specialized actigraphs are not yet widely available, so actigraphy cannot yet be considered an acceptable alternative to PSG for PLMD diagnosis.

PHARMACOLOGICAL TREATMENT OF PERIODIC LIMB MOVEMENT DISORDER

Because this volume is devoted to *behavioral* sleep medicine, a comprehensive and exhaustive evaluation of pharmacological management strategies for PLMD is well beyond the scope of this chapter. However, because pharmacological treatment has remained the *mainstream* approach for this condition, a brief discussion of medication treatment options for PLMD does seem warranted. For a more thorough review of the pharmacology of PLMD, consult additional, more comprehensive discussions of this topic (12, 14).

Table 4.2 provides a summary of the range of medications used for PLMD therapy as well as their therapeutic dosage ranges and common side effects. From a historical perspective, benzodiazepines and opioid compounds were initially the most popular classes of medications used to treat PLMD as well as the related condition, RLS. Among the benzodiazepines, clonazepam seemingly has been the most frequently tested, although temazepam and triazolam have also been used successfully to treat this condition (35–38). The primary benefit of these medications is their consistent effects for improving sleep quality and reducing fragmentation, but their effects on the PLM activity, per se, have varied appreciably across studies (14, 35–38). The efficacy of these medications for treating the daytime symptoms of those with concomitant RLS is also not well established. In contrast, the opioid compounds appear to have clear efficacy with RLS, but their efficacy for PLMD remains questionable. One study (39) showed that oxycodone was effective for reducing PLMs, whereas research (40) with the alternate opioid compound, propoxyphene, showed no reduction in PLMs as a function of treatment. In addition to these two classes of compounds, baclofen and anticonvulsants

Table 4.2   Summary of Medications Most Commonly Used to Treat PLMD

Medication Class	Therapeutic Agent	Dosage (mg)	Common Side Effects
Benzodiazepines	Clonazepam	0.5–2.0	Daytime hangover, tolerance
	Temazepam	15–30	
Dopamine agonists	Pergolide	0.1–0.05	Nausea, orthostatic hypotension, insomnia, daytime fatigue, hallucinations, tolerance
	Bromocriptine	0.1–0.6	
	Pramipexole	0.125–1.0	
Dopamine precursors	Carbidopa/L-dopa	25/100 or 50/200	Same as DA agonists, rebound, and augmentation of RLS
Opiods	Oxycodone	5	Constipation, dependency
	Propoxphene	200	
Anticonvulsants	Carbamazepine	200–400	Nephrotoxicity, daytime somnolence
	Gabapentin	100–400	
Other	Baclofen	20–40	Sedation, insomnia, dizziness

(e.g., carbamazepine, Gabapentin) have been tested with PLM patients. Baclofen appears to reduce PLM-related arousals (41) whereas anticonvulsants have shown limited effectiveness in reducing PLM activity during sleep (42). Nonetheless, given the relative paucity of studies conducted to test these later agents, more research is needed to determine their relative values for PLMD treatment.

Perhaps the most successful PLMD treatment results have been obtained with agents that act on CNS dopamine receptors. These agents have been shown to reduce PLM activity and improve sleep quality as well as ameliorate the daytime symptoms of those PLMD patients with associated RLS (40, 43–44). Within this group, both dopamine precursors (e.g., carbidopa/levodopa compounds) and dopamine receptor agonists (e.g., bromocriptine, pergolide, pramipexole) have been used. Both types of agents represent effective treatments, but the latter compounds appear to have fewer problems associated with their long-term use (14).

Medications are frequently useful in the management of moderate to severe PLMD cases, but the current pharmacotherapies for PLMD represent symptomatic treatments, not cures for this condition. As Table 4.2 also suggests, these agents are not without their side effects. Dopamine precursors and agonists have a range of side effects including orthostatic hypotension, insomnia or daytime fatigue, drug tolerance, GI symptoms, nasal stuffiness, and, occasion-ally, hallucinations (14). In addition, the dopamine precursors (e.g., carbidopa/levodopa compounds) sometimes produce a PLM rebound in the latter half of the night or augmentation of daytime symptoms in those PLMD patients who also have RLS (12, 14). PLMD patients treated with benzo-diazepines often develop tolerance to such medications and/or complain of daytime hangover particularly when treated with the longer acting agents (e.g., clonazepam). Opioids commonly produce constipation, and their extended use may produce dependency, particularly in high-risk groups such as those with substance abuse histories. Finally, the anticonvulsant, carbamazepine, may ad-versely affect kidney function and often is contraindicated in patients with known kidney disease.

ALTERNATE TREATMENTS FOR PERIOD LIMB MOVEMENT DISORDER

Interventions Designed to Reduce Limb Movements

Those who specialize in the treatment of PLMD have generally noted the impor-tance of lifestyle management strategies in the treatment of patients with this condition. Most commonly, sleep hygiene instructions and instructions to avoid provocative substances such as caffeine, alcohol, and nicotine are mentioned as important adjuncts to the medicinal therapies. However, it is not uncommon to encounter PLMD patients who are reticent to engage in ongoing pharmacother-apy for their associated sleep-wake complaints. Some patients indicate strong preferences to avoid medications entirely, whereas other PLMD patients who accept pharmacotherapy appear to be insufficiently treated with medications alone. Given these observations, it is useful to consider the rationales for and ef-fectiveness of alternate PLMD therapies.

One assumption supporting the use of drug-free PLMD therapies is the specu-lation that the underlying pathophysiology leading to sleep-related PLMs can be addressed or rectified via alternate interventions. Ancoli-Israel and colleagues (45–46) speculated that PLMs may arise because of reduced blood flow in the lower extremities because many PLMD patients they encountered complained of cold feet. Based on this speculation, they postulated that thermal biofeedback, de-signed to increase blood flow to the legs and feet, might be a useful treatment for PLMD. Unfortunately, their test of this speculation in a small series of cases failed to support the efficacy of such intervention (46). They did find PLMD pa-tients can learn to increase blood flow in their legs and feet with biofeedback training, but this increased blood flow was not associated with reductions in their PLMD symptoms.

A second alternative treatment evolved from the speculation that PLMs and the hyperreflexia of chronic spasticity as seen in spinal cord-injured patients may share common pathophysiological mechanisms. Specifically, both PLMs and hyperreflexia may result from reduced presynaptic inhibition modulating the effects of afferent signals originating in the spinal cord. Because electrical stimulation has been shown to reduce spasticity, such treatment might be effective in reducing sleep-related PLM activity. Based on this speculation, Kovacevic-Risanovic, Cartwright, and Lloyd (47) attempted to treat a series of eight PLMD patients with 30 minutes of bilateral anterior tibialis electrical stimulation administered via neuromuscular stimulator just before bedtime. Results of this study showed these patients reduced their PLM activity from a pretreatment mean of 44.6 PLMs per hour of sleep to a posttreatment mean of 14 PLMs per hour. Despite these changes, none of the patients' measures of sleep continuity showed statistically significant improvements as a function of this treatment. As a result, it remains questionable whether this approach is useful for addressing the PLM-associated sleep complaints commonly presented by clinical patients.

Interventions Designed to Improve Sleep

In contrast to approaches that focus on the pathophysiology of PLMs, some of the alternative interventions proposed specifically address the sleep complaints associated with PLMD through the use of common behavioral insomnia therapies. There are at least two tenable arguments commonly proposed in support of this type of approach. One argument is based on the speculation that PLMs are epiphenomena (25) arising from sleep disruption due to another cause. If this position is accurate, it is possible that the sleep difficulties of those PLMD patients with insomnia arise from the physiological (e.g., hyperarousal), cognitive (e.g., rumination in bed; dysfunctional beliefs about sleep), and behavioral aberrations (e.g., erratic sleep-wake schedules, daytime napping, allotting too much time in bed) alleged to perpetuate the sleep disturbances noted among primary insomnia sufferers (48–51). Alternately, it seems reasonable to speculate that PLMD patients with insomnia are not exempt from the excessive bedtime arousal, sleep disruptive habits, and cognitive aberrations that perpetuate sleep difficulties in other types of insomnia sufferers. This latter view allows for the possibility that PLMs initiate and contribute to such patients' ongoing sleep difficulties but also speculates that cognitive and behavioral factors play an additional and important role in sustaining their insomnia problems. If either of these speculations is correct, the currently available cognitive and behavioral insomnia therapies (for descriptions, see 48 or 49) should be of some benefit to the subgroup of PLMD patients with chronic insomnia complaints.

Initial support for the presence of potentially sleep-disruptive cognitive and behavioral aberrations among PLMD patients comes from exploratory work conducted in our sleep center. In a retrospective study (52), we obtained age- and gender-matched groups of 10 (8 women, 2 men) primary insomnia sufferers, 10 (7 women, 3 men) PLMD patients with insomnia complaints, and 10 (7 women, 3 men) noncomplaining normal sleepers. The primary insomnia sufferers and PLMD patients were drawn from our center's computerized database of all clinical insomnia patients who had completed a polysomnogram as part of their diagnostic procedures; the normal sleepers were obtained from another study (53) concerned with the home and laboratory sleep patterns of older adults. Subsequent to obtaining these matched groups, we statistically compared their responses to sleep history questionnaire items that assessed their frequency of engaging in a number of poor sleep hygiene practices (e.g., reading, watching TV, worrying, and lying awake for extended periods in bed), their perceived physiological arousal at bedtime, and their perceived level of cognitive rumination in bed.

Results of these comparisons (see Table 4.3) showed that both the primary insomnia sufferers and PLMD patients reported they read in bed more nights per week, experienced more rumination and physiological arousal in bed, and reported a greater proneness to lie awake in bed than did the normal sleepers. However, the PLMD patients and primary insomnia sufferers did not differ significantly from each other on any of these sleep history questionnaire items.

Table 4.3   Comparisons of PLMD Patients with Primary Insomnia Sufferers and Normal Sleepers

Measure	PLMD Patients Mean	SD	Primary Insomnia Mean	SD	Normal Sleepers Mean	SD	$F_{2, 27} =$	$p =$
Age (years)	68.5	3.9	70.2	9.7	67.9	3.4	0.35	.71
Read in bed (nights per week)	3.6[a]	3.6	4.0[a]	3.5	0.5[b]	1.0	4.22	.03
Lie awake in bed (nights per week)	5.8[a]	2.3	6.1[a]	2.2	1.5[b]	1.7	15.09	.0001
Physical arousal (rating)*	6.5[a]	3.3	6.3[a]	3.3	2.1[b]	1.4	7.81	.002
Mental arousal (rating)*	7.9[a]	2.1	8.2[a]	3.0	3.0[b]	1.8	14.97	.0001

*Physical and mental arousal were rated on a 10-point scale with 1 = None and 10 = Extreme. Means that share the same superscript letter are not significantly different from each other; those with different superscript letters are significantly different based on Newman-Kuels post-hoc tests.

These findings suggest the physiological, cognitive, and behavioral aberrations that differentiate primary insomnia sufferers from normal sleepers also may differentiate PLMD patients with insomnia from those without sleep complaints. Because these aberrations are common *targets* of behavioral interventions, it seems reasonable to speculate that such treatments may be beneficial to PLMD patients as well.

To date, a limited number of studies have tested the efficacy of behavioral insomnia therapies for addressing insomnia among PLMD patients. In their landmark study of sleep restriction therapy (SRT), Spielman, Saskin, and Thorpy (54) found that two patients who suffered from both RLS and PLMD showed dramatic improvements in sleep log measures of sleep onset latency, total wake time, total sleep time, and sleep efficiency following a course of SRT. However, this early study included no control group or polysomnographic measures to assess changes in PLM activity. The only randomized clinical trial reported thus far was our study (55), in which we compared the treatment responses shown by PLMD patients receiving either four weekly sessions of cognitive-behavioral insomnia therapy (CBT; $n = 8$) or four weeks of 0.5 to 1.0 mg of clonazepam ($n = 8$). Results of this study, which are summarized in Table 4.4, showed that both groups achieved significant, albeit statistically similar, improvements in sleep log measures of total wake time, total sleep time, and sleep efficiency as well as in their global ratings of nighttime sleep concerns. CBT-treated patients showed a reduction in their reported frequency of daytime napping whereas those treated with clonazepam reported a modest increase in napping from the beginning to the end of treatment. Those receiving clonazepam showed a 44.3% reduction in their PLM-related arousals per hour of sleep whereas the CBT-treated group showed only a 19.8% reduction in PLM-related arousals. Likely because of our small sample sizes, this seemingly marked group difference did not reach statistical significance.

In addition to its limited sample, this latter study included no short- or long-term follow-up assessments to evaluate the relative durability of each modality's treatment effects over time. Also, despite random assignment to treatments, the clonazepam group entered the study with notably more severe PLMD than did the CBT group. Its results nonetheless suggest that behavioral insomnia therapies may have a place in the management of sleep complaints among those insomnia sufferers who meet criteria for PLMD. Although data supporting the long-term efficacy of these treatments for PLMD patients are currently unavailable, their durable treatment effects found for other insomnia subtypes (48–49) give reason for optimism as to their future applications to those with PLMD. It would, thus, seem especially important to test more intensive treatment protocols with adequate long-term follow-up to more thoroughly evaluate the efficacy of the behavioral therapies for PLMD patients.

Table 4.4 Means, Standard Deviations, and Statistics for Improvements Shown by Treatments

Sleep Log Data	Clonazepam Group		CBT Group		Time (Pre- vs. Posttreatment)		Interaction Effects	
	Baseline	Treatment	Baseline	Treatment	$F =$	$p <$	$F =$	$p <$
Total wake time	147.64 (72.2)	80.1 (31.8)	107.9 (52.0)	60.6 (48.2)	17.4	.005	0.5	n.s.
Total sleep time	367.8 (83.4)	427.5 (46.9)	335.8 (70.3)	347.7 (78.7)	5.2	.05	2.3	n.s.
Sleep efficiency percent	71.4 (14.8)	83.6 (7.8)	75.2 (13.1)	84.4 (13.9)	12.6	.005	0.1	n.s.
Insomnia symptom questionnaire (ratings)								
Nighttime sleep concerns	53.5 (15.9)	36.3 (18.7)	49.5 (11.1)	37.5 (22.5)	5.6	.05	0.2	n.s.
Daytime fatigue	45.4 (19.4)	40.3 (21.5)	59.6 (14.0)	54.7 (23.3)	0.7	n.s.	0.0	n.s.
Daytime napping	27.5 (21.2)	37.6 (20.5)	26.2 (23.0)	8.0 (8.4)	0.3	n.s.	4.8	.05
PSG Measures								
Total wake time	106.3 (36.4)	97.7 (31.1)	125.2 (67.5)	88.3 (51.3)	1.9	n.s.	0.7	n.s.
Total sleep time	341.9 (55.5)	379.6 (60.1)	348.0 (58.2)	326.8 (44.6)	0.2	n.s.	1.8	n.s.
PLM movement index (MI)	77.4 (21.6)	63.8 (34.7)	30.7 (15.2)	31.8 (10.7)	0.6	n.s.	1.6	n.s.
PLM arousal index (AI)	37.7 (16.8)	21.0 (22.4)	19.2 (11.4)	15.4 (11.7)	5.0	.05	1.4	n.s.

Note: Values in parentheses are standard deviations. Results shown for sleep log, ISQ, and PSG total sleep and wake times are taken from 2 (CBT vs. clonazepam) × 2 (pre- vs. posttreatment) ANOVAs. For these ANOVAs, the main effect attributable to time (pre- vs. posttreatment) and the interaction term are shown. All main effects comparing treatment groups were nonsignificant and are consequently not shown. One-way repeated measures ANOVAs were used to test for pre- to posttreatment improvements in MIs and AIs across treatment conditions. The "interaction" effects shown for the MI and AI data represent the results of analyses of covariance performed on pre- to posttreatment change scores for MIs and AIs, respectively, adjusted for pretreatment MI and AI values. The ISQ ratings were made on 100-point visual analogue scales with higher scores reflecting greater nighttime sleep concerns, daytime fatigue, and daytime napping.

SUMMARY AND FUTURE DIRECTIONS

PLMD remains a poorly understood and controversial primary sleep disorder. Historically, various forms of pharmacotherapy have received the greatest attention and endorsement for the management of PLMD patients. To date, the dopaminergic agents have shown reasonable promise for amelioration of PLMD symptoms. However, the side effects of these and the other classes of PLMD medications may limit or preclude their use in some patients, whereas other patients may prefer to avoid long-term pharmacotherapy for their sleep-related symptoms. In such cases, alternate, behavioral approaches may be warranted.

Currently, the most promising alternative PLMD treatments are the behavioral therapies most typically used for treating primary insomnia. Perhaps the most convincing and defensible rationale for application of treatments to insomnia sufferers with PLMD is the observation that these patients, like other insomnia sufferers, manifest a host of sleep-disruptive physiological, cognitive, and behavioral aberrations that may be addressed effectively via behavioral techniques. Moreover, the limited research testing such treatments with these patients has provided promising results that suggest such therapies may, indeed, have a role in the management of at least some PLMD patients.

Many questions about the use of behavioral therapies with PLMD patients remain unanswered. Among the more important are these: Can the findings from the previously cited behavioral treatment studies be replicated in larger PLMD samples? How durable are these treatment effects over time among PLMD patients? How effective are the behavioral treatments among PLMD patients who present with severe RLS or who primarily voice concerns about daytime sleepiness or fatigue? Does the effectiveness of behavioral interventions vary as a function of PLMD severity? Are the combined effects of behavioral and pharmacological PLMD interventions superior to either form of treatment used alone? And, are there incremental benefits to be achieved by systematically adding behavioral interventions to pharmacotherapy for a specific subset of PLMD patients? No doubt, many more important questions could be posed. However, it is hoped that the few questions presented along with the material reviewed in this chapter will serve as catalysts for continued interest in the development, testing, and refinement of alternative behavioral therapies for those PLMD patients who present clinically.

REFERENCES

1. Smith, R. C. Relationship of periodic movements in sleep (nocturnal myoclonus) and the Babinski sign. *Sleep* 8: 239–243, 1985.

 2. Radtke, R. A., T. J. Hoelscher, and A. C. Bragdon. Ambulatory evaluation of periodic movements of sleep. In J. S. Ebersole, ed. *Ambulatory EEG Monitoring.* New York, NY: Raven Press. 1989: 317–329.

 3. Symonds, C. P. Nocturnal myoclonus. *Journal of Neurology, Neurosurgery, and Psychiatry* 16: 166–171, 1953.

 4. Martinelli, P., G. Coccagna, and E. Lugaresi. Nocturnal myoclonus, restless legs syndrome, and abnormal electrophysiological findings. *Annuals of Neurology* 21: 515, 1987.

 5. Hening, W., S. Chokroverty, M. Rolleri, and A. Walters. The cortical premovement potential of restless legs syndrome jerks: Differences in potentials before simulated versus symptomatic jerks. *Sleep Research* 20: 355, 1991.

 6. Bucher, S. F., K. C. Seelos, W. H. Oertel, M. Reiser, and C. Trenkwalder. Cerebral generators involved in the pathogenesis of the restless legs syndrome. *Annuals of Neurology* 41: 639–645, 1997.

 7. Watanabe, S., A. Ono, and H. Naito. Periodic leg movements during either epidural or spinal anesthesia in an elderly man without sleep-related (nocturnal) myoclonus. *Sleep* 13: 262–266. 1990.

 8. Jackson, J. Periodic movements of sleep in T10 paraplegic with failure to respond to parlodel. *Sleep Research* 19: 326, 1990.

 9. Dickel, M. J., S. D. Renfrow, T. Moore, and R. B. Berry. Rapid eye movement sleep periodic leg movements in patients with spinal cord injury. *Sleep* 17: 733–738, 1994.

10. Evans, B. Patterns of arousal in comatose states. *Journal of Neurology, Neurosurgery, and Psychiatry* 39: 392–402, 1976.

11. Kjallquist, A., N. Lundberg, and U. Pontren. Respiratory and cardiovascular changes during rapid spontaneous variations of ventricular fluid pressure in patients with intracranial hypertension. *Acta Neurologica Scandinavica* 40: 291–317, 1964.

12. Montplaisir, J., A. Nicolas, R. Godbout, and A. Walters. Restless legs syndrome and periodic limb movement disorder. In M. H. Kryger, T. Roth, and W. C. Dement, eds. *Principles and Practice of Sleep Medicine* (3rd Edition). Philadelphia, PA: W.B. Saunders Company. 2000: 742–752.

13. Coleman, R. M., C. P. Pollak, and E. D. Weitzman. Periodic movements in sleep (nocturnal myoclonus): Relation to sleep disorders. *Annals of Neurology* 8: 416–421, 1980.

14. Hening, W. A., R. Allen, A. S. Walters, and S. Chokroverty. Motor functions and dysfunctions during sleep. In S. Chokroverty, ed. *Sleep Disorders Medicine* (2nd Edition). Woburn, MA: Butterworth-Heinemann. 1999: 441–507.

15. Lavigne, G. J. and J. Y. Montplaisir. Restless legs syndrome and sleep bruxism prevalence and association among Canadians. *Sleep* 17: 739–743, 1994.

16. Ancoli-Israel, S., D. F. Kripke, M. R. Klauber, W. J. Mason, R. Fell, and O. Kaplan. Periodic limb movements in sleep in community-dwelling elderly. *Sleep* 14: 496–500, 1991.

17. Mendelson, W. B. Are periodic leg movements associated with clinical sleep disturbance? *Sleep* 19: 219–223, 1996.

18. Mendelson, W. B. Experiences of a sleep disorders center; 1700 patients later. *Cleveland Clinic Journal of Medicine* 64: 46–51, 1997.

19. Punjab, N. M., D. Welch, and K. Strohl. Sleep disorders in regional centers: A national cooperative study. *Sleep* 23: 471–480, 2000.

20. Coleman, R. M., L. E. Miles, C. C. Guilleminault, V. P. Zarcone Jr., J. van den Hoed, and W. C. Dement. Sleep-wake disorders in the elderly: A polysomnographic analysis. *Journal of the American Geriatrics Society* 29: 289–296, 1981.

21. Phoha, R. L., M. J. Dickel, and S. S. Mosko. Preliminary longitudinal assessment of sleep in the elderly. *Sleep* 13: 425–429, 1990.

22. Bixler, E. O., A. Kales, A. Vela-Bueno, J. A. Jacoby, S. Sarcone, and C. R. Soldatos. Nocturnal myoclonus and nocturnal myoclonic activity in a normal population. *Research in Community Chemical Pathology and Pharmacology* 36: 129–140, 1982.

23. Dickel, M. J. and S. S. Mosko. Morbidity cut-offs for sleep apnea and periodic leg movements in predicting subjective sleep complaints in the elderly. *Sleep* 13: 155–166, 1990.

24. Nicolas, A., P. Lesperance, and J. Montplaisir. Is excessive daytime sleepiness with periodic leg movements during sleep a specific diagnostic category? *European Neurology* 40: 22–26, 1988.

25. Coleman, R. M., D. L. Bliwise, N. Sajbe, L. de Bruyn, A. Boomkamp, M. E. Menn, et al. Epidemiology of periodic movements during sleep. In C. Guilleminault and E. Lugaresi, eds. *Sleep/Wake Disorders: Natural History, Epidemiology and Long-Term Evolution.* New York, NY: Raven Press. 1983: 217–229.

26. Mahowald, M. *Restless Legs Syndrome and Periodic Limb Movements.* Presented as part of the symposium entitled, "Epidemiology of sleep disorders in mid and later life: How do we answer the important questions?" Michael Vitiello, Chair. Annual Meeting of the Associated Professional Sleep Societies, Chicago, IL. 2001.

27. Polysomnography Task Force, American Sleep Disorders Association Standards of Practice Committee. Practice parameters for the indications for polysomnography and related procedures. *Sleep* 20: 406–422, 1997.

28. American Sleep Disorders Association. *The International Classification of Sleep Disorders, Revised: Diagnostic and Coding Manual.* Rochester, MN: American Sleep Disorders Association. 1997.

29. Edinger, J. D., T. J. Hoelscher, M. D. Webb, G. R. Marsh, R. A. Radtke, and C. W. Erwin. Polysomnographic assessment of DIMS: Empirical evaluation of its diagnostic value. *Sleep* 12: 315–322, 1989.

30. Montplaisir, J., S. Boucher, G. Poirier, G. Lavigne, O. Lapierre, and P. Lesperance. Clinical polysomnographic and genetic characteristics of restless legs syndrome: A study of 133 patients diagnoses with new standard criteria. *Movement Disorders* 12: 61–65, 1997.

31. Edinger, J. D., W. V. McCall, G. R. Marsh, R. A. Radtke, C. W. Erwin, and A. Lininger. Periodic limb movement variability in older DIMS patients across consecutive nights of home monitoring. *Sleep* 15: 156–161, 1992.

32. Allen, R. P., P. W. Kaplan, D. W. Buchholz, C. J. Earley, and J. K. Walters. Accuracy of a physical activity monitor (PAM) worn on the ankle for assessment of treatment response for periodic limb movements in sleep. *Sleep Research* 21: 329, 1992.

33. Kazenwadel, J., T. Pollmacher, C. Trenkwalder, W. H. Oertel, R. Kohnen, M. Kunzel, et al. New actigraphic assessment method for periodic leg movements (PLM). *Sleep* 18: 689–697, 1995.

34. Allen, R. P. Activity monitoring to diagnose and evaluate motor abnormalities of sleep. In W. Hening and S. Chokroverty, eds. *Topics in Movement Disorders of Sleep* (Course syllabus: Annual Meeting of the Associated Professional Sleep Societies, San Francisco). Rochester, MN: American Sleep Disorders Association. 1997.

35. Bonnet, M. H. and D. L. Arand. The use of triazolam in older patients with periodic leg movements, fragmented sleep, and daytime sleepiness. *Journal of Gerontology* 45: 139–144, 1990.

36. Mitler, M. M., C. P. Browman, S. Menh, G. Krishnareddy, and R. Timms. Nocturnal myoclonus: Treatment efficacy of clonazepam and temazepam. *Sleep* 9: 385–392, 1986.

37. Ohanna, N., R. Peled, A. H. Rubin, J. Zomer, and P. Lavie. Periodic leg movements in sleep: Effect of clonazepam treatment. *Neurology* 35: 408–411, 1985.

38. Peled, R. and P. Lavie. Double-blind evaluation of clonazepam on periodic leg movements in sleep. *Journal of Neurology, Neurosurgery, and Psychiatry* 50: 1679–1681, 1987.

39. Walters, A. S., M. L. Wagner, W. A. Hening, K. Grasing, R. Mills, S. Chokroverty, et al. Successful treatment of idiopathic restless legs syndrome in a randomized double-blind trial of oxycodone versus placebo. *Sleep* 16: 327–332, 1993.

40. Allen, R. P., P. W. Kaplan, D. W. Buchholz, and J. K. Walters. A double-blinded, placebo controlled study of the treatment of periodic limb movements in sleep using carbidopa/levodopa and propoxyphene. *Sleep* 16: 717–723, 1993.

41. Guilleminault, C. and W. Flagg. Effect of baclofen on sleep-related periodic leg movements. *Annuals of Neurology* 15: 234–239, 1984.

42. Zucconi, M., G. Coccagna, R. Petronelli, R. Gerardi, S. Monodini, and F. Cirignotta. Nocturnal myoclonus in restless legs syndrome: Effect of carbamazepine treatment. *Functional Neurology* 4: 263–271, 1989.

43. Early, C. J. and R. P. Allen. Pergolide and carbidopa/levodopa treatment of restless legs syndrome and periodic leg movements in sleep in a consecutive series of patients. *Sleep* 19: 801–810, 1997.

44. Silber, M. H., J. W. Shepard Jr., and J. A. Wisbey. Pergolide in the management of restless legs syndrome: An extended study. *Sleep* 20: 878–882, 1997.

45. Ancoli-Israel, S., A. R. Seifert, and M. Lemon. Thermal biofeedback and periodic movements in sleep; patients' subjective report and a case study. *Biofeedback and Self Regulation* 11: 177–188, 1986.

46. Knowles, J., S. Ancoli-Israel, R. Gevirtz, and J. S. Poceta. The evaluation of biofeedback in the treatment of periodic limb movement disorder. *Sleep Research* 25: 265, 1996.

47. Kovacevic-Ristanovic, R., R. D. Cartwright, and S. Lloyd. Nonpharmacological treatment of periodic leg movements in sleep. *Archives of Physical Medicine and Rehabilitation* 72: 385–389, 1991.

48. Edinger, J. D. and W. K. Wohlgemuth. The significance and management of persistent primary insomnia: The past present and future of behavioral insomnia therapies. *Sleep Medicine Reviews* 3: 101–118, 1999.

49. Morin, C. M., P. J. Hauri, C. A. Espie, A. J. Spielman, D. J. Buysse, and R. R. Bootzin. Nonpharmacologic treatment of chronic insomnia. *Sleep* 22: 1134–1156, 1999.

50. Morin, C. M., J. Stone, D. Trinkle, J. Mercer, and S. Remsberg. Dysfunctional beliefs and attitudes about sleep among older adults with and without insomnia complaints. *Psychology and Aging* 8: 463–467, 1993.

51. Stepanski, E., F. Zorick, T. Roehrs, D. Young, and T. Roth. Daytime alertness in patients with chronic insomnia compared with asymptomatic control subjects. *Sleep* 11: 54–60, 1988.

52. Edinger, J. D., G. R. Marsh, and A. D. Krystal. Bedtime arousal levels and sleep hygiene practices among older normal sleepers, primary insomnia sufferers, and patients with periodic limb movement disorder. Unpublished pilot study. 1996.

53. Edinger, J. D., A. I. Fins, R. J. Sullivan Jr., G. R. Marsh, D. Dailey, T. V. Hope, et al. Sleep in the laboratory and sleep at home: Comparisons of older insomniacs and normal sleepers. *Sleep* 20: 1119–1126, 1997.

54. Spielman, A. J., P. Saskin, and M. J. Thorpy. Treatment of chronic insomnia by restriction of time in bed. *Sleep* 10: 45–55, 1987.

55. Edinger, J. D., A. I. Fins, R. J. Sullivan Jr., G. R. Marsh, D. S. Dailey, and M. Young. Comparison of cognitive-behavioral therapy and clonazepam for treating periodic limb movement disorder. *Sleep* 19: 442 444, 1996.

Chapter 5

THE SYMPTOMATIC MANAGEMENT OF NARCOLEPSY

ANN E. ROGERS AND JANET MULLINGTON

Narcolepsy is a chronic neurological disorder of unknown etiology, a syndrome more common than Huntington's chorea, multiple sclerosis, or muscular dystrophy (1). For most patients, sleep attacks and excessive daytime sleepiness are the most disabling symptoms of the disorder. Sleep attacks—brief episodes of sleep that may occur many times a day—occur during times of physical inactivity or boredom as well as when least expected: during an exam or business meeting, while waiting for a traffic light to change from red to green, examining patients, or eating a meal (1–3). Some occur without warning while others are preceded by a period of perceptible drowsiness. Following arousal from a sleep attack, the narcoleptic individual usually feels refreshed and often has a refractory period of one to several hours before the next sleep attack. Narcoleptic patients show patterns of waxing and waning of alertness and attention, with periods of lucidity, as well as profound and debilitating sleepiness.

In addition to the excessive daytime sleepiness, nocturnal sleep is often fragmented and shortened. Patients are often aware of waking up several times at night, but this symptom generally appears several years after the onset of excessive daytime sleepiness (4). Rapid eye movement (REM) sleep occurs directly or very rapidly following the initiation of sleep, at times that are not seen in normal sleep-wake patterns, both at the onset of nocturnal sleep and at the start of daytime naps. To meet diagnostic criteria, excessive daytime sleepiness needs to be documented, and in addition, there should be evidence of abnormal timing of REM sleep.

Cataplexy, the sudden bilateral loss of muscle tone with consciousness maintained, that lasts a few seconds to a couple of minutes; symptoms of sleep paralysis, the inability to move voluntary muscles experienced on awakening from sleep; and hypnagogic hallucinations, the experience of visual or auditory hallucination experienced on going to sleep, are all thought to be features of dissociated REM sleep and are all part of the diagnostic profile (5). Severity of cataplexy can range from a mild sensation of muscle weakness in the neck to a complete postural collapse, with a fall to the ground. There is a wide range in frequency of cataplexy, and while some patients may experience cataplexy on a daily basis, others have only one or two episodes during a lifetime. Episodes of cataplexy are almost always precipitated by a sudden emotional stimulus, such as laughter, anger, or surprise.

Sleep paralysis occurs in some narcoleptics during the transition between sleep and wakefulness. When falling asleep or waking up, the individual experiences a temporary paralysis of all striated muscles. The person is unable to move any muscles other than the muscles of respiration and sometimes the ocular muscles. The episode usually lasts a few minutes and may be accompanied by intense fear or hypnagogic hallucinations. Sleep paralysis ends spontaneously or terminates immediately when the individual is touched or spoken to by another person. Like cataplexy, the frequency of these episodes is highly individual; sleep paralysis may occur daily, weekly, or once or twice in a lifetime.

Hypnagogic hallucinations are vivid, lifelike sensory experiences that appear as a person is falling asleep but still conscious. The visual, auditory, or tactile hallucinations occur for approximately 1 to 15 minutes (6).

Narcolepsy usually begins in adolescence with the onset of excessive daytime sleepiness and sleep attacks. Cataplexy and other REM-related symptoms (sleep paralysis and hypnagogic hallucinations) may occur almost immediately or develop 5 to 10 or even 20 years later. The severity of the auxiliary symptoms may wax and wane throughout the patient's life, but excessive daytime sleepiness is chronic and unrelenting. Excessive daytime sleepiness persists into old age but is not exacerbated by the development of age-associated changes in nocturnal sleep (e.g., poorer sleep efficiency, increased awakenings, and decreases in Stage 3/4 sleep; 3, 7, 8). A few patients have even reported less severe daytime sleepiness with increasing age (3, 4, 9), but whether this represents a partial remission or improved coping with the illness is not known.

Up to half of all narcoleptic patients have symptom-related difficulties at work, in marriage, or in their social lives (10). Drowsiness, impaired attention, and poor concentration also interfere with education and employment (2, 11–13). Interpersonal relationships may deteriorate because of sleep attacks or cataplexy during meals, conversations, and even during sexual relations. Friends and family members may refuse to accept narcolepsy as an illness and may attribute the patient's sleepiness to boredom, laziness, or psychological problems (11–13).

ASSESSMENT

Although daytime sleepiness may be assessed in several ways, there are no standardized measures of cataplexy severity. Objective measures of daytime sleepiness include the Multiple Sleep Latency Test (MSLT), the Maintenance of Wakefulness Test (MWT), and 24-hour polysomnographic recordings. Subjective measures of sleepiness, such as the Stanford Sleep Scale (14–15), the Epworth Sleepiness Scale (16), and 24-hour diaries (17), while sometimes useful for assessing baseline levels of sleepiness and evaluating treatment responses, are not sufficient for diagnosing narcolepsy.

The MSLT and MWT are laboratory tests involving five or six 20-minute trials at two-hour intervals throughout the day. During the MSLT, patients are instructed to fall asleep, and their sleep latencies (time it takes to fall asleep) are averaged across the nap trials. Mean sleep latencies of less than five minutes are typical. The presence of two or more SOREMPs (sleep onset REM periods) are suggestive, but not necessarily diagnostic, of narcolepsy. Two SOREMPs, once thought to be a specific diagnostic marker for narcolepsy, have been documented in up to 25% of the patients with sleep apnea and in 17% of normal healthy subjects (18–19). Usually performed to document the diagnosis of narcolepsy, this test measures how fast the person can fall asleep and may not be sensitive to improvements in patients' ability to remain awake. The MWT, which measures how long a patient can stay awake, is sensitive to the effects of treatment (20). It is not clear, however, that statistically significant improvements in sleep latencies on either the MSLT or MWT are predictive of improved functional abilities outside the laboratory setting.

The final objective measure, 24-ambulatory polysomnographic recordings, can be used to record the sleep-wake patterns of narcoleptic patients outside the laboratory setting. This technique, pioneered by Roger Broughton (21–22), is unfortunately rarely used, even for research. As shown in Figure 5.1, 24-hour recordings obtained from treated patients engaged in their usual daily activities can be revealing. The first subject, a 22-year-old college student, exhibited fragmented nocturnal sleep and excessive daytime sleepiness, while the sleep-wake pattern of the second subject, a 36-year-old college professor, resembled those of normal controls (23).

PHARMACOLOGIC MANAGEMENT

Daytime sleepiness must be controlled before most patients with narcolepsy can function adequately at home, while driving, or at work (24). Treatment with

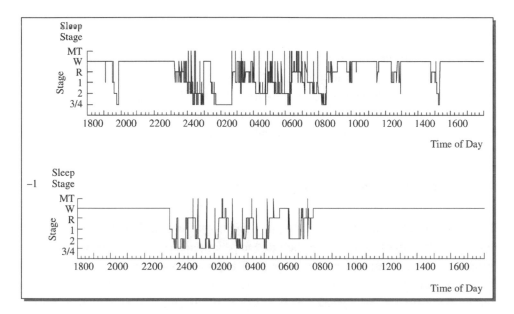

Figure 5.1   Twenty-Four-Hour Ambulatory Polysomnographic Recordings Showing the Sleep/Wake Patterns of Two Treated Narcoleptic Patients

stimulant medications can significantly reduce or eliminate excessive daytime sleepiness (24–25) and improve quality of life (26). Studies have shown increased ability to resist sleep, as measured by the MWT, a test in which the latency to sleep is measured in a comfortable sleep-conducive environment. The ability to resist sleep is significantly increased by stimulant medications (25, 27–29). In addition, daytime performance of narcoleptic patients has been shown to be significantly improved from reaction time (30–31) to simulated driving tasks (32) with the use of stimulant medications.

The current practice parameters for narcolepsy (33) recommend modafinil (usually taken at doses between 100 and 400 mg/day) for the treatment of excessive daytime sleepiness. Stimulant medications, such as methylphenidate (up to 60 mg/day in two to three divided doses), pemoline (0.5 to 3.0 mg/kg/day in one morning dose), and dextroamphetamine (5 to 60 mg/day in two to three divided doses), are still commonly prescribed, although modafinil is usually preferred over traditional stimulants because side effects are less frequent (25, 29, 34, 35). However, not all patients respond to modafinil, particularly those who have been previously treated with amphetamines (29).

Tricyclic antidepressants, such as clomipramine, imipramine, and protriptyline, are usually considered more effective than selective serotonin reuptake inhibitors (SSRIs) for the treatment of cataplexy. Both tricyclic antidepressants and SSRIs are potent REM sleep inhibitors. Anticholinergic side effects may limit their use. Clomipramine and imipramine are tertiary amine tricyclic antidepressants that are normally prescribed in doses of 100 to 200 mg/day. Protriptyline is a secondary amine tricyclic antidepressant. The normally prescribed dose is very low, 10 mg/day. Although pharmacologic treatment is rarely prescribed for the control of other REM dissociation phenomena, treatment of cataplexy usually reduces the severity of hypnagogic hallucinations and sleep paralysis (36).

BEHAVIORAL APPROACHES

Behavioral interventions are very appealing to patient and provider alike, and many practitioners recommend scheduled naps and sleep hygiene strategies in the treatment of narcolepsy. Even if behavioral approaches are not recommended by clinicians, few patients (10% to 15%) rely exclusively on stimulant medications to maintain daytime alertness (37). The majority of patients combine pharmacological therapy with some form of behavioral management, while a substantial number of patients (30% to 54%) report relying exclusively on nonpharmacological measures to combat daytime sleepiness (37–38). Reasons for eschewing stimulant therapy vary widely; patients worry about getting "addicted to stimulants," while others consider that side effects from medications are worse than the symptoms of narcolepsy (39).

Multiple techniques may be employed by narcoleptic patients to maintain alertness and may involve the use of exercise, physical activity, caffeine consumption, eating candy or sugar or avoiding sweets, driving a car with a manual transmission, chewing on ice, and so on (38). Some techniques recommended by patients are fairly benign, for example, splashing cold water on the face, practicing deep breathing/meditation, and avoiding stress. Other techniques such as using an alarm clock (while driving), hurting themselves (while driving), avoiding social situations, and smoking cigarettes have the potential for harm. Some behavioral strategies, for example, scheduling social and business activities to coincide with periods of peak alertness, restricting attendance at evening events, and just giving in and sleeping, suggest a resignation to living with profound sleepiness.

Behavioral techniques are also widely used to control cataplexy. In fact, only one-third of the patients surveyed reported taking anticataplectic medications (38–39). The other patients denied medication use and reported relying exclusively on a variety of behavioral techniques to reduce the severity of this symptom. Some of the techniques to manage cataplexy are similar to those developed to manage excessive daytime sleepiness, for example, napping, getting an adequate amount of sleep at night, restricting sweets, taking vitamin/mineral supplements,

and avoiding stress, while others are related to preventing injury during an epi
sode of cataplexy. Some methods to prevent the occurrence of cataplexy, for example, avoidance of becoming involved, avoiding emotional situations, controlling
their emotions, and so on, can adversely affect interpersonal relationships.

Only napping and sleep hygiene measures have been evaluated by numerous
studies. No other strategies to control excessive daytime sleepiness or cataplexy
have been adequately tested.

EFFICACY OF SLEEP-WAKE SCHEDULING IN THE
TREATMENT OF EXCESSIVE DAYTIME SLEEPINESS

Because nocturnal sleep in narcolepsy is fragmented, some have thought that if it
could be consolidated, the daytime sleepiness would improve. However, efforts
to consolidate nocturnal sleep by using pharmacological aids, such as benzodiazepines or gamma hydroxybutyrate (40–42), failed to improve daytime sleepiness. One study suggests, however, that daytime sleepiness may contribute to
nocturnal sleep disruptions (23). In keeping with the theory that narcoleptic
symptoms are a result of a disorder of a weak circadian drive for wakefulness
(43–44), patients whose daytime sleepiness was eliminated by stimulant medications had nocturnal sleep patterns that were indistinguishable from normal
sleepers, while subjects whose sleepiness was not controlled by stimulants had
fragmented and shortened nocturnal sleep.

In another study, narcoleptic subjects were given 12 hours of nocturnal sleep,
and daytime sleepiness was examined using the MSLT, which measures the
sleep latency in five scheduled nap opportunities per day (45). In this study, average sleep latency increased only 3.6 minutes, resulting in a mean sleep latency
of 7.8 minutes. However, the actual ability of the narcoleptics to resist sleep was
not tested in this study. A sleep hygiene approach was employed in another
study, where subjects followed a home routine schedule, keeping regular times
of nocturnal sleep. This approach reduced perceived symptom severity but did
not reduce the amount of unscheduled daytime sleep in stimulant medicated narcoleptic patients (46).

Both the duration and timing of naps have been evaluated using controlled
studies. Although naps can briefly increase alertness in narcoleptic patients, at
least two studies have shown that the alerting effects are transient. For example,
the alerting effects of both 15-minute and 30-minute naps were lost when narcoleptic subjects were retested 30 minutes after awakening from a nap (47). Although a 120-minute nap produced a statistically significant increase in alertness
as measured by a modified MSLT (more than doubled the mean sleep latency),

scores remained low. And three hours later, unlike sleep-deprived and control subjects, the alerting effects of the nap had disappeared (48).

Very few studies have investigated the efficacy of placement and duration of naps in the alleviation of daytime sleepiness in narcolepsy. In one study (49–51), the efficacy of two different nap schedules was tested, a long and a short nap schedule, and compared with a control condition where subjects were not permitted to sleep during the day but received 100% of their total sleep time in a single nocturnal sleep period. In all three conditions, the total amount of sleep time was based on average sleep amounts per day from ≥ five days of stimulant-free sleep log data. In the long nap condition, subjects were permitted to nap for 25% of their total sleep time, positioned 180 degrees out of phase with the nocturnal mid-sleep time. In the short nap condition, five short naps were spread equidistantly through the waking period, with 5% of total sleep time assigned to each scheduled nap period. The long nap condition led to improved four-choice reaction time performance over the no-nap condition (49) with less sleep inertia and greater subjective benefit (52). The short nap condition did not proffer sustained performance advantage over the no-nap condition, except that the number of incorrect reaction time responses in the short nap condition was significantly lower than in the no-nap condition.

Where feasible, a single long nap may be a desirable strategy for narcoleptic patients who are taking a break from stimulants or for patients who, for whatever reason, want to limit their use of stimulant medications. Of interest, the timing of the highest frequency of spontaneously occurring naps is at least an hour earlier in narcoleptic patients who are stimulant free, recorded in the home environment with ambulatory polysomnographic equipment (44, 49, 53, 54). Based on this information, it would seem potentially most advantageous to schedule a single long nap earlier in the day rather than at the postlunch dip that has been commonly described. No studies have evaluated the benefit of a single nap scheduled at the advanced nap zone for daytime sleep propensity in narcolepsy.

Although these studies demonstrate that extending the sleep period at night and the addition of scheduled nap periods can produce statistically significant increases in daytime alertness, the reliance on behavioral strategies alone may not be practical. Unfortunately, studies evaluating the combination of prescribed sleep periods and stimulant medications are limited. Only two studies, both conducted by Rogers and her colleagues, have compared the efficacy of combining stimulant medication with scheduled sleep to stimulant therapy alone.

During the first study (55), 16 narcoleptic subjects, serving as their own controls, took three 15-minute naps per day but did not alter their (stimulant) medication regime or usual sleeping habits at night. One month later, despite statistically significant increases in mean sleep latencies on the MWT, there was no change in the number of successful trials (20 minutes without sleep). Finally, there was no change in the number of sleep attacks recorded in the subjects' diaries and no significant improvements in symptom severity as measured by the Narcolepsy Symptom Status Questionnaire (NSSQ).

The second study evaluated three different sleep schedules and used ambulatory polysomnographic recordings to objectively measure daytime sleepiness outside the laboratory setting (46). Twenty-nine treated narcoleptic subjects were randomly assigned to one of three treatment groups:

1. Two 15-minute naps per day
2. A regular schedule for nocturnal sleep
3. A combination of scheduled naps and regular bedtimes

Measures of symptom severity and unscheduled daytime sleep were obtained at baseline and at the end of the two-week treatment period, using the NSSQ and 24-hour ambulatory polysomnographic monitoring. No alterations were made in stimulant medications during the study period.

Subjects assigned to the combination therapy group had less daytime sleep and reported less severe symptoms at the end of the two-week treatment period. Although subjects assigned to sleep regular hours at night reported less severe symptoms at the end of the study, their objective level of daytime sleepiness did not change. The addition of two 15-minute naps per day did not alter either the amount of unscheduled daytime sleep or subjective symptom severity. The type of sleep schedule prescribed, however, was less important than the severity of the patients' pretreatment daytime sleepiness. All three sleep schedules produced significant reductions in the amount of unscheduled daytime sleep, if pretreatment levels of daytime sleepiness were high. Subjects with severe daytime sleepiness benefited from the addition of scheduled sleep periods, while those who were only moderately sleepy or able to maintain alertness did not benefit from scheduled sleep periods. Thus, it appears that the efficacy of scheduled sleep periods is highly associated with pretreatment levels of daytime sleepiness.

There are issues of practicality with respect to the scheduling approach to the management of excessive daytime sleepiness in narcolepsy. Patients may be unable to take even one or two 15-minute naps in the workplace. A single long nap, while perhaps the most beneficial, is certainly most difficult to work into the workday. Nonetheless, it may be advantageous to many narcoleptics to plan a sleep-wake schedule. This may be done with the benefit of their own personal sleep log data by charting alert and drowsy periods and relating them to the nap pattern. In this manner, patients can develop a schedule that takes into account their own personal time constraints and best response to napping.

The studies discussed previously show that various schedule manipulations can produce statistically significant improvements in daytime alertness. However, the clinical utility of manipulating sleep schedules remains limited. Adding naps and/or extending or regularizing nocturnal sleep periods can help increase alertness at least for short periods. But patients remain sleepy, even when scheduled sleep periods are combined with stimulant medications.

DIETARY APPROACHES TO THE MANAGEMENT OF EXCESSIVE DAYTIME SLEEPINESS

Although dietary manipulations—for example, restricting intake of simple sugars, use of dietary supplements, and avoiding meals if they need to be alert—are extremely popular among patients, research has not supported the efficacy of these strategies. Nor have numerous reports describing postprandial drowsiness, increased drowsiness after consumption of sugars, carbohydrate cravings, sleep attacks triggered by ingestion of certain foods, and unusual eating patterns among narcoleptic patients (56–58) been substantiated.

Several of the claims mentioned were refuted by Pollak and Green's careful study of the relationship among sleep, eating behavior, and subjective alertness of narcoleptic and control subjects living in a time isolation laboratory (59). In this study, there were no significant differences in the number, frequency, size, or macronutrient composition of the meals consumed by narcoleptic subjects and controls. Narcoleptic subjects consumed more snacks than control subjects, which the researchers attributed to longer periods spent out of bed. Despite increased snacking, narcoleptic subjects consumed the same number of calories and other nutrients as control subjects.

During the scheduled portion of the study, there were meal-associated changes in alertness among the narcoleptic subjects. Subjective ratings of alertness increased 90 to 120 minutes before the meal, peaked at the time of meal onset, then rapidly decreased over a period of 40 to 50 minutes to below premeal baseline. Normal subjects also showed increased alertness before a meal, but their increased alertness continued for more than an hour after the meal. The increased sleep propensity following the meal was not attributed to the effect of the lunch meal itself, but rather to an endogenous circasemidian, or two-per-day sleep rhythm. The time of day when narcoleptic subjects are most likely to be napping is actually earlier in the day than it is for control subjects who are regular nappers (49, 60, 61). Although naps are more likely to follow a meal than precede a meal, naps are no more likely to follow larger meals or meals containing more of any macronutrient (59). Meals followed by naps did not differ in size or macronutrient composition from meals that were not followed by naps.

Caffeine is sometimes recommended as an alternative to traditional stimulant medications or as an adjuvant treatment (62). Caffeine, which can be used to improved alertness in sleep-deprived subjects (63–64), has not been investigated as a treatment for excessive daytime sleepiness in narcoleptic patients. Its alerting effects are limited; it takes six cups of strong coffee to obtain an effect comparable to 5 mg of dexamphetamine (24, 65). Most patients find caffeine ineffective for controlling daytime sleepiness and can easily fall asleep after its ingestion (66). Interestingly, some patients reported improved alertness after consuming caffeine while others reported that avoiding caffeine improved their alertness (38).

Although L-tyrosine, an amino acid precursor to dopamine and norepinephrine, was shown to increase alertness in eight narcoleptic patients (67), other researchers were unable to replicate these findings (68). Nor were manipulations in the dietary intake of precursors of the neurotransmitters, thought to be involved in alertness (norepinephrine), effective in improving the alertness of narcoleptic dogs.

Even if dietary alterations have not been shown to increase daytime alertness, all narcoleptic patients should be encouraged to consume only enough calories to maintain their weight within appropriate levels. Higher than normal rates of Type II diabetes and obesity were observed among Japanese narcoleptic patients almost 20 years ago (69). More recent studies have shown that patients with narcolepsy, on average, have a body mass index (BMI) 10% to 20% greater than matched control subjects (58, 69, 70). However, studies have shown that narcoleptic patients consume fewer calories and carbohydrates than control subjects (71), yet have similar amounts of physical activity over the 24-hour period (72), suggesting narcoleptic patients have a lower metabolic rate (36). The use of medication and/or coexisting depression have also been ruled as factors associated with increased BMI in narcoleptic patients (71). Hypocretins, which affect feeding behavior and energy metabolism, may be involved in this population (36).

OTHER BEHAVIORAL APPROACHES

Several other case studies have reported behavioral treatments for narcolepsy that were reported to be efficacious for controlling excessive daytime sleepiness and/or REM-related symptoms. For example, hypnosis has been reported to be effective for controlling excessive daytime sleepiness (73), cataplexy (74), and sleep paralysis (75). Another clinician reported that progressive muscle relaxation and fluid restriction to improve nocturnal sleep, along with snapping a rubber band against the wrist, was effective for the reduction of daytime sleepiness and the elimination of cataplectic episodes in a 61-year-old patient with multiple medical problems (76). Although these case studies are interesting, there are no rigorous controlled studies that report that hypnosis or progressive muscle relaxation are viable treatments for narcolepsy.

It is well established that bright light can be helpful for shifting circadian rhythms and treating seasonal depression. However, therapy with bright white light (500lx) for four hours per day did not alter subjective or objective symptoms of narcolepsy, leading Hajek and his colleagues (77) to conclude that light therapy was not an appropriate treatment for narcolepsy.

Although limited scientific evidence supports the use of behavioral strategies for the treatment of narcolepsy, they are widely used by patients. Despite a paucity of research, dietary manipulations continued to be recommended. For example, Garma and Marchand (62, p. S100) state in their 1994 article, "good dietary practices are useful in insuring good sleep hygiene," then go on to advise that "morning and midday avoidance of 'sweets' and carbohydrates, especially simple sugars, and large meals will improve alertness in some narcoleptics." Perhaps advocacy of dietary manipulations is due to perception, shared by many patients, that stimulant drugs are ineffective for reducing the severity of daytime sleepiness (37, 38, 78).

However, studies show that stimulant medications are effective in controlling daytime sleepiness in narcolepsy. Laboratory measures of sustained alertness are not brought to normal levels by stimulant medications (79), but ambulatory recordings have shown that approximately 40% of treated narcoleptic patients are able to remain awake throughout the day with low to moderate doses of stimulant medications (23). Because few patients rely exclusively on stimulant medications to control their excessive daytime sleepiness, all patients should be questioned about behavioral strategies used to manage their symptoms and the rationale for selecting these strategies. If patients report difficulties staying awake, especially when driving, their medication regime may need to be modified. Compliance with prescribed therapy should also be assessed, because studies have shown that the majority of narcoleptic patients fail to take their prescribed dosage of stimulant medications (80–81).

Compliance with anticataplectic medications has not been studied. However, there is little evidence to suggest that compliance rates for anticataplectic medications would be higher than those for stimulant medications. Patients of all ages and all educational and socioeconomic levels frequently choose to alter their medications without consulting their health care providers, take their medications at different times than prescribed, and take more or less drugs than prescribed (82–88). Underdosing, not overdosing, is pervasive (84, 86, 87); patients frequently take less medication than prescribed, fail to fill their original prescription or refill their prescriptions in a timely fashion, take drug holidays, or completely stop taking their medications after a few months without consulting their physicians. Approximately one-third of all patients are estimated to be satisfactorily compliant, another third are partially compliant, and the remaining third do not comply at all with treatment (86).

FUTURE DIRECTIONS FOR RESEARCH

Rather than focusing more effort on testing behavioral strategies, perhaps research in the future should focus on examining patient attitudes toward the use of medications and how to help patients accept the need for medications. Issues related to compliance should be explored and strategies developed to help patients take their medications. There is a need to develop ways of combating patient fears about becoming addicted to stimulant medications and their search for a natural remedy. Clinicians need to discuss the difference between drug use and drug abuse and have frank discussion of appropriate uses of stimulants, particularly Ritalin, to combat frequent media claims of overprescribing. If cataplexy occurs, clinicians need to discuss its frequency and the pros and cons to treating this symptom, depending on severity. For medications prescribed for the management of daytime sleepiness or cataplexy, it is important that patients understand safety issues if they choose not to comply with their treatment plan worked out in consultation with their physician. In this regard, it may be useful to examine the utility of working on compliance issues with a structured approach that focuses on what a patient would do if he or she had more time without struggling against sleepiness. While there is no cure for narcolepsy, there are medications that help maintain alertness and eliminate cataplectic attacks.

Recent discoveries have led to renewed optimism for the possibility of a cure for narcolepsy. It has recently been reported that human narcolepsy is associated with a deficiency of the hypocretin (orexin) system (88–90). Despite normal serum levels of Hcrt-1 (hypocretin-1), CSF (cerebro-spinal fluid) levels of Hcrt-1 are low to absent in narcoleptic patients (91, 92). Because serum levels are normal, the deficit does not appear to be caused by damage to neuronal cells in the gut but rather associated with damage to the hypothalamic centers where the peptide receptors are located. Work with animal models further suggests the importance of this system in the development of narcolepsy. For example, a deletion in the Hcrt (hypocretin) receptor-2 gene causes cataplexy in dogs (93), and Hcrt knockout mice exhibit cataplexy or episodes of REM sleep while awake (94).

Currently, stimulant aids are very beneficial in helping narcoleptic patients to maintain wakefulness throughout the day. While these medications do not bring the narcoleptic to the level of normal control subjects with respect to sustained performance, they are more effective than behavioral strategies. New advances in medical technology may one day lead to an effective treatment for narcolepsy, and, at that time, a management approach, with stimulants and/or behavioral strategies, may become obsolete.

REFERENCES

1. National Commission on Sleep Disorders Research. *Report of the National Commission on Sleep Disorders Research* (DHHS Pub. No. 93-XXXX). Washington DC: U.S. Government Printing Office. 1993.

2. Rogers, A. E. Problems and coping strategies identified by narcoleptic subjects. *Journal of Neurosurgical Nursing* 16: 326–334, 1984.

3. Parkes, J. D. *Sleep and Its Disorders.* London, England: W.B. Saunders Company. 1985.

4. Billiard, M., A. Besset, and J. Cadihac. The clinical and polygraphic development of narcolepsy. In C. Guilleminault and E. Lugaresi, eds. *Sleep/Wake Disorders: Natural History, Epidemiology and Long-Term Evolution.* New York, NY: Raven Press. 1983: 171–185.

5. American Academy of Sleep Medicine. *The International Classification of Sleep Disorders: Diagnostic and Coding Manual.* Rochester, MN: American Academy of Sleep Medicine. 2001.

6. Ribstein, M. Hypnagogic hallucinations. In C. Guilleminault, W. C. Dement, and P. Passouant, eds. *Narcolepsy: Advances in Sleep Research* (Volume 3). New York, NY: Spectrum Publications. 1976: 145–160.

7. Stepanski, E., J. Lamphere, P. Badiz, F. Zorick, and T. Roth. Sleep fragmentation and daytime sleepiness. *Sleep* 7: 18–26, 1984.

8. Broughton, W. A. and R. J. Broughton. Psychosocial impact of narcolepsy. *Sleep* 17: S45–S49, 1994.

9. Broughton, R. J. Narcolepsy. In M. J. Thorpy, ed. *Handbook of Sleep Disorders.* New York, NY: Marcel Dekker, Inc. 1990: 197–216.

10. Roy, A. Psychiatric aspects of narcolepsy. *British Journal of Psychiatry* 128: 562–565, 1976.

11. Broughton, R. and Q. Ghanem. The impact of compound narcolepsy on the life of the patient. In C. Guilleminault, W. C. Dement, and P. Passouant, eds. *Narcolepsy:*

Advances in Sleep Research (Volume 3). New York, NY: Spectrum Publications. 1976: 201–220.

12. Broughton, R., Q. Ghanem, Y. Hishikawa, Y. Sugita, S. Nevsimalova, and B. Roth. Life effects of narcolepsy in 180 patients from North America, Asia, and Europe compared to matched controls. *Canadian Journal of Neurological Sciences* 8: 199–204, 1981.

13. Passouant, P. and M. Billiard. The evolution of narcolepsy with age. In C. Guilleminault, W. C. Dement, and P. Passouant, eds. *Narcolepsy: Advances in Sleep Research* (Volume 3). New York, NY: Spectrum Publications. 1976: 179–196.

14. Hoddes, E., W. C. Dement, and V. Zarcone. The development and use of the Stanford Sleepiness Scale (SSS). *Pyschophysiology* 9: 150, 1972.

15. Herscovitch, J. and R. Broughton. Sensitivity of the Stanford Sleepiness Scale to the effects of cumulative partial sleep deprivation and recovery oversleeping. *Sleep* 4: 83–92, 1981.

16. Johns, M. S. A new method for measuring daytime sleepiness: The Epworth Sleepiness Scale. *Sleep* 14: 540–545, 1991.

17. Rogers, A. E., C. Caruso, and M. S. Aldrich. Reliability of sleep diaries for assessment of sleep/wake patterns. *Nursing Research* 42: 368–372, 1993.

18. Biniaurishnille, R. G., J. M. Fry, M. A. DiPhillip, et al. MSLT REM sleep episodes, excessive daytime sleepiness and sleep structure in obstructive sleep apnea. *Sleep Research* 23: 231, 1994.

19. Bishop, C., L. Rosenthal, T. Helmus, et al. The frequency of multiple sleep onset REM periods among subjects with no excessive daytime sleepiness *Sleep* 19: 727–730, 1996.

20. Sangal, R. B., L. Thomas, and M. M. Mitler. Disorders of excessive sleepiness: Treatment improves ability to stay awake but does not reduce sleepiness. *Chest* 102: 699–703, 1992.

21. Broughton, R., W. Dunham, J. Newman, K. Lutley, P. Duschesne, and M. Rivers. Ambulatory 24-hour sleep-wake monitoring in narcolepsy cataplexy compared to matched controls. *Electroencephalography and Clinical Neurophysiology* 70: 473–481, 1988.

22. Broughton, R. and M. Mamelak. Effects of nocturnal gamm-hydroxybutyrate on sleep/waking patterns in narcolepsy-cataplexy. *Canadian Sciences Neurologiques* 7: 23–31, 1980.

23. Rogers, A. E., M. S. Aldrich, and C. C. Caruso. Patterns of sleep and wakefulness in treated narcoleptic subjects. *Sleep* 17: 590–597, 1994.

24. Mitler, M. M., M. S. Aldrich, G. F. Koob, and V. P. Zarcone. Narcolepsy and its treatment with stimulants. *Sleep* 17: 352–371, 1994.

25. U.S. Modafinil in Narcolepsy Multicenter Study Group. Randomized trial of modafinil for the treatment of pathological somnolence in narcolepsy. *Annals of Neurology* 43: 88–97, 1998.

26. Buesterien, K. M., A. E. Rogers, J. A. Walsleben, et al. Health-related quality of life effects of modafinil for the treatment of narcolepsy. *Sleep* 22: 757–767, 1999.

27. Mitler, M. M., R. Hajdukovic, M. Erman, and J. A. Koziol. Narcolepsy. *Journal of Clinical Neuropsychology* 7: 93–118, 1990.

28. Billiard, M., A. Besset, J. Montplaisir, et al. Modafinil: A double-blind multicentric study. *Sleep* 17: S107–S112, 1994.

29. Broughton, R. J., J. A. E. Fleming, C. F. P. George, et al. Randomized, double-blind, placebo-controlled crossover trial of modafinil in the treatment of excessive daytime sleepiness in narcolepsy. *Neurology* 49: 444–451, 1997.

30. Boivin, D. B., J. Montplaisir, D. Petit, C. Lambert, and S. Lubin. Effects of modafinil on symptomatology of human narcolepsy. *Clinical Neuropharmacology* 16: 46–53, 1993.

31. Besset, A., M. Tafti, E. Villemin, and M. Billiard. Effects du modafinil (300 mg) sur le sommeil, la somnolence et la vigilance du narcoleptique. *Neurophysiologie Clinique* 23: 47–60, 1993.

32. Mitler, M. M., R. Hajdukovic, and M. K. Erman. Treatment of narcolepsy with methamphetamine. *Sleep* 16: 306–317, 1993.

33. Littner, M., S. F. Johnson, W. V. McCall, et al. Practice Parameters for the treatment of narcolepsy. An update for 2000. *Sleep* 24: 451–466, 2001.

34. Fry, J. M. Treatment modalities for narcolepsy. *Neurology* 50(Suppl. 1): S43–S48, 1998.

35. Nishino, S. and E. Mignot. Pharmacological aspects of human and canine narcolepsy. *Progress in Neurobiology* 52: 27–28, 1997.

36. Overeem, S., E. Mignot, J. G. van Dijk, and G. J. Lammers. Narcolepsy: Clinical features, new pathophysiological insights, and future perspectives. *Journal of Clinical Neuropsychology* 18: 78–105, 2001.

37. Daniels, E., M. A. King, I. E. Smith, and J. M. Shneerson. Health-related quality of life in narcolepsy. *Journal of Sleep Research* 10: 75–81, 2001.

38. Cohen, F. L., W. M. Nehring, and L. Cloninger. Symptom description and management in narcolepsy. *Holistic Nursing Practice* 10: 45–53, 1996.

39. Alaia, S. L. Life effects of narcolepsy: Measures of negative impact, social support and psychological well-being. *Loss, Grief, and Care* 5: 1–22, 1992.

40. Montplaisir, J. and R. Godbout. Nocturnal sleep of narcoleptics: Revisited. *Sleep* 9: 159–161, 1986.

41. Scrima, L., P. G. Hartman, F. R. Johnson, Jr., and F. C. Hiller. Efficacy of gamma-hydroxybutyrate versus placebo in treating narcolepsy-cataplexy: Double blind subjective measures. *Biological Psychiatry* 26: 331–341, 1985.

42. Thorpy, M. J., M. Snyder, F. S. Aloe, P. S. Ledereich, and K. E. Starz. Short-term triazolam use improves nocturnal sleep of narcoleptics. *Sleep* 15: 212–216, 1992.

43. Danz, B., D. M. Edgar, and W. C. Dement. Circadian rhythms in narcolepsy: Studies in 90 minute day. *Electroencephalography Clinical Neurophysiology* 40: 24–35, 1994.

44. Broughton, R., S. Krupa, B. Boucher, M. Rivers, and J. Mullington. Impaired circadian waking arousal in narcolepsy-cataplexy. *Sleep Research Online* 1: 159–165, 1998.

45. Yuchiyama, M., G. Mayer, and K. Meirer-Ewart. Differential effects of extended sleep in narcoleptic patients. *Electroencephalography Clinical Neurophysiology* 91: 212–218, 1994.

46. Rogers, A. E., M. S. Aldrich, and X. Lin. A comparison of three different sleep schedules for reducing daytime sleepiness in narcolepsy. *Sleep* 24: 1–7, 2001.

47. Roehrs, R., F. Zorick, R. Wittig, C. Paxton, J. Sicklesteel, and T. Roth. Alerting effects of naps in patients with narcolepsy. *Sleep* 9: 191–194, 1986.

48. Helmus, T., L. Rosenthal, C. Bishop, T. Roehrs, M. L. Syron, and T. Roth. The alerting effects of short and long naps in narcoleptic, sleep-deprived, and alert individuals. *Sleep* 20: 251–257, 1997.

49. Mullington, J. and R. Broughton. Scheduled naps in the management of daytime sleepiness in narcolepsy-cataplexy. *Sleep* 16: 444–456, 1993.

50. Fitzpatrick, J. and M. J. Donovan. A follow-up study of the reliability and validity of the motor activity rating scale. *Nursing Research* 28: 179–181, 1979.

51. Broughton, R. and J. Mullington. Chronobiological aspects of narcolepsy. *Sleep* 17: S35–S44, 1994.

52. Mullington, J. and R. Broughton. Daytime sleep inertia in narcolepsy-cataplexy. *Sleep* 16: 444–456, 1993.

53. Murray, J. The use of health diaries in the field of psychiatric illness in general practice. *Psychological Medicine* 15: 827–840, 1985.

54. Dement, W. C. and W. P. Baird. *Narcolepsy: Care and Treatment for the Primary Care Physician Whose Patient is Afflicted with Narcolepsy.* Stanford, CA: American Narcolepsy Association. 1976.

55. Rogers, A. E. and M. S. Aldrich. Do Regularly Scheduled Naps Reduce Sleep Attacks and Excessive Daytime Sleepiness Associated with Narcolepsy? *Nursing Research* 42: 111–117, 1993.

56. Zarcone, V. Narcolepsy. *New England Journal of Medicine* 288: 1156–1166, 1973.

57. Kales, A. and J. Kales. Sleep disorders: Recent findings in the diagnosis and treatment of disturbed sleep. *New England Journal of Medicine* 290: 487–499, 1974.

58. Bell, I. R. Diet history in narcolepsy. In C. Guilleminault, W. C. Dement, and P. Passouant, eds. *Narcolepsy: Advantages in Sleep Research* (Volume 3). New York, NY: Spectrum Publications. 1976: 221–228.

59. Pollak, C. P. and J. Green. Eating and its relationships with subjective alertness and sleep in narcoleptic subjects living without temporal cues. *Sleep* 13(6): 467–478, 1990.

60. Mullington, J., J. Newman, W. Dunham, and R. Broughton. Phase timing and duration of naps in narcolepsy-cataplexy: Preliminary findings. In J. Horne, ed. *Sleep '90.* Bochum, Germany: Pontengal. 1990: 158–160.

61. Mullington, J. and R. Broughton. Does a chronobiologic defect exist in narcolepsy? In K. Meier-Ewert and M. Okawa, eds. *Sleep-Wake Disorders.* New York, NY: Plenum Press, 1998: 91–103.

62. Garma, L. and F. Marchand. Nonpharmacological approaches to the treatment of narcolepsy. *Sleep* 17: S97–S102, 1994.

63. Wright, K. P., Jr., P. Badia, B. L. Myers, and S. C. Plenzler. Combination of bright light and caffeine as a countermeasure for impaired alertness and performance during extended sleep deprivation. *Journal of Sleep Research* 6: 26–35, 1997.

64. Panetar, D., U. McCann, G. Kamimori, et al. Caffeine reversal of sleep deprivation effects on alertness and mood. *Psychopharmacology* 112: 359–365, 1993.

65. Parkes, J. D. and M. Dahlitz. Amphetamine prescription. *Sleep* 16: 201–203, 1993.

66. Thorpy, M. J. and M. Goswami. Treatment of narcolepsy. In M. J. Thorpy, ed. *Handbook of Sleep Disorders.* New York, NY: Marcel Dekker, Inc. 1990: 235–258.

67. Mouret, J., P. Lemoine, P. Sanchez, N. Robelin, J. Taillard, and F. Canini. Treatment of narcolepsy with L-tyrosine. *Lancet* 2: 1458–1459, 1988.

68. Guilleminault, C., R. Stoohs, and A. Clerk. Daytime somnolence: Therapeutic approaches. *Neurophysiology Clinics* 23: 23–33, 1993.

69. Honda, Y., Y. Doi, C. Ninomiya, and O. Ninomiya. Increased frequency of noninsulin-dependent diabetes mellitus among narcoleptic patients. *Sleep* 9: 254–259, 1986.

70. Schuld, A., J. Hebebrand, F. Geller, and T. Pollmacher. Increased body-mass index in patients with narcolepsy. *Lancet* 355: 1274–1275, 2000.

71. Lammers, G. J., H. Pijl, J. Iestra, J. A. Langius, G. Baunk, and A. E. Meinders. Spontaneous food choice in narcolepsy. *Sleep* 19: 75–76, 1996.

72. Middlekoop, H. A., G. J. Lammers, B. J. Van Hilten, C. Ruwhof, H. Pijl, and H. A. Kamphuisen. Circadian distribution of motor activity and immobility in narcolepsy: Assessment with continuous motor activity monitoring. *Psychophysiology* 32: 286–291, 1995.

73. Schneck, J. M. Hypnotherapy for narcolepsy. *International Journal of Clinical and Experimental Hypnosis* 28: 95–100, 1980.

74. Price, R. Hypnotherapy in the control of cataplexy in a narcoleptic subject. *American Journal of Clinical Hypnosis* 29: 201–205, 1987.

75. Nardi, T. J. Treating sleep paralysis with hypnosis. *International Journal of Clinical and Experimental Hypnosis* 9: 358–365, 1981.

76. Kolko, D. J. Behavioral treatment of excessive daytime sleepiness in an elderly woman with multiple medical problems. *Journal of Behavior Therapy and Experimental Psychiatry* 15: 341–345, 1984.

77. Hajek, M., K. Meier-Ewart, A. Wirz-Justice, et al. Bright white light does not improve narcoleptic symptoms. *European Archives of Psychiatry and Neurological Sciences* 238: 203–2976, 1989.

78. Schumacher, A., S. L. Merritt, and F. L. Cohen. The effect of drug therapy on the perceived symptom and ADL experiences of narcoleptics. *Journal of Neuroscience Nursing* 29: 15–23, 1997.

79. Mitler, M. M. Evaluation of treatment with stimulants in narcolepsy. *Sleep* 17: S103–S106, 1994.

80. Rogers, A. E., M. S. Aldrich, A. M. Berrios, and R. S. Rosenberg. Compliance with stimulant medications in narcolepsy. *Sleep* 20: 28–33, 1997.

81. Rogers, A. E., C. Cantor, and S. Marcus. Compliance with stimulant medications in patients with narcolepsy: Measurement with a MEMS TrackCap. *Sleep* 2001. (Abstract).

82. Sleator, E. K. Measurement of compliance. *Psychopharmacology Bulletin* 21(3): 1089–1093, 1985.

83. Simons, M. R. Nursing interventions related to compliance. *Nursing Clinics of North America* 27: 477–485, 1992.

84. Kauffman, R. E., D. Smith-Wright, C. A. Reese, R. Simpson, and F. Jones. Medication compliance in hyperactive children. *Pediatric Pharmacology* 1: 231–237, 1981.

85. Firestone, P. Factors associated with children's adherence to stimulant medication. *American Journal of Orthopsychiatry* 52(3): 447–457, 1982.

86. Urquhart, J. Variable patient compliance in ambulatory trials-nuisance, threat, opportunity. *Journal of Antimicrobial Chemotherapy* 32: 643–649, 1993.

87. Cramer, J. A., R. H. Mattson, M. L. Prevey, R. D. Scheyer, and V. L. Ouellette. How often is medication taken as prescribed? A novel assessment technique. *Journal of the American Medical Association* 261: 3273–3277, 1989.

88. Silber, M. H. and D. B. Rye. Solving the mysteries of narcolepsy: The hypocretin story. *Neurology* 56: 1616–1618, 2001.

89. Lin, L., M. Hungs, and E. Mignot. Narcolepsy and the HLA region. *Journal of Neuroimmunology* 117: 9–20, 2001.

90. Melberg, A., B. Ripley, L. Lin, J. Hetta, E. Mignot, and S. Nishino. Hypocretin deficiency in familial symptomatic narcolepsy. *Annals of Neurology* 49: 136–137, 2001.

91. Dalal, M. A., A. Schuld, M. Haack, et al. Normal plasma levels of orexin A (hypocretin-1) in narcoleptic patients. *Neurology* 56: 1749–1750, 2001.

92. Nishino, S., B. Ripley, S. Overeem, et al. Low CSF hypocretin (orexin) and altered energy homeostasis in human narcolepsy. *Annals of Neurology* 50: 381–388, 2001.

93. Lin, L., J. Faraco, R. Li, et al. The sleep disorder canine narcolepsy is caused by a mutation in the hypocretin (Orexin) receptor 2 gene. *Cell* 98: 365–376, 1999.

94. Chemelli, R. M., J. T. Willie, C. M. Sinton, et al. Narcolepsy in orexin knockout mice: Molecular genetics of sleep regulation. *Cell* 98: 437–451, 1999.

Chapter 6 ———————————————————

TREATMENT EFFICACY OF BEHAVIORAL INTERVENTIONS FOR OBSTRUCTIVE SLEEP APNEA, RESTLESS LEGS SYNDROME, PERIODIC LEG MOVEMENT DISORDER, AND NARCOLEPSY

TRACY F. KUO AND CLETE A. KUSHIDA

This chapter reviews treatment studies of behavioral interventions for obstructive sleep apnea syndrome (OSAS), restless legs syndrome (RLS), periodic limb movement disorder (PLMD), and narcolepsy. Individual study results on efficacy are reviewed. For each study, the design, subject characteristics, prescribed behavioral treatment, and findings are briefly described. Studies in which effect sizes could be derived from the published data are summarized in tables. The efficacy of cognitive-behavioral therapy for primary and secondary insomnia is detailed in Chapter 10.

The extent to which the treatment normalizes sleep and neuropsychological and other impaired daytime functions should be a major consideration in determining efficacy (1). Sleep variables have been the primary outcome measure for most outcome studies on behavioral interventions. Treatment benefits for reversing neuropsychological and other daytime impairments are understudied.

OBSTRUCTIVE SLEEP APNEA SYNDROME (OSAS)

The primary goal of any treatment for OSAS is to eliminate sleep-disordered breathing (i.e., abolishing all abnormal respiratory events including snoring, hypopneas, and apneas). Measures of sleep-disordered breathing (SDB) include the apnea-hypopnea index (AHI), indexes of oxygen desaturation, respiratory event-related arousals, and daytime symptoms (1). Most of the existing behavioral intervention studies have used the AHI as the primary outcome measure.

Behavioral treatment options for OSAS include diet and exercise for weight loss and sleep-positional therapy (2–7). Small sample sizes and lack of randomization or a control group in study design pose limitations to allow for establishing causal links between treatments and outcome. Existing studies, overall, nevertheless, showed that these nonsurgical and nonmedical behavioral modalities resulted in some clinical improvement for most patients. Bariatric surgical weight loss and rapid weight loss through inpatient stay or medically supervised very low calorie fasting (8–10) are considered medical therapies and thus are not covered in this chapter.

A few case reports suggest some benefits with sleep hygiene practice (e.g., avoidance of alcohol) and myofunctional therapy (e.g., exercises to tone upper airway muscles). At this time, published long-term data on the effects of such behavioral interventions are sparse.

Obesity is a major risk factor for OSAS. The contribution of obesity to the pathogenesis of OSAS has been estimated at 30% to 67% (11). A case report by Browman et al. (12) characterized the relationship between apnea and body weight as a logarithmic function. A modest initial decrease in weight was associated with a disproportionately larger decrease in the number of apnea events. Although the etiologic mechanisms of promoting sleep apnea are not well understood, several mechanisms are thought to explain the relationship between obesity and OSAS. Obesity reduces upper airway caliber through increased deposition of adipose tissue (13–16). Obesity appears to alter upper airway compliance and change the biomechanical relationships of the upper airway muscles (14, 17). Hypotonality of the airway dilating muscles is associated with obesity and predisposes the airway to collapse. Obesity and the tendency to sleep in a supine position can also lead to reduced residual lung volume and thus increase the impact of SDB (i.e., greater degrees of desaturation and more respiratory event-related arousals). Weight loss reduces the amount of adipose tissue in the oropharynx (18) thus improves airway caliber, reduces airway collapsibility, increases residual volume in the lungs, and reduces respiratory effort (14, 19).

Association of Weight Loss and Obstructive Sleep Apnea Syndrome

Weight loss is considered a conservative intervention for OSAS. Some patients with OSAS are cured by significant and maintained weight loss. Given that weight gain and obesity are major risk factors for the development of OSAS, weight control should be an integral part of a patient's clinical management plan.

Losing weight is difficult, and keeping the weight off is even more challenging. A substantial proportion of dieters are able to achieve some short-term success, but only a small percentage maintains sustained success (12, 20). A meta-analysis of 29 studies on long-term weight loss maintenance reported > 3 kg (> 3% reduction of initial body weight) in an average individual five years after completing structured weight loss programs (21). Long-term maintenance is possible through continued care and sustained effort to avoid excess caloric intake (22–23). A multidisciplinary team consisting of a physician, nurse, dietitian, and peer group constitutes the most effective approach in facilitating long-lasting weight control (24). Weight regain can be minimized if patients maintain frequent, regular contact with their provider to reinforce compliance (25) and if they engage in regular physical activity for two to three hours a week (26).

Specific to OSAS patient population, several studies with small sample sizes ($N < 30$) have evaluated the effect of varying degrees of weight loss on the indexes of SDB. While most of these studies were uncontrolled and varied in the nature of the weight loss program, patient characteristics, the severity of SDB and obesity at baseline, and the length of follow-up, almost all showed that weight loss improved SDB to some extent in some patients (15, 17, 27).

Weight Change Is Associated with Reduction in the Severity of Sleep-Disordered Breathing (SDB)

A longitudinal prospective cohort study by Peppard and colleagues (28) established that body weight change is positively related to change in the AHI. A total of 690 randomly selected employees of Wisconsin were evaluated by polysomnography twice, separated by a four-year interval. Forty-six participants had moderate to severe (AHI $\geq$ 15) SDB at baseline. At follow-up, 17 (out of the 45) participants' AHIs had dropped below 15, and they had lost an average of 3.1 ±6.2 kg. Of the 644 participants who did not have moderate to severe SDB, 39 manifested moderate to severe SDB at follow-up. These 39 participants gained an average 3.9 ±6.8 kg of body weight. The study found that for a small weight increment or decrement, each percentage change in weight was associated with an approximate 3% change in the AHI. For example, a 10% weight gain predicted an approximately 32% increase in the AHI, and a 10% weight loss was associated with a 26% decrease in the AHI. The results of this study suggest that modest weight loss is likely to reduce the severity of SDB and the risk of developing clinically significant OSAS. Conversely, preventing weight gain may protect a person from developing clinically significant OSAS.

Efficacy of Weight Loss as a Treatment for Obstructive Sleep Apnea Syndrome

Table 6.1 on pages 140–143 provides a summary of behavioral weight loss intervention studies. Twenty-three overweight OSAS patients (age 46.4 ±9.2 years; BMI 37.5 ±9.8 kg/m^2) who were free of cranialfacial malformations were studied by Pasquali et al. (29) to examine the effects of weight loss on SDB. Weight loss was achieved through diet therapy, which consisted of either low (800 to 1,800 kcal/day) or very low calorie (320 to 500 kcal/day) diets for 3 to 14 months (mean 5.6 ±3.0 months). Treatment goal was to lose ≥50% of the excess weight, using BMI of 25 as a normal reference value. Posttreatment polysomnogram was performed at least two to four weeks after weight stabilization. A mean of 15.9% of weight loss (BMI dropped from 37.5 ±9.8 to 30.9 ±5.0 kg/m^2) was accompanied by a mean 50% ±46% reduction in the AHI (from 66.5 ±23.0 at baseline to 33.0 ±26.2/h). Oxygenation was improved as well, from baseline minimum oxygen saturation of 81.9 ±6.9% at baseline to 87.6 ±3.9%. There was a significant correlation ($r = -0.55$) between weight loss and change in the AHI.

Lojander and associates (30) studied the effect of a one-year nurse-administered weight reduction program in 24 (23 men; age 48 ±7 years) newly diagnosed OSAS patients. Two patients were lost to follow-up at one year. The program began with a six-week very low calorie diet (VLCD; 500 kcal/day) followed by normal food low in calories. Patients also had 12 group meetings targeting behavioral modifications. The number of oxygen desaturation events of ≥4% per hour (ODI-4) and visual analogue (0 = none; 100 = very severe) assessed daytime sleepiness were the primary outcome measures. Mean BMI dropped from 36 ±3.0 kg/m^2 (weight 110 ±11 kg) at baseline to 31 ±3 kg/m^2 (weight 97 ±11 kg) at the end of the six-week VLCD and was maintained (31 ±7 kg/m^2; weight 99 ±12 kg) at one year. Respiration was improved as evidenced in a reduction of ODI-4, which was 30 ±20/hr at baseline, 13 ±12/hr at the end of the six-week VLCD, and 12 ±14/hr at one year. Weight loss was also associated with decrease in daytime sleepiness. Sleepiness rating dropped from 47 ±30 at baseline to 28 ±22 at the end of the six-week VLCD and to 37 ±34 at one year. Overall, the percent of weight loss maintained (approximately 10% of baseline body weight and 33% [11 kg] of excess weight) was associated with approximately 60% reduction in the AHI. Reduction in ODI-4 was significantly corrected ($r = 0.34$) with the reduction in the BMI.

Norman et al. (31) reported data on nine subjects (eight men; age 48 ±9 years; BMI 31.2 ±4.6 kg/m^2) with OSAS (AHI 21.7 ±9.0/hr, range 10.1 to 35/hr). The study specifically examined the effect of exercise conditioning in patients with mild to moderate OSAS. Five subjects concurrently used CPAP regularly

Table 6.1 Efficacy of Behavioral Weight Loss Intervention for Treating OSAS

	Study Design	N M/F	Intervention	Outcome Pre-/Posttreatment	Effect Size[a]	Comments Clinical Significance
Pasquali et al. (1990)[b]	Within subject pre- and posttreatment comparisons	23 22/1	Very low calorie diet (n=6). Hypocaloric diet (n=17).	AHI: 66.5/33.0 MinO$_2$sat: 81.9/87.6 Wt: 105.1/86.7 BMI: 37.5/30.9	−1.46 +0.83 −0.68 −0.67	Eight subjects had RDI < 10 posttreatment. Average weight loss for these eight was 20% (26.6 kg) of baseline weight.
Lojander et al. (1998)[c]	Within subject pre- and posttreatment comparisons	24 23/1	One-year program. Very low calorie diet (first six weeks). Low calorie diet (week 7 on). Behavioral modification (12 group sessions).	Pre/VLCD/1-year ODI4: 30/13/12 VAS sleepiness: 47/28/37 Wt: 110/97/99	−0.85/−0.90 +0.63/+0.33 −1.18/−1.0	Subjects varied in the amount of weight loss required to achieve clinical significant reduction of OSAS.
Norman et al. (2000)[d]	Within subject pre- and posttreatment comparisons	9 8/1	Six months moderate intensity aerobic exercise and attempt to lose weight.	AHI: 21.7/11.8 ODI4: 6.5/1.7 Wt: 110.9/104.7 BMI: 31.2/29.6	−1.1 −0.35 −0.52 −0.35	Six achieved RDI < 10. Average weight loss = 6% of baseline weight (6.2 kg).

Study	Design	N; M/F	Intervention	Results	Effect size	Comments
Noseda et al (1996)[e]	Within subject pre- and postattempted weight loss	39 35/5	CPAP with dietary restriction to lose weight for one year.	AHI: 66.5/50.3 MinO$_2$sat: 62/78 Wt: 108.3/99.7	−0.56 +1.0 −0.30	Three patients whose baseline BMI >40 had bariatric surgery. At one year, four patients had RDI < 10, with associated mean 24% weight loss.
Schwartz et al. (1991)[f]	Between group comparisons	26 26/0	13 patients attended weight loss program and 13 received usual care.	Weight loss group: usual care group. Non-REM RDI: 83.3/32.5:85.5/81.4 Pcrit: 3.1/−2.4:5.2/4.2 BMI: 42.0/34.7:38.2/38.3	−1.64:−0.22 −1.31:−0.43 −1.03:+0.02	When Pcrit fell below −4cm H$_2$O, RDI generally dropped below 20/h. The RDI of six patients in weight loss group dropped below 20.
Smith et al. (1985)[g]	Randomized control trial	23 19/4	15 patients received weight loss intervention and 13 patients were controls.	Weight loss group: control group. Non-REM AI: 55.0/29.2:66.3/70.8 REM AI: 57.0/37.6:48.3/48.3 Max decrease in SO$_2$ in non-REM: 28.0/17.0:21.8/26.4 Max decrease in SO$_2$ in REM: 35.3/27.4:25.5/27.0 Weight: 106.2/96.6:118.8/120.2	Unable to compute effect sizes.	Patients whose body weight was 10% to 15% greater than ideal body weight showed significant improvement in SDB following modest weight loss.

(continued)

Table 6.1 *Continued*

	Study Design	N M/F	Intervention	Outcome Pre-/ Posttreatment	Effect Size[a]	Comments Clinical Significance
Monasterio et al. (2001)[h]	Randomized control trial	125 102/23	59 patients received conservative therapy (CT; weight loss and sleep hygiene) and 66 patients received conservative therapy plus CPAP six-month follow-up.	Weight loss group: Weight loss + CPAP group AHI: 21/17:20/6 BMI: 29.5/28.5:29.4/29.5	−0.67:−2.33 −0.30:+0.03	Conservative therapy patients lost significantly more weight than patients who receive CT + CPAP. Average weight loss in the CT group at six months was 2.7 ± 4.3 kg.
Sampol et al. (1998)[i]	Clinical series, comparisons between baseline and two follow-ups	67 59/8 22 20/2	Weight loss program was not detailed. Second evaluation occurred 11.5 ± 6.1 months after baseline. Third evaluation occurred 94.3 ± 27.4 months after baseline.	AHI ≥ 10 group: AHI: 52.3/44.2 BMI: 31.5/25.9 AHI < 10 group: AHI: 44.3/3/26.4 BMI: 32.8/27.2/30.8	−0.35 −1.12 −1.49/−0.64 −1.22/−0.43	Data are presented in the order of baseline, first follow-up and second follow-up. Following weight loss, AHI of 67 patients remained ≥ 10 and AHI of 34 patients dropped below 10.

Study	Design	N	M/F	Treatment	Measures	Effect size[a]	Notes
Rajala et al (1991)[j]	Clinical series, comparisons between baseline and posttreatment	27	13/14	Dietary weight loss was not detailed. Patients were re-evaluated at one year.	ODI4: 45.8/31.6 BMI: 50.7/44.1	−1.64 −0.79	Data reported here are eight who received dietary regimen. No patient was cured (ODI < 10).
Braver et al (1995)[k]	Comparisons between baseline and combination of nasal spray plus position therapy and nasal spray plus position therapy plus weight loss	19	19/0	Asymptomatic men. Six-month behavioral weight loss program including behavioral modification and diet.	BL/S+P/S+P+WL Snoring index: 379/328/232 AHI: 18/14/12 Wt: 109/101	−0.24/−0.70 −0.15/−0.22 −0.49	12 out of 9 subjects lost weight. Data reported here are on the nine subjects.

[a] Effect size (if possible to derive from published data) is computed by the difference between the means of the control and the treatment conditions divided by the standard deviation of the control condition. AHI = Apnea hyponea index (per hr); AI = Apnea index (per hr); BMI = Body mass index (kg/m^2); $MinO_2sat$ = Minimum oxygen saturation (%); ODI4 = Oxygen desaturation of 4% index (per hr); Pcrit = Upper airway critical pressure (cm H_2O); RDI = Respiratory disturbance index (per hour); SO_2 = Oxygen hemoglobin saturation (%); Wt = Weight (kg).

[b] 18% of weight loss was associated with 50% reduction in the AHI.

[c] 10% of weight loss was associated with 60% reduction in the ODI4 at one year.

[d] Exercise training with 6% of weight loss was associated with 46% reduction in the AHI.

[e] 8% of weight loss was associated with 24% reduction in the AHI.

[f] In the weight loss group, 18% weight loss was associated with 61% reduction in the RDI.

[g] In the weight loss group, 9% weight loss was associated with 40% reduction in the AI.

[h] In the conservative therapy group, 3.3% drop in the BMI was associated with 19% reduction in the AHI.

[i] At 4 to 23 months follow-up, 17% to 18% drop in BMI was associated with16% to 93% reduction in the AHI; At 61 to 132 months follow-up, 6% of weight loss maintenance was associated with 40% reduction in the AHI.

[j] 13% reduction in BMI was associated with 31% reduction in the ODI.

[k] 7% reduction in body weight was associated with 33% reduction in the AHI and 39% reduction in snoring index.

throughout the study period. The structured exercise intervention lasted six months and was primarily a low-impact moderate intensity (60% to 85% maximum heart rate reserve) aerobic program of 30- to 45-minute duration. Subjects had three supervised sessions every week for the first four months followed by a once-weekly supervised session plus twice-weekly unsupervised sessions. The treatment program also included a one-time dietary counseling with a dietician at entry into the study. Subjects were given instructions to eat a balanced diet using the food pyramid paradigm and to reduce caloric intake and portion sizes to lose 0.5 to 1.0 kg body weight per week. Average weight loss was 6.2 kg (equivalent to 5.6% reduction in body weight), from 110.9 ±12.0 kg at baseline to 104.7 ±12.3 kg (BMI 29.6 ±4.4 kg/m^2) posttraining. The combined effect of minimal weight loss and physical conditioning was associated with a 46% reduction in the AHI (11.8 ±6.8/hr). There was no differential treatment response between the five CPAP users and the four nonusers. In terms of clinical significance, two subjects were "cured" posttraining because their AHIs dropped below study entry criteria (> 5/hr). Four subjects had an AHI between 5 and 10, and the AHI dropped below 20 for all subjects. Other improvements following treatment included global measures of sleep (e.g., increased total sleep time and sleep efficiency, decreased number of arousals), resting systolic and diastolic blood pressure, anthropometric measures (e.g., neck girth, waist-to-hip ratio), subjective daytime sleepiness, mood, and quality of life. The decrease in the AHI, however, was not significantly correlated ($r = 0.35$) with weight loss. These findings suggest that for persons with mild to moderate OSAS, physical conditioning may have an additional or synergistic benefit with weight loss. Exercise may also lead to global improvement of sleep and well-being.

In a case series, Noseda and colleagues (32) followed 39 (35 were men; age not reported) OSAS patients who were CPAP compliant to assess the effect of attempted weight loss on the severity of SDB. Thirty-three patients attended a dietary clinic to facilitate weight loss, and three of the four patients whose BMI was > 40 kg/m^2 underwent bariatric surgery. Excluding the three patients who had gastroplasty, mean weight dropped from 102.6 ±18.4 kg at baseline to 99.2 ±17.5 kg one year later (mean for the entire group was 108.3 ±29.0 kg at baseline and 99.2 kg at one year, an 8.4% weight loss). Weight loss was associated with a significant reduction (24%) in the AHI, which dropped from 66.5 ±28.7 to 50.3 ±38.4/hr. The decrease in the AHI was significantly correlated ($r = 0.47$) with the reduction in BMI. Although patients continued to have severe SDB after losing a modest amount of weight, the findings suggest that weight loss can improve SDB to some degree.

Smith and colleagues (33) reported significant decrease in apnea frequency and oxygen desaturation in mild to moderately obese OSAS patients following weight loss. Although, this study had a small sample size, it is one of the very few published controlled trials. Participants were randomly assigned to either the control group ($N = 8$; 7 men; age 53.3 ±2 years, weight 118.8 ±7.4 kg) or the weight loss group ($N = 15$; 12 men; age 58.8 ±2.5 years; weight 106.2 ±7.3 kg). Patient characteristics of the two groups were matched for age, weight, and severity of SDB. While no special diets or behavioral modifications were prescribed, patients in the weight reduction group were instructed to cut down caloric intake to lose 0.45 to 0.9 kg body weight per week. Patients were routinely followed every two to three months until they had lost at least 5% of total body weight. Control group subjects were followed until their weight had stabilized for at least one month. Time lag between baseline and reevaluation was 5.3 ±1.6 months for the weight loss group and 8.5 ±3.5 months for the control patients. At follow-up, control patients did not lose weight and showed no changes in SDB or oxygenation. In contrast, the weight loss group on average lost 9.6 kg (9% body weight) and showed a significant decrease in both non-REM sleep and REM sleep apnea index (AI). The AI dropped from 55.0 ±7.5/hr to 29.2 ±7.1/hr for non-REM sleep and from 57.0 ±3.2 to 37.6 ±5.7/hr for REM sleep. The AI of 8 of the 13 patients who lost weight dropped below 20, and 4 patients showed near elimination of apneic events. Improvement was evident as well for oxygenation in the weight loss group. Maximum percent of arterial oxygen desaturation dropped from 28.0 ±4.5 to 17.0 ±3.6% in non-REM sleep and from 35.3 ±5.7 to 27.4 ±4.4% in REM sleep. This study showed that modest weight loss led to significant improvement in SDB. Such benefits of weight loss were evident in patients with varying severity of SDB and baseline body weight.

The extent to which weight loss improves upper airway collapsibility and SDB severity was studied by Schwartz et al. (14). Newly diagnosed OSAS patients were invited to join either a weight loss group or a usual care control group. The two groups were matched by age, sex, and weight. In addition to receiving the usual follow-up care at the sleep clinic as the usual care group (13 men; age 43.9 ±10.5 years; weight 121.7 ±16.3 kg), the weight loss group (13 men; age 46.9 ±8.9 years; weight 129.1 ±19.6 kg) attended weekly sessions of intensive counseling and behavior modification targeting losing 15% body weight. Usual follow-up included provision of general advice as to the importance of losing weight, avoiding alcohol and sedatives, and specific recommendation to use CPAP. No specific strategies for weight loss were given to patients in the usual care group. Reevaluation was performed 16.9 ±10 months and 18.4 ±9.5 months later for the weight loss group and the usual care group, respectively. Thirteen of the 23 patients who elected to join weight loss programs met the minimum 5% body weight loss requirement to be restudied. Compared to the usual care control group, which maintained a stable weight, the weight loss group showed significantly improved resistance to upper airway collapse. The BMI in the weight loss group decreased from 42.0 ±7.1 to 34.7 ±5.1 kg/m², which was associated with decreased disordered breathing index (83.3 ±31.0 versus 32.5 ±35.9/hr) and increased upper airway critical pressure (3.1 ±4.2 versus −2.4 ±4.4 cm H_2O). Findings of the study indicate that for persons who are able to lose moderate amount of weight, their upper airway can become less vulnerable to collapse and they can have significantly fewer SDB events.

A handful of studies (34–35) employed weight loss as a conservative control treatment to evaluate CPAP efficacy. The efficacy of weight loss can be appreciated by comparing measures of weight and SDB pre- and posttreatment within the control group. A study by Redline et al. was a randomized trial involving persons with mild to moderate (respiratory disturbance index [RDI] 5 to 30/hr) disease. Unfortunately, data on weight was not reported at follow-up. A study by Monasterio and associates (35) did report information on weight to allow quantifying the degree of weight loss in relation to change in SDB. Subjects were a consecutive series of patients who were randomly assigned to receive either conservative therapy ($N = 59$; 54 were men; age 54 ±9 years) or conservative therapy plus CPAP ($N = 66$; age 53 ±9 years). The conservative therapy consisted of a program for weight loss and instructions to obtain adequate sleep and to avoid sedatives, alcohol, and supine sleeping position. A second polysomnogram was performed to assess SDB at six months after baseline. Patients who received the conservative therapy lost minimal weight (3% body weight; BMI dropped from 29.5 ±3.3 kg/m² at baseline to 28.5 ±3.5 kg/m²) at six-month follow-up. The small amount of weight loss, nevertheless, was associated with a small improvement in the AHI (21 ±6 to 17 ±10/hr). The conservative therapy patients showed improvement comparable to that of the CPAP group on steer-clear tasks and on cognitive tests of memory and executive function.

Long-term benefit of dietary weight loss for OSAS was examined by Sampol and associates (25). A larger sample size and having two follow-up evaluations subsequent to baseline are strengths of this study. Overweight clinic patients with OSAS were followed to evaluate whether the benefit of weight loss is sustained over time. Patients were initially managed by a weight reduction program, which included a low calorie diet (1,000 kcal per day), encouragement to increase physical activity, and periodic clinic follow-up to reinforce compliance. Of a series of 315 patients, 104 patients (51%) were successful in achieving weight loss of > 10% of initial body weight. A second diagnostic polysomnogram was performed on 101 of these 104 patients. The AHIs of 67 patients (59 were men; mean age 53.2 ±8.7 years) remained ≥ 10 per hour. The BMI of these 67 patients dropped from 31.5 ±5.0 to 25.8 ±2.9 kg/m², which was associated with a 15% decrease in the AHI (52.3 ±23.2 to 44.2 ±25.6/hr). Of the other 34 patients whose AHIs had dropped below 10 per hour, 25 reported that they had stopped snoring completely and amelioration of daytime sleepiness. These 34 patients were considered "cured" and only 24 (22 men; mean age 49.6 ±5.9 years) had a third polysomnogram. The mean decrease in BMI that led to a cure was 5.6 ±2.5 (BMI at baseline was 32.8 ±4.6 kg/m^2 and 27.2 ±3 kg/m^2 at the second evaluation). The time elapse between diagnosis and the first follow-up was 11.5 ±6.1 months and 94.3 ±27.4 months for the long-term follow-up. At long-term follow-up, as a group, patients regained some weight (BMI = 30.8 ±5.5 kg/m^2) and their SDB got worse (AHI = 26.4 ±26.2/hr). No correlation was observed between changes in BMI and the AHI, which was probably attributable to wide individual variability in the relationship between the amounts of weight loss or gain and the degrees of change in SDB severity. Seven of the 13 patients who maintained the weight loss remained cured (AHI = 3.1 ±3.1/hr at third evaluation). Eight of the 11 patients who had regained weight experienced recurrence of OSAS (AHI = 44.3 ±23.3/hr at third evaluation). The findings highlighted the variability in individuals' response to weight loss. This study also showed that although almost half of the patients who lost weight remained cured at long-term follow-up, relapse of OSAS in the long term is frequent among those previously cured by dietary weight loss. Regaining weight is associated with reemergence of clinical significant OSAS.

Rajala et al. (36) characterized the effect of weight loss in 27 morbidly obese patients (13 men; age 36.9 ±8.2 years; BMI 50.2 ±6.2 kg/m^2). Fourteen patients had gastroplasty, eight patients received intensive dietary regimen, and the remaining five were treated conservatively. Data were available on eight (seven were men) nonsurgically treated patients. At one-year follow–up, these eight subjects achieved a 13% decrease in BMI (50.7 ±8.4 at baseline and 44.1 ±6.4 kg/m^2 at follow-up). Their oxygen desaturation index dropped from 45.8 ±27.9 to 31.6 ±26.2/hr. Findings suggest that moderate weight loss in morbidly obese patients can lead to substantial improvement in SDB. Some weight loss, however, is not sufficient to produce significant clinical improvement to be used as the primary treatment in morbidly obese patients with severe OSAS.

Studying a group of obese OSAS patients (> 130% above ideal body weight), Kiselak et al. (37) found that dietary weight loss led to significant reduction in the RDI, blood pressure, soft palate width, and snoring frequency, and improved lung vital capacity and functional residual capacity. Nineteen patients (nine were men; age 43 ±11 years; 183 ±23% above ideal body weight) enrolled in a weight management program consisting of one week of caloric monitoring, 12 weeks of a protein-sparing modified fast, 6 weeks of gradual reintroduction to foods, 7 weeks of a balanced calorie-restricted diet, cognitive-behavioral therapy group sessions, a weekly exercise program, and nutritional education. Reevaluation by in-home ambulatory monitoring was performed 18 to 20 weeks after initiation of the weight loss program, during the balanced diet phase. Data were available on 14 out of 19 participants. Average weight loss was 27.2 ±2.5 kg, which was associated with significant decrease in the RDI (mean decrease = 16.6 ±7.3/hr), blood pressure (mean decrease = 10.1 ±3.2 mm), increased vital capacity (by 218 ±9 ml) and functional residual capacity (by 317 ±12 ml), and decreased soft palate width (by 1.39 ±0.48 mm). Percent of weight loss and percent of decrease in the RDI following weight loss could not be computed because pre- and posttreatment data were not reported.

Braver et al. (38) investigated the efficacy of combined weight loss, positional therapy, and nasal spray on SDB. Data on each individual subject were reported. Patients were 19 asymptomatic male heavy snorers (age 42 ±12.0 years) whose baseline weight, BMI, and AHI were 112 ±4 kg, 36 ±1.1 kg/m^2, and 18 ±7 per hour. The behavioral weight loss program lasted six months and consisted of 24 weekly group sessions in which self-monitoring, self-reinforcement, cognitive modification, and problem-solving skills were taught. On average, participants lost 3.6 kg (3%) of body weight. The combination of weight loss with concurrent nasal spray and sleep position therapy was associated with a 27% reduction in the AHI (from 18 ±7/hr to 13 ±6/hr). Of the 19 subjects, 12 lost weight and 7 gained weight. Excluding the 7 who gained weight, the average weight loss in the 12 subjects (age 46.9 ±12.1 years; baseline weight = 109.3 ±16.0 kg) was 8.0 ±2.0 kg, equivalent to a 7.2% drop of initial body weight. In this subset of weight loss successful patients, the AHI and snoring index dropped from 17.9 ±26.5 to 12 ±23.3/hr and 379 ±208 to 232 ±203/hr, respectively. Weight loss resulted in additional and significant reduction in snoring above and beyond that produced by nasal spray and position therapy combination (snoring index was 328 ±214 on nasal spray plus position therapy). Three subjects who lost an average of 7.6 kg showed virtual elimination of snoring. This study showed that even a small degree of weight loss was associated with improvement in snoring. The combination of weight loss with other behavioral intervention may result in clinically significant improvement in SDB.

Collectively, existing studies showed that weight loss has a beneficial effect on SDB. Weight loss might be efficacious, at least in the short term. Even a small degree of weight loss was associated with decreased snoring, frequency of apneas and hypopneas, oxygen desaturation, and collapsibility of the airway. Weight control should be an important part of an OSAS patient's treatment plan. Avoiding weight gain is an important preventive measure for developing clinically significant OSAS. Long-term benefits of this intervention remained to be established.

Efficacy of Sleep Positional Training as a Treatment for Obstructive Sleep Apnea Syndrome

Sleep Position and Obstructive Sleep Apnea Syndrome

The relationship between sleep position and SDB has been explored by many investigators (39–42), including a series of studies by Cartwright and associates

(43–48) and Oksenberg et al. (49–51). The frequency and severity of SDB is influenced by body position in 50% to 60% of patients. The AHI in OSAS patients was found to be twice as high during the time they spent sleeping in the supine position compared to the time they spent in the lateral position (43, 49). *Positional sleep apnea syndrome* was termed to describe the phenomena in which the AHI during supine sleep is two or more times the AHI during sleep in the lateral position (47). The upper airway is most vulnerable to collapse in the supine sleep position (42, 52) resulting in worse degree of oxygen desaturation and higher occurrence of SDB events. Interventions that decrease time spent in the supine sleep position, therefore, should have therapeutic benefit through diminishing the impact of obesity on the residual capacity of the lung and reducing the effort required for the mechanics of respiration. Positional therapy is probably an adequate conservative intervention for nonobese patients who demonstrate position-dependent SDB and who do not manifest significant associated pathologies (e.g., oxygen desaturation, cardiac arrhythmias, excessive daytime sleepiness; 2–3, 5, 7).

Methods and devices to avoid the supine sleep position include the tennis ball technique (53), backpack and softball (54), foam rubber wedges (55) or sandbag (38) placement, position monitoring device with alarm (45–46, 56), and sleeping in an elevated upright position (39). Table 6.2 provides a summary of the position therapy studies.

Cartwright and colleagues (45) used a gravity-activated position monitor alarm that emitted an auditory signal when the patient was in the supine position for more than 15 seconds. This device was used to train 10 male patients (age 48.5 ±10.1 years, 30.6 ±19.4% above ideal body weight; AHI 54.7 ±36.8/hr) to avoid the supine sleeping position. Wearing the position monitoring device significantly increased the proportion of the total sleep time (from 48.6 ±37.5 to 97.9 ±5.7%) that patients spent asleep in the lateral positions. This intervention was associated with decreases in the AHI (from 54.7 ±36.8 at baseline to 21.4 ±31.6/hr) and the number of oxygen desaturation events (from 238.8 ±177 at baseline to 86.7 ±152.3 events). After one night of positional training with the device in the laboratory, the patients were instructed to continue to practice sleeping in the lateral positions at home, on their own without the device. At follow-up reevaluation three months later, the patients were given only presleep verbal instructions to maintain a lateral sleep posture. Polysomnography results showed that as a group, the AHI (32.8 ±25.9/hr) remained significantly improved from baseline, and patients were able to avoid the supine position (24.1 ±31.8 versus 51.4 ±37.5% of total sleep time). For those patients who were unable to maintain the supine position for the majority of their total sleep time, their AHIs were higher (39 versus 27/hr) compared to the AHIs of patients who slept mainly in the lateral position. This study suggests that positional training is a promising noninvasive,

Table 6.2 Efficacy of Position Therapy for OSAS

	Study Design	N M/F	Intervention	Outcome Pre-/Posttreatment	Effect Size[a]	Comments Clinical Significance
Cartwright et al. (1985)[b]	Within subject, comparisons of baseline and training night, and three-month follow-up	10 10/0	One-night sleep positional training to avoid supine position. Reevaluated three months later without wearing the position alarm.	Baseline/position training/3-mo FU AHI: 54.7/21.4/32.8 O₂Desat events: 239/87/157 % sleep time in supine: 54.4/2.1/24.1	−0.90/−0.60 −0.86/−0.89 −1.31/−0.73	Four patients were able to maintain the side sleep posture during the whole night at follow-up. Lower response rate in obese patients.
Cartwright et al. (1991)[c]	Randomized trial Eight-week treatment Baseline compared with follow-up	60 60/0 15 per condition	Four treatment conditions: Tongue retaining device (TRD), posture alarm (PA), TRD + PA, good health habits (HH).	PA: HH groups Baseline/follow-up AHI: 33.3/20.8:26.7/7.7	−0.58:−1.43	Data reported here are on the PA and HH groups. AHI of eight patients in the PA group and nine patients in the HH group dropped below five.
Mcevoy et al. (1986)[d]	Within subject pre and posttreatment comparisons	13 13/0	Sleep in a 60-degree upright posture half of the night and the other half in supine.	RDI: 68.4/46.8 AI: 48.9/19.6 NREM MinO₂sat: 64.8/80.8		Unable to compute effect sizes. The AI in 9 of 13 patients was reduced by >50%.

| Jokic et al. (1999)[e] | Randomized, crossover design Comparisons between baseline and CPAP and position therapy | 13 | 12/1 | Two weeks of CPAP and two weeks of position therapy. Position therapy consisted of softball inside a backpack to prevent supine sleep position. | BL/CPAP/Position therapy AHI: 17.9/3.4/9.5 % sleep time in supine: 25.6/not reported/2. | −1.02/−0.59 | Positional therapy and CPAP have similar efficacy in improving daytime sleepiness, mood, and cognitive functioning. CPAP is more effective in reducing the AHI and oxygen desaturation. |

[a]Effect size (if possible to derive from published data) is computed by the difference between the means of the control and the treatment conditions divided by the standard deviation of the control condition. AHI = Apnea hyponea index (per hr); MinO$_2$sat = Minimum oxygen saturation (%).
[b] Avoidance of supine sleep position is associated with 61% reduction in the AHI during training night and 40% at follow-up.
[c] Avoidance of supine sleep position is associated with 38% to 71% reduction in the AHI.
[d] Sleeping in 50% upright position is associated with 32% reduction in the RDI and 60% reduction in the AI.
[e] Positional therapy was associated with 47% reduction in the AHI and 92% reduction in percent of sleep time spent in the supine position.

inexpensive treatment either as an interim, single therapy, or in combination with other therapies for the management of OSAS. Learning from one-night positional training was maintained at three months in some patients.

In a subsequent study by Cartwright et al. (46), the sleep-positional training device was compared with a tongue-retaining device (TRD) designed to prevent tongue retrolapse when the patient is in the supine position. This study is one of the few randomized trials that also reported the extent to which patients are able to implement beneficial behavioral changes on their own. Sixty male patients (mean age 48.7, mean 28.5% above ideal body weight) who had two or more times the rate of SDB events during supine sleep than that of during lateral sleep were randomly assigned to receive one of the four treatments (TRD, posture alarm, TRD plus posture alarm, or good health habit-only group) for eight weeks. Good health habit instructions include losing weight by diet, exercising at least 20 minutes a day, avoiding alcohol after 6 P.M., sleeping on the side, and avoiding the back sleep position. These recommendations were given to all study patients. Data reviewed here focus on the posture alarm and good health habit-only groups. The AHI of the posture group improved from 33.25 ±21.3/hr at baseline to 20.83 ±29.25/hr at eight-week follow-up, and even greater magnitude of improvement was observed in the good health habit group, from 26.69 ±13.31 to 7.72 ±9.91/hr. One possible explanation is that patients in the latter group lost weight (3.17 lbs) and the former group did not (gained 0.75 lb). The health habit-only group also showed ability to avoid the supine position comparable to the group that was provided the monitoring alarm. The findings certainly support therapeutic benefit of avoiding the supine position. More importantly, findings show that patients can take charge of their own care, if instructed in the habit changes important to their health. Eleven patients in the health habit group lost weight in eight weeks. All patients in this group improved, and 10 of the 15 did not sleep in the supine position at all when restudied, which shows they learned to avoid this posture on their own.

McEvoy and associates (39) investigated the therapeutic benefit of sleeping sitting up at a 60-degree angle as compared to lying supine in 13 OSAS male patients (age 48.9 ±13.9 years; weight 106.8 ±17.4 kg). To test the effect of sleep position, an overnight polysomnographic study was divided into two halves. In one half, the patient lay supine with his or her head supported by a pillow. In the other half, the patient sat in bed slightly reclined with head and trunk raise at a 60-degree angle. The order was counterbalanced. Compared to supine sleep, the 60-degree sleep position was associated with a reduction in the AHI (48.9 ±5.4/hr versus 19.6 ±6.9/hr). The apnea indexes in 9 of 13 patients were reduced by more than 50% by the postural intervention. Obese patients and patients who show greater degree of hypoxemia had greater response to this intervention than nonobese patients.

Sleeping in the upright position did not disrupt sleep architecture. This study shows that significant reduction of SDB can be facilitated by the adoption of a more upright sleep posture.

The extent to which lateral sleep position improves SDB was examined by Braver and Block (55). Twenty asymptomatic male snorers (age 42 ±11.7 years; BMI 35.7 ±5.1 kg/m^2) were studied. They underwent a baseline polysomnogram, followed by three more nights in which patients received nasal spray, lateral sleep position, or nasal spray plus lateral sleep position intervention. The order of treatment condition was randomized. The lateral sleep position was maintained with the use of foam rubber wedges both behind and in front of the subject. Discussion here focuses on sleep position intervention as compared to baseline. Approximately 19% reduction in the AHI was associated with sleep position intervention (14.1 ±28.3 versus 17.5 ±29.1/hr at baseline). Snoring, however, was not improved by the intervention because the snore index remained the same as baseline (355.9 ±206 versus 355.8 ±206).

Efficacy of positional treatment was compared with CPAP therapy by Jovic and colleagues (54) in a randomized, single blind, crossover trial. Thirteen patients (12 were men; age 51 ±9 years; BMI 30 ±4 kg/m^2; baseline AHI 16.9 ±8.0) received two weeks of CPAP and two weeks of positional therapy with no washout period. Avoidance of the supine sleep position was achieved through positioning a backpack (10 × 5.5 inches) with a softball inside. One of the unique features of this study was that it included evaluation of daytime sleepiness and neuropsychological testing. Positional intervention resulted in significant reduction in sleep time spent in the supine position (2 ±3% versus 26 ±16% at baseline). Compared with CPAP treatment, positional therapy was associated with similar improvement in sleep architecture and arousal frequency (arousal index = 15 ±1.8 SEM for CPAP and 19.4 ±1.9 SEM/hr for position therapy). CPAP had a slight but significant advantage over positional therapy in reducing the AHI (15 ±1.8 SEM versus 19.4 ±1.9 SEM per hour). Compared to baseline AHI (16.9 ±8.0), while both treatments resulted in reduction in the AHI, CPAP produced greater reduction than position therapy. Improvement of comparable magnitude was observed in terms of daytime sleepiness, measures of mood, and cognitive test performance. This study demonstrated that positional intervention does provide some benefits, some of which may be comparable to that provided by CPAP therapy. Positional therapy may be an effective alternative treatment to CPAP, at least for the short term for persons with positional-dependent OSAS.

Although there are only a handful of studies on the efficacy of positional therapy, findings consistently support the therapeutic benefits of this intervention for persons with positional sleep apnea syndrome. This treatment modality is relatively inexpensive and easy to implement.

Cervical Positional Therapy

Kushida and associates (57) tested the efficacy of a custom-designed cervical pillow. The potential benefit of this treatment was based on prior observations that head position modifies upper airway resistance, with less resistance noted when the person's head was extended (58–59). The cervical pillow was made of urethane foam with an overlying "memory foam," and the pillow was designed to extend the head in posture similar to that used in cardiopulmonary resuscitation to create an open airway. Twelve sleep clinic patients (ages 24 to 67 years) with mild to severe OSAS were studied. Patients spent two consecutive nights in the laboratory for baseline; then, they used the cervical pillow at home for five days before returning for two more nights in the laboratory. All subjects reported subjective improvement in the depth and restfulness of their sleep with use of the cervical pillow. In terms of objective benefits, this intervention was effective only in patients with mild disease (RDI 5 to 20/hr) and not in patients with moderate (RDI 20 to 40/hr) or severe (RDI > 40) disease. The RDI of the mild OSAS patients dropped from 14.7 to 10.5 per hour and remained about the same in the moderate patients (30.1 versus 37/hr) and severe patients (56.9 versus 56.5/hr). More studies are needed to establish the efficacy of this intervention.

Myofunctional Therapy

Myofunctional therapy targets improving the tone of the upper airway muscles, thereby improving sleep-disordered breathing. While this intervention approach can be theoretically appreciated, it has not been tested. One group of investigators (60) had suggested the potential of using oromuscular function evaluation to identify OSAS patients who might benefit from therapeutic exercise training.

Sleep Hygiene

Although OSAS patients are usually given the advice to maintain good sleep hygiene, there are no published studies reporting on the efficacy of sleep hygiene as a single intervention for OSAS. Given that alcohol, sedatives, tranquilizers, narcotics, and other central nervous system suppressants induce hypotonality of the upper airway musculature during sleep, these substances, obviously, should be avoided to prevent exacerbation of SDB (4, 61–62). By the same logic, cessation of smoking tobacco or other substances should prevent further compromising of the airway because these substances can irritate the airway mucosa and cause congestion and increased nasal inspiratory resistance (4).

While there are no studies showing that the patient's SDB is significantly improved by eliminating evening alcohol ingestion, several studies demonstrated that alcohol ingestion near bedtime exacerbates SDB. Adverse effects included increase in number of apneas in OSAS patients (63), asymptomatic male snorers' developing apnea (64), and significant increase in the number and severity of hypoxic events in OSAS patients (65). Alcohol's effect on breathing during sleep appears more profound than those of the benzodiazepines (62). Abstinence from alcohol before bedtime is, therefore, an important part of therapy.

The advice to avoid sleep deprivation came from reports, for example (66), that found sleep deprivation increases the severity of obstructive sleep apnea. There is no study that shows that consistently obtaining adequate sleep improves SDB.

RESTLESS LEGS SYNDROME AND PERIODIC LIMB MOVEMENT DISORDER

Current evidence reveals that pharmacotherapy, in particular dopaminergic agents, are the most efficacious treatments for the restless legs syndrome (RLS) and periodic limb movement disorder (PLMD; 67). To date, there are no empirically validated nonpharmacological treatments for these sleep disorders. There are, however, a few reports indicating some benefits with behavioral interventions. Existing reports are hampered by small sample sizes and the lack of employing adequate controls. Table 6.3 summarizes studies on behavioral interventions for RLS and PLMD.

A case report by Ancoli-Israel and colleagues (68) suggested some benefits of thermal feedback for PLMS. The authors theorized that inadequate peripheral blood circulation, as manifested in the complaint of cold feet, contributes to the etiology of PLMD. The hypothesis was tested on one patient by assessing the extent to which thermal biofeedback training, combined with autogenic training for relaxation, increased foot temperature and reduced periodic leg movements. The subject demonstrated an average increase of 8° F following 25 training sessions. The number of periodic limb movements was dramatically reduced from 61.7 per hour of sleep to 3.6 per hour of sleep. Although the treatment effect is impressive, the durability of treatment benefit is unknown. The intervention did not result in an increased total sleep time or a substantial decrease in the arousal index.

A randomized controlled trial (69) comparing a group receiving thermal biofeedback training versus wait-list controls found that thermal biofeedback training was superior in reducing the periodic limb movement (PLM) index. PLM index reduced from 66 to 59 per hour (11% reduction) in the biofeedback group and no change (35 to 36) in the wait-list group (69).

Table 6.3 Efficacy of behavioral interventions for RLS and PLMD

	Study Design	N	Intervention	Outcome	Effect Size*	Comments
Edinger, Fins, Sullivan, Marsh, Dailey, & Young (1996)	Randomized control trial	16	Four-week Clonazepam (0.5–1.0 mg) versus CBT.	Pre- vs. posttreatment: Movement index CZP: 77.4 (21.6):21.0 (22.2) CBT: 30.7 (15.2):31.8 (10.7) Arousal Index: CZP: 37.7 (16.8):21.0 (22.4) CBT: 19.2 (11.4):15.4 (11.7)	0.63 −0.07 0.99 −0.33	Both treatment improved sleep. CZP produced greater reduction in the movement index and arousal index.
Montagna, Sassoli de Bianchi, Zucconi, Cirgnotta, & Lugaresi (1984)	Within subject pre- and posttreatment comparisons	6	Clonazepam (1mg) versus vibration therapy.	Compared to baseline CZP: 28.5% improved VT: 10.7% improved		Subjective ratings.
Ancoli-Israel, Seifert, & Lemon (1986)	Within subject pre- and posttreatment comparisons	1	25 sessions of thermal biofeedback training to increase foot temperature.	Mean PLM index Pre tx = 61.7 (2.7) Post tx = 3.6 (3.6) Mean Arousal index Pre tx = 59.5 (13.5) Post tx = 41.5 (2.5)	21.5 1.3	Treatment led to dramatic reduction in the number of PLM.

*Effect size (if possible to derive from data reported in the given article) is computed by the difference between the means of the control group and the treatment group divided by the standard deviation of the control group. CBT = Cognitive-behavioral therapy; CZP = Clonazepam; PLM = Periodic limb movements.

The effect of a 30-minute stimulation of the dorsiflexors of the feet and toes before bedtime was investigated in eight nonmedicated patients with PLMD (70). All subjects were treated with a neuromuscular stimulator delivering a pulse train (on for 1.5 seconds and off for 1.8 seconds). A single nocturnal polysomnogram after treatment showed that all patients responded to stimulation, with reduction of leg movements from an average pretreatment PLM index of 44.6 per hour to a posttreatment PLM index of 14 per hour. Improvement was seen during NREM sleep. Indexes of sleep continuity did not change, although there was a trend toward improved consolidation of sleep with stimulation.

Comparing the short-term effect of a cognitive-behavioral therapy (CBT) and conventional pharmacotherapy (clonazepam) among a group of 16 insomniacs with PLMD, Edinger and colleagues (71) reported that clonazepam was more effective in reducing the periodic limb movement arousal index and arousal index than CBT at the end of a four-week trial. While both groups showed some improvement in global measures of sleep, the movement arousal index dropped from 77.4 ±21.6 to 30.7 ±15.2 in those who received clonazepam as compared to minimal reduction, from 19.2 ±11.4 to 15.4 ±11.7, in the CBT group. Findings suggested that CBT is not an effective treatment for PLMD.

Clonazepam was also found to be more effective in a case series of six patients (72). The study compared the efficacy of clonazepam with vibratory stimulation of the leg in reducing leg dysthesia and improving subjective sleep quality in patients with RLS. Patients were treated with vibratory simulation for a week, which involved applying a small, battery-operated mechanical vibrator to the lower limbs for at least 15 minutes at bedtime. Patients' ratings of leg dysthesia remained essentially unchanged from the baseline when they were on vibration therapy. Findings suggested lack of benefit for vibration therapy.

Regular moderate exercise has been suggested to alleviate RLS symptoms, whereas inactivity, excessive exercise, and sleep deprivation may aggravate them (73). Adequate sleep hygiene including adopting regular and sufficient sleep hours; avoiding daytime naps, tapering physical activity before bedtime, and avoiding caffeine, alcohol, or heavy meals in the hours before bedtime are recommended. No studies, however, have formally tested the efficacy of such practice. Some individuals, especially those whose symptoms emerge with the early night drop in body temperature, often benefit from a hot bath before bedtime (73–74).

NARCOLEPSY

The behavioral management of narcolepsy aims to decrease sleepiness by eliminating factors and situations in which sleep deprivation occurs, increase wakefulness, and forestall unplanned sleep attacks. Specific behavioral interventions include scheduled naps, regular sleep-wake schedules, the avoidance of frequent time zone changes and shift work, and sleep hygiene practices (75–76). The behavioral approaches, as a single treatment, are not adequate. For this reason, they have been incorporated into general management strategies and as an adjunct to pharmacotherapy for the treatment of narcolepsy (77). Table 6.4 summarizes studies of behavioral interventions for narcolepsy.

Scheduled Daytime Naps

There are only a few published studies reporting the efficacy of behavioral interventions. These studies have found that naps decrease sleepiness in patients with narcolepsy (78–80). Short naps as little as 15 minutes have been shown to effectively reduce sleepiness and thereby improve ability to stay awake (78, 81). Existing studies, with a few exceptions, are case series with small sample sizes. More research is needed to investigate the frequency and duration of naps that result in maximal reduction of excessive daytime sleepiness.

Mullington and Broughton (79) reported the efficacy of three schedules in eight drug-free narcoleptic subjects (ages 19 to 55): no nap, a single long nap (duration = 25% of customary total sleep time; mean = 129 min) in the afternoon placed 180° out of phase with the nocturnal midsleep time, and multiple short naps (duration = 25% of customary total sleep time positioned equidistantly throughout the day, with the third nap set at 180° out of phase; mean duration = 26 min). The investigators found that the single long nap condition produced the greatest improvement (11%) in reaction time performance compared to the no nap condition, despite the fact that sleep per 24 hours was held constant. In addition, the number of unscheduled sleep episodes was substantially fewer in the long nap condition compared to no nap condition (4.3 ±2.6 versus 7.1 ±4.0).

Roehrs and colleagues (78) investigated the duration of naps that produced the maximal alerting effects in 45 patients with narcolepsy (19 women, 26 men; mean age 46). Patients were randomly assigned to three conditions: a 15-minute nap period followed by a sleep latency test 15 minutes later (15–15), a 30-minute nap period followed by a sleep latency test 15 minutes later (30–15), a 15-minute nap period followed by a sleep latency test 30 minutes later (15–30). They found that 15-minute and 30-minute naps were equally effective, as evidenced by increased sleep latencies on the Multiple Sleep Latency Test (MSLT), in improving wakefulness in narcoleptic patients. Sleep latencies increased from 3.0 ±1.6 minutes to 8.6 ±6.2 minutes in the 15–15 condition. Patients who had a 30-minute nap and tested 15 minutes after the nap (30–15 condition) showed

Table 6.4 Efficacy of Behavioral Interventions for Narcolepsy

	Study Design	N	Intervention	Outcome	Effect Size*	Comments
Roger & Aldrich (1993)	Case series, comparison across three treatment conditions	16	One-month, three scheduled 15-minute naps.	MWT: pre/post 7.4 ±6.0/10.0 ±5.8 EDS Subjective ratings: pre/post	0.43	
Mullington & Broughton (1993)	Case series, comparisons across three treatment conditions	8	Two days each. No nap, one long nap, and five short naps, order counterbalanced.	Unscheduled sleep episodes: no nap/long nap/short naps 7.1 ±4.0/4.3 ±2.6/6.5 ±6.0	LN: 0.7 SN: 0.15	

*Effect size (if possible to derive from data reported in the given article) is computed by the difference between the means of the control group and the treatment group divided by the standard deviation of the control group. MWT = Maintenance of wakefulness test.

improved sleep latencies from 3.1 ±1.4 to 7.6 ±6.4 minutes. The alerting benefit of the nap, however, was short-lived. These findings led authors to conclude that longer nap duration provided no additional increase in alertness; therefore, patients with narcolepsy should take naps of no more than 15 minutes. They also concluded that napping cannot be considered as a primary treatment.

Rogers and Aldrich (82) investigated the effectiveness of three regularly scheduled 15-minute naps daily in 16 (9 female, 7 male, ages 21 to 65) narcoleptic patients. An individualized nap schedule was given to each patient, who was instructed to nap for 15 minutes, three times a day following the schedule and using an alarm clock to time the naps. After one month on this therapy, mean sleep latency on the Maintenance of Wakefulness Test (MWT) significantly increased from 7.4 ±6.0 minutes to 10.0 ±5.8 minutes. Nap therapy was more helpful for persons who manifested high frequency of sleep attacks than those whose alertness was within normal limits.

Volks and associates (83) studied 14 patients with narcolepsy who were randomly assigned to stay in bed during the day or sit at a table. Patients were free to nap ad lib. Sleep during the day in the continuous bed rest condition was two to three times more (34% of the time) than that of the seated condition (13.5%). Daytime propensity to sleep was related to the body position and somatic activity. For clinical application, advising patients with narcolepsy to avoid recumbent postural position and inactivity may help them be more resistant to falling asleep inadvertently.

In a case report, Kolko (84) noted that sensory stimulation via snapping a rubber band against the wrist was an effective countermeasure to reduce sleep attacks in a 61-year-old woman with narcolepsy. Treatment gain was maintained at 6- and 12-month follow-up.

SUMMARY AND CONCLUSION

Behavioral interventions, especially weight loss and positional therapy, may serve well in the conservative management for patients with mild to moderate OSAS. Existing data indicate that behavioral strategies can probably provide some symptomatic acute relief of discomfort associated with PLMD but not sufficient to produce clinically significant improvement. Behavioral management in the way of scheduled naps can substantially reduce daytime sleepiness and thus should be an integral part of the patient's treatment. More studies are needed to establish long-term benefits of behavioral treatments and the extent to which behavioral strategies as adjunctive treatment to optimize medical therapy for intrinsic sleep disorders.

REFERENCES

1. Series, F. Evaluation of treatment efficacy in sleep apnea hypopnea syndrome. *Sleep* 19: S71–S76, 1996.

2. Fairbanks, D. N. Nonsurgical treatment of snoring and obstructive sleep apnea. *Otolaryngology: Head and Neck Surgery* 100(6): 633–635, 1989.

3. Aubert, G. Alternative therapeutic approaches in sleep apnea syndrome. *Sleep* 15(6 Suppl.): S69–S72, 1992.

4. Westbrook, P. and R. Millman. Controversies in the treatment of snoring and obstructive sleep apnea. In N. Saunders and C. Sullivan, eds. *Sleep and Breathing*. New York, NY: Marcel Dekker, Inc. 1994: 529–555.

5. Levy, P., J. L. Pepin, P. Mayer, B. Wuyam, and D. Veale. Management of simple snoring, upper airway resistance syndrome, and moderate sleep apnea syndrome. *Sleep* 19(9 Suppl.): S101–S110, 1996.

6. Kryger, M. Management of obstructive sleep apnea-hypopnea syndrome. In M. H. Kryger, T. Roth, and W. C. Dement, eds. *Principles and Practice of Sleep Medicine*. Philadelphia, PA: W.B. Saunders Company. 2000: 940–954.

7. Magalang, U. and M. Mador. Behavioral and pharmacologic therapy of obstructive sleep apnea. In T. Lee-Chiong, M. Sateia, and M. Carskadon, eds. *Sleep Medicine*. Philadelphia, PA: Hanley and Belfus, Inc. 2002: 389–396.

8. Harman, E. M., J. W. Wynne, et al. The effect of weight loss on sleep-disordered breathing and oxygen desaturation in morbidly obese men. *Chest* 82(3): 291–294, 1982.

9. Suratt, P. M., R. F. McTier, et al. Changes in breathing and the pharynx after weight loss in obstructive sleep apnea. *Chest* 92(4): 631–637, 1987.

10. Rubinstein, I., N. Colapinto, et al. Improvement in upper airway function after weight loss in patients with obstructive sleep apnea. *American Review of Respiratory Diseases* 138(5): 1192–1195, 1988.

11. Peiser, J., P. Lavie, et al. Sleep apnea syndrome in the morbidly obese as an indication for weight reduction surgery. *Annals of Surgery* 199(1): 112–115, 1984.

12. Browman, C. P., M. G. Sampson, et al. Obstructive sleep apnea and body weight. *Chest* 85(3): 435–438, 1984.

13. Horner, R. L., R. H. Mohiaddin, et al. Sites and sizes of fat deposits around the pharynx in obese patients with obstructive sleep apnoea and weight matched controls. *European Respiratory Journal* 2(7): 613–622, 1989.

14. Schwartz, A. R., A. R. Gold, et al. Effect of weight loss on upper airway collapsibility in obstructive sleep apnea. *American Review of Respiratory Diseases* 144(3 Pt 1): 494–498, 1991.

15. Loube, D. I., A. A. Loube, et al. Weight loss for obstructive sleep apnea: The optimal therapy for obese patients. *Journal of American Dietetic Association* 94(11): 1291–1295, 1994.

16. Mortimore, I. L., I. Marshall, et al. Neck and total body fat deposition in nonobese and obese patients with sleep apnea compared with that in control subjects. *American Journal of Respiratory and Critical Care Medicine* 157(1): 280–283, 1998.

17. Strobel, R. J. and R. C. Rosen. Obesity and weight loss in obstructive sleep apnea: A critical review. *Sleep* 19(2): 104–115, 1996.

18. Shelton, K., H. Woodson, et al. Pharyngeal fat in obstructive sleep apnea. *American Review of Respiratory Diseases* 148: 462–466, 1993.

19. Suratt, P. M., R. F. McTier, et al. Collapsibility of the nasopharyngeal airway in obstructive sleep apnea. *American Review of Respiratory Diseases* 132(5): 967–971, 1985.

20. Kajaste, S., T. Telakivi, et al. Effects of a weight reduction program on sleep apnea: A two-year follow-up. *Sleep Research* 1991(20A): 332, 1991.

21. Anderson, J. W., E. C. Konz, et al. Long-term weight-loss maintenance: A meta-analysis of U.S. studies. *American Journal of Clinical Nutrition* 74(5): 579–584, 2001.

22. Bjorvell, J. and S. Rossner. A ten-year follow-up of weight change in severely obese subjects treated in a combined behavioral modification program. *International Journal of Obesity and Related Metabolic Disorders: Journal of the International Association for the Study of Obesity* 16: 623–625, 1992.

23. Latner, J. D., A. J. Stunkard, et al. Effective long-term treatment of obesity: A continuing care model. *International Journal of Obesity and Related Metabolic Disorders* 24(7): 893–898, 2000.

24. Saskin, P. Obstructive sleep apnea: Treatment options, efficacy, and effects. In M. Pressman and W. Orr, eds. *Understanding Sleep: The Evaluation and Treatment of Sleep Disorders*. Washington, DC: American Psychological Association. 1997: 283–297.

25. Sampol, G., X. Munoz, et al. Long-term efficacy of dietary weight loss in sleep apnoea/hypopnoea syndrome. *European Respiratory Journal* 12(5): 1156–1159, 1998.

26. Pavlou, K. N., S. Krey, et al. Exercise as an adjunct to weight loss and maintenance in moderately obese subjects. *American Journal of Clinical Nutrition* 49: 1115–1123, 1989.

27. Wittels, E. H. and S. Thompson. Obstructive sleep apnea and obesity. *Otolaryngologic Clinics of North America* 23(4): 751–760, 1990.

28. Peppard, P. E., T. Young, et al. Longitudinal study of moderate weight change and sleep-disordered breathing. *Journal of the American Medical Association* 284(23): 3015–3021, 2000.

29. Pasquali, R., P. Colella, et al. Treatment of obese patients with obstructive sleep apnea syndrome (OSAS): effect of weight loss and interference of otorhinolaryngoiatric pathology. *International Journal of Obesity and Related Metabolic Disorders* 14(3): 207–217, 1990.

30. Lojander, J., P. Mustajoki, et al. A nurse-managed weight reduction program for obstructive sleep apnoea syndrome. *Journal of Internal Medicine* 244(3): 251–255, 1998.

31. Norman, J. F., S. G. Von Essen, et al. Exercise training effect on obstructive sleep apnea syndrome. *Sleep Research Online* 3(3): 121–129, 2000.

32. Noseda, A., C. Kempenaers, et al. Sleep apnea after 1 year domiciliary nasal-continuous positive airway pressure and attempted weight reduction. Potential for weaning from continuous positive airway pressure. *Chest* 109(1): 138–143, 1996.

33. Smith, P. L., A. R. Gold, et al. Weight loss in mildly to moderately obese patients with obstructive sleep apnea. *Annals of Internal Medicine* 103(6 Pt 1): 850–855, 1985.

34. Redline, S., N. Adams, et al. Improvement of mild sleep-disordered breathing with CPAP compared with conservative therapy [see comments]. *American Journal of Respiratory and Critical Care Medicine* 157(3 Pt 1): 858–865, 1998.

35. Monasterio, C., S. Vidal, et al. Effectiveness of continuous positive airway pressure in mild sleep apnea-hypopnea syndrome. *American Journal of Respiratory and Critical Care Medicine* 164(6): 939–943, 2001.

36. Rajala, R., M. Partinen, et al. Obstructive sleep apnoea syndrome in morbidly obese patients. *Journal of Internal Medicine* 230(2): 125–129, 1991.

37. Kiselak, J., M. Clark, et al. The association between hypertension and sleep apnea in obese patients. *Chest* 104(3): 775–780, 1993.

38. Braver, H. M., A. J. Block, et al. Treatment for snoring. Combined weight loss, sleeping on side, and nasal spray. *Chest* 107(5): 1283–1288, 1995.

39. McEvoy, R. D., D. J. Sharp, et al. The effects of posture on obstructive sleep apnea. *American Review of Respiratory Diseases* 133(4): 662–666, 1986.

40. Phillips, B. A., J. Okeson, et al. Effect of sleep position on sleep apnea and parafunctional activity. *Chest* 90(3): 424–429, 1986.

41. Katz, A. and D. S. Dinner. The effect of sleep position on the diagnosis of obstructive sleep apnea: A word of caution. *Cleveland Clinic Journal of Medicine* 59(6): 634–636, 1992.

42. Penzel, T., M. Moller, et al. Effect of sleep position and sleep stage on the collapsibility of the upper airways in patients with sleep apnea. *Sleep* 24(1): 90–95, 2001.

43. Cartwright, R. D. Effect of sleep position on sleep apnea severity. *Sleep* 7(2): 110–114, 1984.

44. Cartwright, R. D. Predicting response to the tongue retaining device for sleep apnea syndrome. *Archives of Otolaryngology* 111(6): 385–388, 1985.

45. Cartwright, R. D., S. Lloyd, et al. Sleep position training as treatment for sleep apnea syndrome: A preliminary study. *Sleep* 8(2): 87–94, 1985.

46. Cartwright, R., R. Ristanovic, et al. A comparative study of treatments for positional sleep apnea. *Sleep* 14: 546–552, 1991.

47. Cartwright, R. D., F. Diaz, et al. The effects of sleep posture and sleep stage on apnea frequency. *Sleep* 14(4): 351–353, 1991.

48. Cartwright, R. Effect of sleep position on sleep apnea severity. *Sleep* 17: 110–114, 1994.

49. Oksenberg, A., D. S. Silverberg, et al. Positional vs. nonpositional obstructive sleep apnea patients: Anthropomorphic, nocturnal polysomnographic, and multiple sleep latency test data. *Chest* 112(3): 629–639, 1997.

50. Oksenberg, A., I. Khamaysi, et al. Association of body position with severity of apneic events in patients with severe nonpositional obstructive sleep apnea. *Chest* 118(4): 1018–1024, 2000.

51. Oksenberg, A., I. Khamaysi, et al. Apnoea characteristics across the night in severe obstructive sleep apnoea: Influence of body posture. *European Respiratory Journal* 18(2): 340–346, 2001.

52. Lloyd, S. R. and R. D. Cartwright. Physiologic basis of therapy for sleep apnea. *American Review of Respiratory Diseases* 136(2): 525–526, 1987.

53. Berger, M., A. Oksenberg, et al. Avoiding the supine position during sleep lowers 24 h blood pressure in obstructive sleep apnea (OSA) patients. *Journal of Human Hypertension* 11(10): 657–664, 1997.

54. Jokic, R., A. Klimaszewski, et al. Positional treatment vs. continuous positive airway pressure in patients with positional obstructive sleep apnea syndrome. *Chest* 115(3): 771–781, 1999.

55. Braver, H. M. and A. J. Block. Effect of nasal spray, positional therapy, and the combination thereof in the asymptomatic snorer. *Sleep* 17(6): 516–521, 1994.

56. Badia, P., J. Harsh, et al. Behavioral control of abnormal breathing in sleep. *Journal of Behavioral Medicine* 11(6): 585–592, 1988.

57. Kushida, C. A., S. Rao, et al. Cervical positional effects on snoring and apneas. *Sleep Research Online* 2(1): 7–10, 1999.

58. Hellsing, E. Changes in the pharyngeal airway in relation to extension of the head. *European Journal of Orthodontics* 11(4): 359–365, 1989.

59. Jan, M. A., I. Marshall, et al. Effect of posture on upper airway dimensions in normal human. *American Journal of Respiratory and Critical Care Medicine* 149(1): 145–148, 1994.

60. Murthy, H., C. Kushida, et al. Oromuscular correlates of patients with the obstructive sleep apnea syndrome. *Sleep* 22(Suppl.): S193, 1999.

61. Remmers, J. E. Obstructive sleep apnea. A common disorder exacerbated by alcohol. *American Review of Respiratory Diseases* 130(2): 153–155, 1984.

62. Roth, T., T. Roehrs, et al. Pharmacological effects of sedative-hypnotics, narcotic analgesics, and alcohol during sleep. *Medical Clinics of North America* 69(6): 1281–1288, 1985.

63. Issa, F. G. and C. E. Sullivan. Alcohol, snoring and sleep apnea. *Journal of Neurology, Neurosurgery, and Psychiatry* 45(4): 353–359, 1982.

64. Mitler, M. M., A. Dawson, et al. Bedtime ethanol increases resistance of upper airways and produces sleep apneas in asymptomatic snorers. *Alcoholism: Clinical and Experimental Research* 12(6): 801–805, 1988.

65. Scrima, L., M. Broudy, et al. Increased severity of obstructive sleep apnea after bedtime alcohol ingestion: Diagnostic potential and proposed mechanism of action. *Sleep* 5(4): 318–328, 1982.

66. Leiter, J. C., S. L. Knuth, et al. The effect of sleep deprivation on activity of the genioglossus muscle. *American Review of Respiratory Diseases* 132(6): 1242–1245, 1985.

67. Chesson, A. L., Jr., M. Wise, et al. Practice parameters for the treatment of restless legs syndrome and periodic limb movement disorder. An American Academy of Sleep Medicine Report. Standards of Practice Committee of the American Academy of Sleep Medicine. *Sleep* 22(7): 961–968, 1999.

68. Ancoli-Israel, S., A. Seifert, et al. Thermal biofeedback and periodic movements in sleep: Patients' subjective reports and a case study. *Biofeedback Self Regulation* 11: 177–188, 1986.

69. Knowles, J., S. Ancoli-Israel, et al. The evaluation of thermal biofeedback in the treatment of periodic limb movement disorder. *Sleep Research* 25: 265, 1996.

70. Kovacevic-Ristanovic, R., R. Cartwright, et al. Nonpharmacologic treatment of periodic leg movements in sleep. *Physical Medical Rehabilitation* 72: 385–389, 1991.

71. Edinger, J., A. Fins, et al. Comparison of cognitive-behavioral therapy and clonazepam for treating periodic limb movement disorder. *Sleep* 19: 442–444, 1996.

72. Montagna, P., L. Sassoli de Bianchi, et al. Clonazepam and vibration in restless legs syndrome. *Acta Neurologica Scandinavica* 69: 428–430, 1984.

73. Hening, W., R. Allen, et al. The treatment of restless legs syndrome and periodic limb movement disorder: An American Academy of Sleep Medicine review. *Sleep* 22: 970–999, 1999.

74. Mosko, S. S. and K. L. Nudleman. Somatosensory and brainstem auditory evoked responses in sleep-related periodic leg movements. *Sleep* 9(3): 399–404, 1986.

75. Garma, L. and F. Marchand. Nonpharmacological approaches to the treatment of narcolepsy. *Sleep* 17(8 Suppl.): S97–S102, 1994.

76. Silber, M. Sleep Disorders. *Neurologic Clinics* 19(1): 173–185, 2001.

77. Cohen, F. Narcolepsy: A review of a common, lifelong sleep disorder. *Journal of Advanced Nursing* 13: 546–556, 1988.

78. Roehrs, T., F. Zorick, et al. Alerting effects of naps in narcolepsy. *Sleep* 9: 194 199, 1986.

79. Mullington, J. and R. Broughton. Scheduled naps in the management of daytime sleepiness in narcolepsy-cataplexy. *Sleep* 16: 444–456, 1993.

80. Helmus, T., L. Rosenthal, et al. The alerting effects of short and long naps in narcoleptic, sleep deprived, and alert individuals. *Sleep* 20: 251–257, 1997.

81. Guilleminault, C., R. Stoohs, et al. Daytime somnolence: Therapeutic approaches. *Neurophysiol Clinique* 23: 23–33, 1993.

82. Rogers, A. and M. Aldrich. The effect of regularly scheduled naps on sleep attacks and excessive daytime sleepiness associated with narcolepsy. *Nursing Research* 42: 111–117, 1993.

83. Volk, S., H. Schulz, et al. The influence of two behavioral regimens on the distribution of sleep and wakefulness in narcoleptic patients. *Sleep* 13: 136–142, 1990.

84. Kolko, D. J. Behavioral treatment of excessive daytime sleepiness in an elderly woman with multiple medical problems. *Journal of Behavior Therapy and Experimental Psychiatry* 15(4): 341–345, 1984.

SECTION IV

Behavioral Sleep Medicine

Chapter 7 ──────────────────────────────

BEHAVIORAL-COGNITIVE SCIENCE: THE FOUNDATION OF BEHAVIORAL SLEEP MEDICINE

KENNETH L. LICHSTEIN AND SIDNEY D. NAU

BEHAVIORAL SLEEP MEDICINE AS A SCIENTIFIC DISCIPLINE

The antecedent near-namesake discipline, behavioral medicine, provides guidance for the sculpting of the new discipline, behavioral sleep medicine (BSM). When behavioral medicine was formalized and the parameters of the field defined at the Yale conference in 1977 (1), one of the main purposes was to distinguish the field by the adoption of exacting scientific standards. Franz Alexander (2) and others had already established the field of psychosomatic medicine, which studied the interplay between psychological and medical forces in health and illness. However, this earlier group too often seemed content to rely on theory and philosophy to draw conclusions, rather than scientific method, and this casual respect for science (mixed with occasional contempt) helped instigate the defection known as behavioral medicine.

The role of psychological phenomena in sleep also boasts a long history, but at least part of this tradition derives from clinical experience and faith-based theory more than science. Freud's *Interpretation of Dreams* (3) is now a century old, and its truths are still wanting scientific validation.

BSM seeks the respect born of scientific validity. Methods and assertions derived from nonscientific traditions serve only to mitigate respect for this emerging field and hamper the progress of basic knowledge and clinical efficacy.

This chapter provides an overview of theory in behavioral-cognitive science, the principles on which BSM interventions are most often based. The review emphasizes clinically relevant aspects of theory, followed by examples of clinical applications of these theories in the BSM domain.

All of these theories share one common characteristic: Experimental data support their validity.

BEHAVIORAL-COGNITIVE MODELS

Classical Conditioning

This section and the next on operant conditioning are based on standard learning theory texts. For a more detailed rendition of conditioning, see these texts (4–6).

Discovered while Pavlov was studying the physiology of digestion in dogs, classical conditioning concerns itself with unlearned and autonomically mediated thoughts and emotions elicited by environmental events. Such involuntary acts are referred to as *respondents* or *reflexes*. Conditioning is initiated by a stimulus that owns a natural relationship with the individual, termed an *unconditioned stimulus* (US). Events such as physical trauma or sexual stimulation are US because they evoke reflexive, unconditioned responses (UR) such as fear and arousal, respectively. When a second stimulus having no prior US properties with respect to the UR of interest occurs by plan or coincidence in temporal proximity to the US, usually preceding the US, it will acquire US-like properties, termed *conditioned stimulus* (CS), and evoke responses similar to the UR, termed *conditioned responses* (CR). The US or the CS may be circumscribed or comprise a cluster of events, and the UR and CR may be simple or multifaceted. Stimulus generalization commonly occurs whereby the CR is elicited by novel CS that bears some similarity to the original CS.

Depending on the intensity of the US and the readiness of the person to emit the UR, a single CS-US pairing may be sufficient to establish conditioning. Alternatively, dozens of pairings may be required. Once established, a CS will continue to produce a CR only as long as the individual perceives a connection between the CS and US. Thus, the power of the CS to control the individual derives from the expectation that the CS signals that the US is near at hand. Occasional pairings of the CS with the US may be sufficient to sustain the influence of the CS. Repeated presentations of the CS, unaccompanied by the US, will eventually result in extinction of the CR, and the CS will return to its formerly neutral status. An extinguished CS may spontaneously recover and produce a CR, but such occurrences are unpredictable and short lived. Diminished potency of the CS may be expedited by pairing it with a novel US that evokes a UR incompatible with the original UR.

By these processes, individuals may acquire maladaptive beliefs and emotions associated with events or situations perceived as benign by people who do not share a common idiosyncratic conditioning history. In the course of human events, the source of such undesired beliefs and emotions may be reduced to obscurity. Recollection of the original CS-US training experience may fade, and stimulus generalization may convert innocent stimuli into CS. Lack of knowledge of the origin of conditioning notwithstanding, corrective classical conditioning experiences can be expected to be efficacious.

Operant Conditioning

In contrast to classical conditioning, this model (also known as *instrumental conditioning*) focuses on voluntary behaviors usually associated with skeletal muscles (biofeedback is an exception). The behaviors are emitted by the individual and operate on the environment. These operants, according to founder B. F. Skinner, are controlled by a combination of antecedent and consequent stimuli.

A behavioral consequence is rewarding if the behavior preceding it subsequently increases in frequency. This consequence is termed *reinforcer*. Similarly, a *punisher* will lead to a decrease in frequency of the behavior it follows. There are two varieties of reinforcers: A positive reinforcer onsets following the emission of a behavior, and a negative reinforcer, usually an aversive stimulus, terminates when the behavior of interest onsets. There are also two varieties of punishers: (1) a negative contingency onsetting immediately following a behavior or (2) a positive stimulus terminating with the onset of a behavior.

Complex behavior may involve long chains of responses. At times, reinforcement is available for selected responses in the sequence. In some circumstances, the completion of a response serves as the reinforcer for the behavior that preceded it in the chain. In episodic reinforcement, a single reinforcer is received at the completion of a long sequence of behaviors.

Antecedent stimuli, or setting conditions, that are regularly associated with subsequent reinforcers summon operants. Their presence signals that if a specified behavior is produced, there is an elevated likelihood that reinforcers will follow. These are called *discriminative stimuli,* S^D. Stimuli that are either associated with punishing consequences or the absence of positive contingencies are termed S^Δ and predict that the behavior is less likely to occur in their presence.

Any of the four contingency patterns can occur in five types of scheduling patterns. We present a brief overview by showing how scheduling works with positive reinforcement of a given behavior, getting a youngster to go to sleep peacefully. A continuous schedule means that every instance of cooperative bedtime behavior is reinforced. The reinforcement can take an unlimited number of forms typified by social approval, food treats, or a point system that contracts for accumulated points traded for prized activities. If every instance of appropriate behavior is not reinforced, an intermittent schedule is used, and four of these are characterized by interval or ratio patterns. Interval schedules may be fixed, meaning that reinforcement occurs following the first appropriate response after a fixed time interval has elapsed, or variable, meaning reinforcement is delivered after intervals of varying duration. Ratio schedules may also be fixed or variable. A fixed ratio (FR) scale will deliver a reinforcement after a fixed number of appropriate responses has occurred. For example, an FR3 schedule would reinforce the youngster every third night of peaceful bedtime behavior. A variable ratio schedule would produce a reinforcer after a varying number of appropriate responses.

Different schedules vary in their effectiveness, depending on the frequency and malleability of the target behavior and the availability and potency of reinforcers. Generally, a continuous schedule is preferred initially to establish the goal behavior; then reinforcers are gradually delivered less often, thus converting to a variable ratio schedule. In general, variable schedules are more effective in sustaining behaviors than fixed or continuous schedules.

We consider two final operant conditioning concepts: shaping and extinction. If the goal behavior does not currently exist in the behavioral repertoire of the individual, it cannot be reinforced. Shaping identifies some part of the goal behavior to reinforce, and, subsequently, successive approximations of the goal behavior are reinforced, so that the goal behavior is finally produced by increments. In the case of the recalcitrant youngster, forlorn parents may have to reinforce going to his room and playing at the requested time as a first step toward going to sleep at the specified time. Extinction refers to withdrawal of reinforcement, which will eventually lead to the disappearance of conditioned behaviors, unless the behavior is self-gratifying or naturally occurring reinforcers have emerged. Extinction will lead to behavioral reduction most quickly following a continuous reinforcement schedule and most slowly following a variable schedule.

Social Cognitive Theory

Like classical and operant conditioning before it, social cognitive theory was invented primarily by one individual, Albert Bandura. His theory of human behavior grew out of his classic work on modeling affects on aggression in his Bo-Bo doll experiments (7), evolved into a broader theoretical system called *social learning theory* (8), and matured further by incorporating self-efficacy theory and other cognitive dimensions into what Bandura called *social cognitive theory* (9). This section is based on the 1986 text.

As with any theoretical system of human behavior, social cognitive theory rests on a series of assumptions that guide its inquiry and application. These can be summarized by the concept of *triadic reciprocity.* "Behavior, cognitive and other personal factors, and environmental events" (9) act on one another to shape personality and its behavioral expression. This view assumes a number of "capabilities" that enable people to benefit from triadic reciprocity:

- *Symbolizing capability:* People can judge their experiences and environment by symbolic representation of relationships and expectations of consequences to determine future action without having to rely on empirical testing of such action.

- *Forethought capability:* The ability to conceptualize a future time perspective enables people to evaluate courses of action based on anticipated outcomes.

- *Vicarious capability:* Knowledge of others' experience can have the equivalent impact on shaping the direction of behavior as direct experience.

- *Self-regulatory capability:* People exercise volition in selecting environments, establishing standards, and creating incentives, such that self-directedness emerges as one more determinant of behavior.

- *Self-reflective capability:* Having embarked on a behavioral/emotional/cognitive course of action, people scrutinize and revise their activities based on judgments they render on their own conduct.

Triadic reciprocity capabilities are embedded in the ability to experience and profit from a variety of specific behavioral-cognitive strategies. A summary of the most relevant of these to BSM follows.

Observational Learning

Modeling and vicarious learning are often-used synonyms for observational learning. Observing others often produces symbolic encoding of procedural elements that may subsequently produce enactment of the behavior in the observer. The model may engage in the desired behavior, may be a pictorial representation of behavior, or may consist only of verbal description.

Successful modeling requires four processes: attention (perceiving the model), retention (encoding procedures), production (translating encoded behavior into performance), and motivation (perceived advantages to enactment). The observer must attend to the modeled behavior; encode behavioral sequences into memory; rehearse either behaviorally, visually, or verbally to perfect the goal behavior; and then reproduce it at a future time. Modeling strategies that use physical or verbal cues to emphasize salient elements of the modeled behavior increase the likelihood of successful reproduction. Observational learning is not restricted to behavior. Values, concepts, and emotions may be transmitted by this mechanism as well.

Modeling may aid acquisition of novel behaviors or may inhibit or encourage behaviors existing within the repertoire of the observer. Drawing on a cognitive interpretation of operant theory, Bandura and others have shown that the positive and negative consequences befalling the model raise or lower the likelihood of subsequent enactment of the modeled behavior. However, individuals are capable of discriminating between observed consequences and anticipated consequences so that experiencing vicarious punishment administered to a model will compete in some settings with self-conceived incentives, resulting in reproduction of the previously punished behavior.

Incentive Motivators

Social cognitive theory embraces the operant notion that behavior is mediated by consequences, but casts this mechanism within a broad social cognitive context. Once individuals are mature enough to encode anticipated consequences, the necessary constraints of immediacy are diminished. Thus, unreinforced behavior may be maintained for extended periods of time when sustained by anticipation of desired distant outcomes.

The nature of reinforcement includes customary operant consequences such as positive social attention, valued objects (e.g., money), and opportunities (e.g., also known as the Premack Principle). Supplementing external sources of reinforcement, social/cognitive processes may establish social status, satisfaction of personal values, achieving personal goals, and vicarious reinforcement (i.e., consequences accruing to a model) as effective consequences. Parallel processes deter behavior when associated with actual or perceived punishment.

In the social cognitive model, personal standard setting assumes added importance. Individuals judge the success and associated reinforcement value of attainments against internally generated standards. Setting meaningful, but attainable, standards increases the likelihood of positive self-appraisals of performance that will promote satisfaction and continued achievement, compared to discouragement and behavioral suppression resulting when success standards are set beyond reach. Similarly, establishing proximal subgoals provides frequent opportunity for self-enhancement compared to limiting oneself to distal goals. This may be viewed as the social cognitive counterpart to operant shaping.

Self-Efficacy

This integrative concept is perhaps the crowning achievement of Bandura's social cognitive theory. *Self-efficacy* refers to self-knowledge or self-appraisal about an individual's ability to perform. Self-efficacy is largely dependent on possessing a collection of cognitive, behavioral, and social skills and organizing these into a coordinated action plan.

Self-efficacy varies with respect to three dimensions. The *level* of self-efficacy may permit simple, complex, or demanding tasks. The *generality* of self-efficacy may be narrow (i.e., task specific) or broad (i.e., easily generalizable to novel situations). The *strength* of self-efficacy may be weak and easily debilitated by attainment failures or may be strong and lead to perseverance in overcoming obstacles.

The strength of an individual's competencies and self-efficacy appraisal interact with the person's judgment about the outcome of his or her efforts to facilitate or discourage action. A person may possess strong cognitive, behavioral, and social competencies, but self-efficacy will suffer if these are self-appraised as low. Low self-efficacy, independent of strength of competencies, predicts the absence of action. High self-efficacy predicts action only when combined with a valued outcome expectation. Low self-efficacy combined with high outcome expectation is not likely to produce action because the individual anticipates failure in attempts to achieve the valued goal. When high self-efficacy and high expectancy outcome motivate action, self-efficacy will be reappraised based on the quality of performance. Overall, accurate appraisals of both self-efficacy and of outcome expectations lead to better decision making in withholding or proceeding with action.

Individuals given to underevaluating their self-efficacy are likely to limit themselves to a constricted range of opportunities. Individuals who persist in overevaluating their self-efficacy are likely to experience repeated discouragement or harm. Optimally, self-efficacy should be set at or slightly above an individual's competencies so that opportunities are maximized and competencies are challenged to grow.

Four factors contribute to the evolution of self-efficacy in an individual. *Performance* success or failure provides the most convincing feedback and will strengthen or shrink self-efficacy, respectively. *Vicarious experience* gained by observing the success or failure of others deemed similar to oneself will correspondingly influence that individual's own self-efficacy. *Encouragement* from others may instigate action under conditions of ambivalent self-efficacy. Last, information from *somatic feedback* may be interpreted as triumphant or fearful and alter self-efficacy appraisal accordingly.

Cognitive Science

Unlike unified, systematic theories of behavior such as operant and classical conditioning, cognitive science covers a more diverse terrain and more closely resembles a collection of independent observations than a unified theory. Though cognitive therapists routinely assume their methods derive from basic science, the path from science to practice is not without transformations and gaps. Cognitive science is most strongly related to the cognitive processes contributing to psychopathology but provides less guidance in devising interventions to alter and replace dysfunctional cognitions.

Most cognitive therapy articles describe the process of altering self-defeating thoughts but provide little information on the origins of the therapy in cognitive science. The link between cognitive therapy and cognitive science is at times taken for granted and at other times described in somewhat fuzzy terms (10). A series of chapters in Clark and Fairburn (11) is the most comprehensive accounting of the cognitive science basis of cognitive therapy that we have found. This review relies most heavily on the Clark and Fairburn chapters, supplemented by other contributions.

One additional cautionary note: No area of science can boast unanimous agreement. Because cognitive science lacks an overriding theoretical structure that guides the majority of theories, lack of unanimity is perhaps more apparent here than in other areas. For purposes of this chapter, we present consensus views, but conflicting conceptualizations, oftentimes reasonably well founded, do exist for some of the constructs.

At the heart of the matter is a series of assumptions that have, for the most part, been supported by laboratory demonstrations (11):

- There is reciprocity between emotion and cognition. Emotions both arise from cognitions and generate cognitions, which then fuel the emotion.
- Faulty cognitions produce negative, dysfunctional emotions.
- Faulty cognitions may be altered either by substituting constructive cognitions or by corrective behavioral experience.
- Correcting faulty cognitions will instigate desired emotional change.

Basic Cognitive Premises

That aspect of cognitive science relating to clinical change comprises a series of assumptions and principles, which then form the basis of cognitive interventions. In brief, systematic bias in "interpretation, attention, and memory" initiate and sustain emotional dysfunction (12). These sources of bias are now summarized.

Schema or schemata are stable cognitions that help organize perceptions, process information, and formulate attitudes within experiential domains (13–15). Schema result from early experience and are most problematic when they are few in number, inflexible, and negatively biased. Negativistic schema bias our view of the world and spawn dysfunctional cognitions that give rise to emotional distress. Schema may appear as elaborate cognitive systems or simply dysfunctional beliefs, and these comprise the cornerstone of Beck's cognitive theory of depression.

Mind-in-place refers to a collection of schemata forming a mind-set or generalized world view (12). This conceptualization is part of a larger cognitive model referred to as *interacting cognitive subsystems*.

Each of us has numerous minds that we put in place at different times, creating a shifting series of modes of interacting with the environment. We may have one mind-in-place at work, another with our children, and another with our friends. Some individuals become stuck in one mind-in-place and do not exhibit the adaptability needed for psychologically healthy functioning. For example, individuals wedded to a depressogenic mind-in-place would be dependent on schemata that filter information to sustain the depressive mind-set. Teasdale presented data showing that behavioral experience contradictory to the prevailing mind-in-place is most effective in creating a broader perspective and in facilitating the retrieval of more varied and functional alternative minds-in-place. As an example, planning mastery experiences for an individual with a low self-confidence mind-in-place may be instrumental in shifting that mind-set.

Information processing distortions characterize depression and anxiety disorders. Common distortions found in depression are termed arbitrary influence (drawing unsupported conclusions), magnification (exaggerating the significance of an event), and overgeneralization (drawing general, stable conclusions from isolated incidents) (13, 15). Typical of these processes is attentional bias given an array of information and biased interpretation of ambiguous visceral and environmental stimuli (16). In both cases, cognition is attracted to content congruent with the individual's distress.

Memory bias toward information that is supportive of emotional distress is common to individuals with persistent psychological problems. Low mood is self-perpetuating in that it elevates the likelihood of both storing negative events and retrieving negative memories (15–16).

Bower (17) emphasized the emotion-causing cognition path. Under the umbrella of associative network theory, he described a series of brilliant experiments that demonstrated the self-perpetuating characteristics of emotional influences affecting biases in both information processing and memory described previously. Using state-dependent learning as a basic model, he showed that memories acquired during an emotional state, for example, depression, were more likely to be recalled when depression recurred. Similar processes steer interpretation of interpersonal relations and social judgment to be confirmatory of a person's mood.

Memory inhibition processes may be highly relevant to clinical practice as a strategy for counteracting memory bias effects (18). Basic research has shown that instructions to forget can induce impaired recall, and this memory impairment is further promoted if new material is learned in its place.

Metacognition refers to evaluating an individual's own cognitions (15). Judging his or her own negativistic thoughts or distressing condition can introduce its own effect of escalating worry. Wells and Matthews (19) detailed metacognition potential for harm in consuming cognitive resources and inducing performance deficits.

Distraction or diverting attention from negative thoughts is likely to produce comparable reduction in the emotions associated with those thoughts (15).

Automatic processing refers to unintended, uncontrollable cognitive processes. They often assume a ruminative, obsessive quality and are stubbornly resistant to intervention because they are highly practiced and are seemingly insulated from volition (16). Any of these cognitive modes or their combination may attain automatic status.

Self-Regulation

The domain of self-regulation, also known as self-control, emerged around 1970 from the synergy of several independent forces, including the rise of cognitive therapy (20) and extensions of operant conditioning (21). Continuing to the present, this area is a loose conglomeration of theories and procedures that still lacks a single, unifying definition (see 22 for an overview). But if we must have a definition, Heatherton and Baumeister (23) provided an adequate one that is unparalleled in its efficiency—"self-regulation involves any effort on the part of an agent to alter its own responses" (p. 91). Some common ingredients present in most views of what constitutes self-regulation include:

1. Observed behavior cannot be accounted for by external influences.
2. Some elements of cognition or volition appear to explain the behavior.

Typical Self-Regulation Processes

Mechanisms typifying self-regulation models have common components and a predictable sequence:

1. The individual recognizes that an altered course of behavior is desired and perceives that environmental influences are not facilitative of this goal.
2. Environmental barriers may take several forms.
   —Available environmental reinforcers, including social support and valued contingencies, are insufficient to promote the course of action.
   —There may be discouragements to behavior. Punishing consequences and/or physical barriers may dissuade the planned behavior. Alternatively, the individual's behavioral history may leave him or her poorly equipped for success.
   —The individual is inclined to withhold behavior despite easily accessible, endearing reinforcers.
3. The individual produces internally generated *goals, methods* of achieving these, and *incentives* such as self-satisfaction or pride.

4. An action plan that is incongruous with environmental demands is performed, altered, or resisted.

Conditions 1 and 2 are routinely encountered by all of us and usually lead to
abandonment of the course of action under consideration. Steps 3 and 4 distinc-
tively characterize self-regulation and often invite descriptors such as *courage,*
perseverance, and *ingenuity.* Because by definition, self-regulatory courses of
action defy environmental influences, should the action plan fail, the individual
risks assignment of a negative interpretation ascribed by either himself or herself or others that replaces these laudatory descriptors with recklessness, stub-
bornness, and haphazardness, respectively.

Sampling of Self-Regulation Models

Kanfer's (21) three-stage model remains today one of the most frequently cited
self-control strategies for change:

- Stage 1, *self-monitoring:* The individual collects salient information relating to setting events, behavioral options, and consequences.
- Stage 2, *self-evaluation:* Performance is monitored and compared against
  initial goals and standards. This step may be repeated as performance is re-
  fined and/or goals or standards are revised.
- Stage 3, *self-reinforcement:* On successful performance, the individual self-
  administers internal or external reinforcing consequences.

Bandura's (9) social cognitive theory embraced self-regulatory capability
and endorsed a three-stage model similar to Kanfer's. The main distinction is
that Bandura's model has a much stronger cognitive bent, including the integration of Bandura's related theories of modeling and self-efficacy. For example, stage 2, called by Bandura *judgmental process,* emphasizes internal
standards for determining the adequacy of behavior, modeling mechanisms for
establishing standards, generation of generalized standards from delimited experience, and establishing an individual's own behavior as a reference point for
recalibrating standards.

Biofeedback captures the quintessence of self-regulation and is distinguished
by its focus on *involuntary,* autonomic functions (24–25). The essential elements
of biofeedback are:

1. Detection and amplification of a physiological signal
2. Converting the signal to an easily interpreted analogue, such as a visual or
   auditory display

3. Immediate presentation of the analogue information to the individual for use in self-regulation of the physiological response

Biofeedback was introduced in the 1960s, and though the underlying mechanism of action leading to self-control has never been clearly articulated, it has demonstrated efficacy in basic research with both animal and human subjects. Biofeedback has successfully been adapted to clinical applications for the purpose of inducing desired physiological states and modulating physiological irritants.

EXAMPLES OF PAST AND POTENTIAL APPLICATIONS OF BEHAVIORAL-COGNITIVE SCIENCE IN BEHAVIORAL SLEEP MEDICINE

This section draws on case studies and clinical trials to illustrate applications of behavioral-cognitive science in BSM. This section is not intended to be a comprehensive review of BSM, but rather touches on highlights to illustrate the enactment of the theories discussed to this point in the chapter.

We would be remiss in failing to acknowledge a clinically meaningful caveat. Neither intervention procedures nor patient complaints are always designed to fit neatly into a single theory to satisfy orthodox views. Procedural complexity may often reflect the combined influence of several theoretical perspectives in a given treatment plan, and multiple comorbidity existing in patients may require simultaneous interventions and/or tailored interventions that stray from their original theoretical purity. Further, when a new behavioral treatment is introduced, the inventor may describe a linkage with theory, yet in some cases, the choice of best theoretical home for a new treatment inspires debate and evolves in different directions over time.

Classical Conditioning

The use of behavior therapy to treat anxiety symptoms often adheres to a classical conditioning framework. The elements of classical conditioning habit formation are commonplace but not necessarily obvious. Careful evaluation may reveal potent examples of classical conditioning effects on problem behavior and emotions that would be amenable to classical conditioning-based treatment.

Patient resistance to continuous positive airway pressure (CPAP) treatment for obstructive sleep apnea often provides an opportunity for the application of classical conditioning therapy. Illustrative of the concept of stimulus generalization is the case of CPAP phobia we encountered in our Insomnia Clinic (a misnomer for a behavioral sleep medicine clinic). Mrs. Jones (fictitious name) was in a serious car wreck (US) and was trapped in the car, producing a claustrophobic response (UR). Subsequently, confined areas (CS) evoked negative emotions associated with the auto accident (CR). The CPAP mask (CS) also evoked such conditioned emotional reactions (CR), preventing successful treatment of her sleep apnea. In vivo desensitization consisting of gradual mask exposure while deeply relaxed (incompatible UR) abated this aversion, eliminated the CS properties of the CPAP mask, and apnea treatment proceeded as planned.

Operant Conditioning

The importance of operant concepts is interwoven in the history of behavior therapy, including the management of sleep behavior. Therapist awareness of planned and incidental reinforcers, schedules of reinforcement, shaping new behaviors, and so on are all important tools in the BSM armamentarium.

Several basic aspects of operant conditioning can be effectively orchestrated to address children's avoidance of sleeping alone. In treating a child's fear of being alone at bedtime, Ferber (26) instructed parents to gradually shape the goal behavior, starting with fixed interval reinforcement for successive approximations of sleeping alone. As the child's ability to sleep alone strengthens, the parents are told to gradually lengthen the delay (i.e., extinction) in giving their attention to the negative behavior of crying when left alone to sleep. Diligent parents can expect rapid progress from this approach.

Perhaps the most widespread application in all of learning theory in BSM is embodied in stimulus control treatment of insomnia. Introduced by Bootzin (27), this approach remains one of the most widely used and most effective interventions for this disorder. Stimulus control comprises restricting bedroom use to sleep by eliminating wake time in bed and other nonsleep activities from the bedroom.

Bootzin advanced an operant analysis of the mechanism of influence of stimulus control. The bedroom had become an S^Δ for sleep through associations with wakefulness and arousing stimuli. To establish the bedroom as an S^D for sleep, nonsleep activities are banned from the bedroom. If the individual attempts sleep and it does not come within 15 to 20 minutes, he or she must exit the bedroom. In time, the constellation of stimuli comprising the bedroom signal imminent sleep as the bedroom acquires S^D properties. Eventually, approaching the bedroom at bedtime elicits attitudes and physiological responses consistent with a sleep S^D. Subsequent sleep experiences reinforce this process.

Positional therapy for position-related snoring and obstructive sleep apnea can also be conceptualized as an operant conditioning procedure. The typical approach to positional therapy involves the attachment of some object, such as a tennis ball, to the back area of the sleep clothes between the shoulder blades to discourage supine sleep. Sleep position is an instrumental behavior to attain desired rewards (improved sleep and daytime functioning by decreasing sleep apnea and/or snoring plus the possibility of increasing bed partner companionship). If expected outcomes are not forthcoming, the behavior will likely extinguish.

Social Cognitive Theory

Applications of this paradigm in BSM are scarce, but we believe there is much untapped potential here.

New patients in sleep disorders centers frequently receive advance information about the sleep evaluation process from more experienced patients while sitting in the waiting area. Newly diagnosed obstructive sleep apnea patients may have CPAP treatment graphically described to them by CPAP users. The utility of such happenstance vicarious learning for acceptance and adherence to treatment varies with the treatment experience and communication skills of the "helper" patient. With increasing frequency, sleep centers use staged introductions, brochures, and videotapes to more effectively control the quality of information transmitted by patient education vehicles for observational learning.

There have been a few limited excursions exploring the role of self-efficacy in insomnia. Three investigators found successful insomnia treatment was accompanied by elevated self-efficacy concerning ability to sleep (28–30). Watts, East, and Coyle (31) found mixed levels of self-efficacy concerning sleep among untreated people with insomnia. The potential role of self-efficacy manipulations instigating sleep improvement has not been tested.

Cognitive Science

Insomnia has profited greatly from cognitive science-based interventions, but not so other areas of BSM.

Mainly during the late 1970s and early 1980s, there was a spate of well-controlled studies evaluating paradoxical instruction treatment of insomnia (32–37). This treatment instructs clients to *try to stay awake at bedtime* to relieve them of the worry and performance anxiety fueling their insomnia.

In more recent years, cognitive therapy for insomnia has been shown to be highly therapeutically effective (38), and Harvey (39) has proposed a comprehensive cognitive theory of insomnia drawing on varied dimensions of cognitive science to explain the clinical phenomena. The term *cognitive therapy* is sometimes used interchangeably with *cognitive-behavior therapy,* and the latter term usually functions as a synonym for comprehensive behavior therapy of insomnia. A typical cognitive-behavior therapy package includes stimulus control treatment, sleep restriction therapy, relaxation methods, and formal cognitive therapy.

The cognitive therapy part draws on the cognitive therapy model for depression (13). It is a structured, psychoeducational intervention based on the assumption that negative emotions, maladaptive behaviors, and physiological symptoms associated with psychological disorders are largely the result of dysfunctional cognitions. In the context of insomnia treatment, this approach seeks to moderate dysfunctional beliefs and attitudes (both automatic thoughts and schemas) about sleep.

Worry about sleep is recognized as a hallmark of persistent insomnia, perhaps the most universal distinguishing characteristic that separates "poor sleepers" from "good sleepers." Excessively worrying about the ability to fall asleep or the consequences of a poor night's sleep (40–41), sometimes referred to as an *exacerbation cycle,* exemplifies metacognition. The individual's reflection on his or her own disorder, sometimes attaining obsessive status while generating supplemental anxiety, serves to worsen the very disorder that the individual wishes to ameliorate.

Some simple cognitive strategies may prove useful in combating such metacognition. Practicing "detached mindfulness" (19) permits individuals to recognize problems and faults as a tool for self-correction rather than promoting further self-victimization. Power (18) described "planned forgetting." In bedtime anxiety, for example, it might prove useful to instruct patients to try to discard unpleasant bedtime memories and, in their place, dwell on positive memories related to sleep.

There has also been a fair amount of basic research investigating cognitive influences in insomnia. Exemplifying this literature, people with insomnia perceive cognitive arousal as the preeminent cause of their sleep disturbance (42); they report greater problem-solving thoughts, listening to noises, thinking about not sleeping, reappraisal strategies, and worry at bedtime than normal sleepers (43–44); they exhibit an attentional bias toward sleep-related cues (45); and they exhibit cognitive hypersensitivity to disturbing stimuli at bedtime (46).

Self-Regulation

Self-regulation techniques have enjoyed broad acceptance among mental health practitioners (47), but have achieved more limited application within BSM.

By far, the most frequent application of self-regulation in BSM is represented by biofeedback for insomnia. Electromyographic biofeedback has demonstrated promising results (48–52), and though it has attracted less interest, electro-encephalographic biofeedback has also registered successes (53–54).

The area of parasomnias has attracted self-regulation approaches. Kohen, Mahowald, and Rosen (55) employed a self-regulation model, sometimes supplemented with medication, to successfully treat 11 children with night terrors. Treatment was composed of relaxation training, self-hypnosis, and suggestions of empowerment and personal control. Seven of the children were administered no medication and achieved excellent results.

Training insomnia patients in sleep hygiene behaviors (such as limiting napping, not exercising shortly before bedtime) is conceptually a self-regulation approach. Patients are taught basic knowledge about sleep to promote better self-regulation of sleep-promoting and sleep-disruptive behaviors (56).

In addition, sleep hygiene changes are generally objective, quantifiable, and compatible with basic features of behavioral treatment. For example, sleep hygiene interventions often include baseline assessment for individualization of recommendations, continuous monitoring, and frequent adjustment of treatment in response to the outcomes obtained. As with any behavioral approach, the clinical value of sleep hygiene instruction is based on teaching new behaviors and appraising these against measurable standards. This psychoeducational approach could thus benefit from the spectrum of operant, cognitive, and social cognitive strategies outlined earlier.

CONCLUSIONS: STRENGTHS, WEAKNESSES, AND FUTURE DIRECTIONS

Behavioral-cognitive science is woven throughout BSM and informs effective BSM interventions. But BSM has yet to exhaust potential clinical applications of psychological science.

Use of classical and operant conditioning procedures in BSM is common but still probably underused. Areas that seem ripe for pioneering new strategies of these sorts include manipulating the distribution and content of activities to better manage circadian rhythm dysfunction; expanded efforts with sleep irregularity in infants, young children, and teens; and time management for older adults confronting diminished sleep need and disruptive napping habits.

Cognitive science has received robust acceptance within the insomnia domain, but not elsewhere in BSM. Areas of potential utility that have yet to be tested include managing obstacles to adherence and relapse prevention in a variety of sleep disorders.

Social cognitive theory is nearly untapped within BSM, and the related strategy of self-regulation has diminished in popularity in recent decades. Kanfer's (21) self-regulation model has enjoyed widespread application within psychology, but has yet to be adopted in the sleep arena. There are opportunities for important pioneering work here from these several approaches. Self-efficacy and self-regulation manipulations could contribute to adherence strategies, dampening disruptive sleep cognitions, circadian rhythm management, and sleep hygiene implementation.

There are mainstream behavioral-cognitive interventions that do not fit neatly into behavioral-cognitive theory. Most prominent among these are sleep restriction (57) and relaxation (58).

Sleep restriction treatment of insomnia has achieved a high success rate, particularly among older adults (59). The treatment consists of limiting the time spent in bed per night to the actual amount of time asleep determined during baseline assessment. No theoretical framework was offered by Spielman et al. It does exhibit many characteristics in kind with stimulus control and, therefore, may have operant conditioning influences at play. For example, both treatments restrict awake time in bed and strengthen the S^D properties of the bedroom. In addition, much reinforcement accrues to those who succeed with sleep restriction procedures (or stimulus control) when they learn new behaviors that lead to more consolidated sleep, improved sleep quality, and improved daytime experience.

The invention of relaxation/meditation predates behavioral-cognitive science by several thousand years. However, this approach could be recast with little effort into a modern mold. Relaxation is the primary deconditioning agent in systematic desensitization (60) and might provide the same function in the bedroom; relaxation (US) produces a relaxed response in the presence of the bedroom (UR), replacing arousing conditioned responses (CR). Further, relaxation practice creates a soothing cognitive set, directly competing with disruptive cognitions.

Alternatively, is much gained by taking effective behavioral methods—sleep restriction and relaxation, for example—and forcing them into behavioral-cognitive theory? BSM should not feel estranged from procedures that do not boast a clear theoretical basis. High-achieving empiricism is reinforcing to the therapist and client alike.

There are, however, at least two advantages to having knowledge of scientific theory and applying it to BSM. First, theory that has been proven in the lab owns some insight into the lawfulness of human behavior, and such theory will likely elevate the probability of success of novel treatments derived from it. Second, knowledge of theory is among the most effective bases for tailoring treatments to clients, trouble-shooting solutions for refractory clients, and extending and re-fining existing treatments.

REFERENCES

1. Schwartz, G. E. and S. M. Weiss. Yale Conference on Behavioral Medicine: A proposed definition and statement of goals. *Journal of Behavioral Medicine* 1: 3–12, 1978.

2. Alexander, F. *Psychosomatic Medicine: Its Principles and Applications.* New York, NY: W.W. Norton. 1950.

3. Freud, S. The interpretation of dreams. In J. Strachey, ed. and trans. *The Standard Edition of the Complete Psychological Works of Sigmund Freud* (Volumes 4 & 5). London, England: Hogarth Press. 1953. (Original work published 1900).

4. Kanfer, F. H. and J. S. Phillips. *Learning Foundations of Behavior Therapy.* New York: John Wiley. 1970.

5. Hilgard, E. R. and G. H. Bower. *Theories of Learning* (4th Edition). Englewood Cliffs, NJ: Prentice-Hall. 1975.

6. Millenson, J. R. and J. C. Leslie. *Principles of Behavioral Analysis* (2nd Edition). New York: Macmillan. 1979.

7. Bandura, A., D. Ross, and S. A. Ross. Transmission of aggression through imitation of aggressive models. *Journal of Abnormal and Social Psychology* 63: 575–582, 1961.

8. Bandura, A. *Social Learning Theory.* New York: General Learning Press. 1971.

9. Bandura, A. *Social Foundations of Thought and Action: A Social Cognitive Theory.* Englewood Cliffs, NJ: Prentice-Hall. 1986.

10. Teasdale, J. D. Emotion and two kinds of meaning: Cognitive therapy and applied cognitive science. *Behavior Research and Therapy* 31: 339–354, 1993.

11. Clark, D. M. and C. G. Fairburn, eds. *Science and Practice of Cognitive Behavior Therapy.* Oxford, England: Oxford University Press. 1997.

12. Teasdale, J. D. The relationship between cognition and emotion: The mind-in-place in mood disorders. In D. M. Clark and C. G. Fairburn, eds. *Science and Practice of Cognitive Behavior Therapy.* Oxford, England: Oxford University Press. 1997: 67–93.

13. Beck, A. T., A. J. Rush, B. F. Shaw, and G. Emery. *Cognitive Therapy of Depression.* New York: Guilford Press. 1979.

14. Rush, A. J. Cognitive therapy of depression: Rationale, techniques, and efficacy. *Psychiatric Clinics of North America* 6: 105–127, 1983.

15. Gelder, M. The scientific foundations of cognitive behavior therapy. In D. M. Clark and C. G. Fairburn, eds. *Science and Practice of Cognitive Behavior Therapy.* Oxford, England: Oxford University Press. 1997: 27–46.

16. Mathews, A. Information processing biases in emotional disorders. In D. M. Clark and C. G. Fairburn, eds. *Science and Practice of Cognitive Behavior Therapy.* Oxford, England: Oxford University Press. 1997: 47–66.

17. Bower, G. H. Mood and memory. *American Psychologist* 36: 129–148, 1981.

18. Power, M. J. Cognitive science and behavioral psychotherapy: Where behavior was, there shall cognition be. *Behavioral Psychotherapy* 19: 20–41, 1991.

19. Wells, A. and G. Matthews. Modeling cognition in emotional disorder: The S-REF model. *Behavior Research and Therapy* 34: 881–888, 1996.

20. Bandura, A. *Principles of Behavior Modification.* New York: Holt, Rinehart and Winston. 1969.

21. Kanfer, F. H. The maintenance of behavior by self-generated stimuli and reinforcement. In A. Jacobs and L. B. Sachs, eds. *The Psychology of Private Events: Perspectives on Covert Response Systems.* New York: Academic Press. 1971: 39–59.

22. Karoly, P. Self-control theory. In W. T. O'Donohue and L. Krasner, eds. *Theories of Behavior Therapy: Exploring Behavior Change.* Washington, DC: American Psychological Association. 1995: 259–285.

23. Heatherton, T. F. and R. F. Baumeister. Self-regulation failure: Past, present, and future. *Psychological Inquiry* 7: 90–98, 1996.

24. Blanchard, E. B. and L. H. Epstein. *A Biofeedback Primer.* Reading, MA: Addison-Wesley. 1978.

25. Gatchel, R. J. and K. P. Price, eds. *Clinical Applications of Biofeedback: Appraisal and Status.* New York: Pergamon Press. 1979.

26. Ferber, R. *Solve Your Child's Sleep Problems.* New York: Simon & Schuster. 1985.

27. Bootzin, R. R. Stimulus control treatment for insomnia. *Proceedings of the 80th Annual Convention of the American Psychological Association* 7: 395–396, 1972.

28. Espie, C. A. and W. R. Lindsay. Paradoxical intention in the treatment of chronic insomnia: Six case studies illustrating variability in therapeutic response. *Behavioral Research and Therapy* 23: 703–709, 1985.

29. Lacks, P. *Behavioral Treatment of Persistent Insomnia.* Elmsford, NY: Pergamon Press. 1987.

30. Engle-Friedman, M., R. R. Bootzin, L. Hazlewood, and C. Tsao. An evaluation of behavioral treatments for insomnia in the older adult. *Journal of Clinical Psychology* 48: 77–90, 1992.

31. Watts, F. N., M. P. East, and K. Coyle. Insomniacs' perceived lack of control over sleep. *Psychology and Health* 10: 81–95, 1995.

32. Ascher, L. M. and J. S. Efran. Use of paradoxical intention in a behavioral program for sleep onset insomnia. *Journal of Consulting and Clinical Psychology* 46: 547–550, 1978.

33. Relinger, H., P. H. Bornstein, and D. M. Mungas. Treatment of insomnia by paradoxical intention: A time-series analysis. *Behavior Therapy* 9: 955–959, 1978.

34. Turner, R. M. and L. M. Ascher. Controlled comparison of progressive relaxation, stimulus control, and paradoxical intention therapies for insomnia. *Journal of Consulting and Clinical Psychology* 47: 500–508, 1979.

35. Ascher, L. M. and R. M. Turner. Paradoxical intention and insomnia: An experimental investigation. *Behavior Research and Therapy* 17: 408–411, 1979.

36. Fogle, D. O. and J. A. Dyal. Paradoxical giving up and the reduction of sleep performance anxiety in chronic insomniacs. *Psychotherapy: Theory, Research and Practice* 20: 21–30, 1983.

37. Lacks, P., A. D. Bertelson, L. Gans, and J. Kunkel. The effectiveness of three behavioral treatments for different degrees of sleep onset insomnia. *Behavior Therapy* 14: 593–605, 1983.

38. Morin, C. M., J. Savard, and F. C. Blais. Cognitive therapy. In K. L. Lichstein and C. M. Morin, eds. *Treatment of Late-Life Insomnia.* Thousand Oaks, CA: Sage. 200: 207–230.

39. Harvey, A. G. A cognitive model of insomnia. *Behaviour Research and Therapy* 40: 869–893, 2002.

40. Kales, A., A. B. Caldwell, T. A. Preston, S. Healey, and J. D. Kales. Personality patterns in insomnia: Theoretical implications. *Archives of General Psychiatry* 33: 1128–1134, 1976.

41. Spielman, A. J. and P. B. Glovinsky. Introduction: The varied nature of insomnia. In P. J. Hauri, ed. *Case Studies in Insomnia.* New York, NY: Plenum Press. 1991: 1–15.

42. Lichstein, K. L. and T. L. Rosenthal. Insomniacs' perceptions of cognitive versus somatic determinants of sleep disturbance. *Journal of Abnormal Psychology* 89: 105–107, 1980.

43. Harvey, A. G. Presleep cognitive activity: A comparison of sleep-onset insomniacs and good sleepers. *British Journal of Clinical Psychology* 39: 275–286, 2000.

44. Harvey, A. G. I can't sleep, my mind is racing! An investigation of strategies of thought control in insomnia. *Behavioral and Cognitive Psychotherapy* 29: 3–11, 2001.

45. Taylor, L. M., C. A. Espie, and C. A. White. Attentional bias in people with acute versus persistent insomnia secondary to cancer. *Behavioral Sleep Medicine* in press.

46. Lichstein, K. L. and J. Fanning. Cognitive anxiety in insomnia: An analogue test. *Stress Medicine* 6: 47–51, 1990.

47. Karoly, P. and F. H. Kanfer, eds. *Self-Management and Behavior Change: From Theory to Practice.* New York: Pergamon Press. 1982.

48. Raskin, M., G. Johnson, and J. W. Rondestvedt. Chronic anxiety treated by feedback-induced muscle relaxation: A pilot study. *Archives of General Psychiatry* 28: 263–267, 1973.

49. Freedman, R. and J. D. Papsdorf. Biofeedback and progressive relaxation treatment of sleep-onset insomnia: A controlled, all-night investigation. *Biofeedback and Self-Regulation* 1: 253–271, 1976.

50. Haynes, S. N., H. Sides, and G. Lockwood. Relaxation instructions and frontalis electromyographic feedback intervention with sleep-onset insomnia. *Behavior Therapy* 8: 644–652, 1977.

51. Nicassio, P. M., M. B. Boylan, and T. G. McCabe. Progressive relaxation, EMG biofeedback and biofeedback placebo in the treatment of sleep-onset insomnia. *British Journal of Medical Psychology* 55: 159–166, 1982.

52. Sanavio, E., G. Vidotto, O. Bettinardi, T. Rolletto, and M. Zorzi. Behavior therapy for DIMS: Comparison of three treatment procedures with follow-up. *Behavioral Psychotherapy* 18: 151–167, 1990.

53. Bell, J. S. The use of EEG theta biofeedback in the treatment of a patient with sleep-onset insomnia. *Biofeedback and Self-Regulation* 4: 229–236, 1979.

54. Hauri, P. J., L. Percy, C. Hellekson, E. Hartmann, and D. Russ. The treatment of psychophysiologic insomnia with biofeedback: A replication study. *Biofeedback and Self-Regulation* 7: 223–235, 1982.

55. Kohen, D. P., M. W. Mahowald, and G. M. Rosen. Sleep-terror disorder in children: The role of self-hypnosis in management. *American Journal of Clinical Hypnosis* 34: 233–244, 1992.

56. Riedel, B. W. Sleep hygiene. In K. L. Lichstein and C. M. Morin, eds. *Treatment of Late-Life Insomnia*. Thousand Oaks, CA: Sage. 2000: 125–146.

57. Spielman, A. J., P. Saskin, and M. J. Thorpy. Treatment of chronic insomnia by restriction of time in bed. *Sleep* 10: 45–56, 1987.

58. Lichstein, K. L. *Clinical Relaxation Strategies*. New York: John Wiley. 1988.

59. Wohlgemuth, W. K. and J. D. Edinger. Sleep restriction therapy. In K. L. Lichstein and C. M. Morin, eds. *Treatment of Late-Life Insomnia*. Thousand Oaks, CA: Sage. 2000: 147–166.

60. Wolpe, J. *The Practice of Behavior Therapy* (2nd Edition). New York: Pergamon Press. 1973.

Chapter 8 ⎯⎯⎯⎯⎯⎯⎯⎯⎯⎯⎯⎯⎯⎯⎯⎯⎯⎯⎯⎯⎯⎯⎯⎯

EVALUATION OF INSOMNIA

ARTHUR J. SPIELMAN, DEIRDRE CONROY, AND PAUL B. GLOVINSKY

Sleep is the outcome of many physiological and psychological processes work-ing together. Its presence can be blocked or cut short by any number of factors. This idea may appear strange to good sleepers, who tend to think of sleep as merely a byproduct of staying awake. Certainly, sleep does seem inevitable after prolonged wakefulness. This "knockout sleep" does in fact result from a relatively simple recipe. However, consistent sleep, reliably arriving night after night irrespective of the day's events, is not so easy to come by. It requires not only physical recumbence, but also mental quiescence, satiety, comfort, and a sense of safety. It depends on a cascade of hormonal releases in synchronized step with a strongly articulated temperature cycle. When sleep is disrupted, the causes of insomnia may lie in any of these domains. Like waves sloshing in a pool, a disturbance in one area can set off disruption in another. By the time a clinician becomes involved, the context of the insomnia may resemble a froth of variables. Amid this confusion, effective evaluation must resort to both sys-tematic inquiry and clinical art.

This complexity does not mean that one evaluative approach is as good as an-other or that clinicians are reduced to haphazard guessing. Researchers have identified factors that are commonly associated with poor sleep. A comprehen-sive insomnia evaluation covers these areas in a systematic fashion even when they do not appear to be contributing to the understanding of the disorder on first glance, whether from the clinician's or from the patient's point of view.

Various assessment methods have been devised to survey these potential causes. Symptom checklists for clinical depression, questionnaires to uncover poor sleep hygiene, and sleep logs to portray details of the sleep schedule are ex-amples of tools that are based on the scientific understanding of the causes of in-somnia. Similarly, the clinician's history is directed toward particular cognitive features that are known to contribute to sleep disturbance—for example, the racing mind, the distorted beliefs about sleep, and the vicious cycle of worrying about sleeplessness. Touching on these well-worn signposts, the inquiry usually yields sufficient understanding to prepare the way for satisfactory treatment.

However, the path to understanding cannot always rely on expectations raised from normative studies. The patient's idiosyncratic perceptions, the personal meanings assigned to symptoms, the changes in self-image engendered by living with a chronic problem—these are the kinds of overlays that can transform the manifestation of insomnia. For example, two individuals might easily trace the onset of their sleep disorder to a major stress such as divorce. For one individual, the sleep problem remains tethered to circumstances, mitigated by an implicit understanding that with the passage of time and the building of a new life, sleep should eventually improve. For the second sufferer, the loss of control experienced on a near nightly basis is totally astounding. Its effects will not stay bound to the divorce but instead take on a life of their own, oftentimes persisting well past the apparent resolution of the trauma. To effectively treat these two patients, the clinician must be appreciative of the varied psychological meanings contained in a symptom and understanding of the interplay between the patient's evolving self-concept and behavioral change. In this thicket of interaction, it is most helpful to adopt a clinical stance that engages the patient as a collaborator in the investigation. The model of the detached clinical observer and the passive patient will not take either very far.

This chapter reviews well-established areas of inquiry, highlighting their usefulness in structuring the collaboration between clinician and patient. These evaluation techniques broadly indicate fruitful directions to pursue. Grounded in this straightforward approach, we then convey some of the subtler, more intuitive means of untangling the web of insomnia.

A FEW INSOMNIA COMPLAINTS ARE ASSOCIATED WITH MANY INSOMNIA DIAGNOSES

There are just a few ways in which patients complain of their insomnia (see Table 8.1), yet there are diverse causes of sleeplessness. The same presenting complaint of "trouble falling asleep," for example, may be due to disparate conditions such as a circadian rhythm disorder (delayed sleep phase disorder), learned associations (psychophysiological insomnia, sleep onset association disorder), and psychiatric disorders (major depressive disorder, generalized anxiety disorder).

In a single patient, factors primarily responsible for difficulty initiating sleep may vary across nights, and the severity of the resultant disturbance also

Table 8.1   Typical Complaints of Insomnia

Difficulty falling asleep

Difficulty staying asleep

Waking too early

Too little sleep

Light, unrefreshing sleep

Sleep is unpredictable

Work schedule interferes with sleep

Need drugs to sleep

Note: Adapted from "The Clinical Evaluate as Guide to Understanding the Nature of Insomnia: The CCNY Semi-Structured Interview for Insomnia," by A. J. Spielman and M. A. Anderson, in S. Chokroverty, eds. *Sleep Disorders Medicine* (2nd Edition), 1999, Boston, MA: Butterworth-Heinemann, pp. 385–426.

fluctuates. Confronted with seemingly endless variability in their experience, patients often throw up their hands and assume that their sleep is random—that there is no rhyme or reason to its vicissitudes. Implicit in this attitude is the sense that it does not really pay to make systematic changes in their behavior. A thorough evaluation aims to connect, in the patient's view, his or her complaint with the branching nexus of mechanisms that are responsible for it (see Table 8.2). This requires tolerance of complexity and an appreciation of the imperfect linkages between cause and effect when it comes to human behavior.

EVALUATION STARTS BEFORE THE FIRST VISIT— SELF-REPORT INSTRUMENTS

Materials sent to the patient when the initial appointment is made do more than gather information. They also serve to inform the patient of what a comprehensive evaluation really entails. The questions should appear far ranging—so much so that in some cases, they may hardly seem connected with the complaint. "Why should my afternoon coffee break make a difference?" one patient might think. "What could a broken nose sustained years ago have to do with sleep disturbance?" wonders another.

Patients must in many cases agree to reopen their inquiry. After living with insomnia for weeks, months, or years, many have solidified a formulation and excluded some causes of the difficulty through trial and error. It is the rare clinician who has not heard from many patients, for example, that their sleep disturbances are absolutely unaffected by caffeine consumption. Similarly, through awful

Table 8.2 *International Classification of Sleep Disorders* **Diagnostic Categories That Present with the Complaint of Insomnia**

Categories	Classification Number
Dyssomnias	
Intrinsic Sleep Disorders	
Psychophysiological insomnia	307.42-0
Sleep state misperception	307.49-1
Idiopathic insomnia	780.52-7
Periodic limb movement disorder	780.52-4
Restless legs syndrome	780.52-5
Extrinsic Sleep Disorders	
Inadequate sleep hygiene	307.41-1
Environmental sleep disorder	780.52-6
Altitude insomnia	289.0
Adjustment sleep disorder	307.41-0
Limit-setting sleep disorder	307.42-4
Sleep-onset association disorder	307.42-5
Food allergy insomnia	780.52-2
Hypnotic-dependent sleep disorder	780.52-0
Stimulant-dependent sleep disorder	780.52-1
Alcohol-dependent sleep disorder	780.52-3
Circadian Rhythm Sleep Disorders	
Time-zone change syndrome (jet lag)	307.45-0
Shift work sleep disorder	307.45-1
Irregular sleep-wake pattern	307.45-3
Delayed sleep phase syndrome	780.55-0
Advanced sleep phase syndrome	780.55-1
None-24-hour sleep-wake disorder	780.55-2
Sleep Disorders Associated with Medical/Psychiatric Disorders	
Associated with mental disorders	290-319
Associated with neurological disorders	320-389
Associated with other medical disorders	Various (086-729)

Note: Adapted from *International Classification of Sleep Disorders, revised: Diagnostic and Coding Manual* by American Sleep Disorders Association, 1997, Rochester, MN: American Sleep Disorders Association.

experience, many insomniacs arrive at their initial consultation fully convinced that they are unable to sleep without the aid of medications.

The effort the patient spends on questionnaires, symptom checklists, and sleep logs does save time at the first visit. However, a score on a scale or a sleep schedule pattern is far from an adequate assessment. The data provided by the

Table 8.3 Self-Report Instruments to Be Completed before the Initial Interview

Depression scale (3–4)
Anxiety scale (5–6)
Cognitive beliefs (7)
Sleep hygiene questionnaire (8–9)
Sleep log (7–11)

Note: Numbers in parentheses refer to references at the end of the chapter that contain examples of instruments.

self-report is merely a starting point to direct the clinician's attention to particular areas. The domains that we recommend be surveyed by self-report— psychiatric symptoms, sleep schedule, and habits and practices of everyday living—are major contributing factors to insomnia in well more than half of the cases (see Table 8.3). These domains may be covered by a wide array of instruments with proven utility and ready availability.

Evaluation of Depression

Depression is commonly found in individuals with insomnia and, as such, the possibility of depression needs to be thoroughly evaluated. The detection of depression is more crucial than ever with the availability of a number of effective therapeutic modalities. Depression inventories and rating scales have long played a role in clinical practice and psychiatric research (3–4). These same instruments are well suited to characterize and quantify the presence of depression within the context of sleep disturbance.

The presence of depressive symptoms does not settle the issue of what has caused insomnia in a given patient. Sleep loss itself produces effects that are also part of the depressive syndrome, such as sadness, reduced motivation, and functional impairments. It is a difficult task to tease apart causality. The patient and the clinician are often unsure as to how much sleep loss contributes to depression versus how much the insomnia is stemming from depression.

We recommend avoiding premature closure on this issue. An inclusive attitude, open both to the presence of depression independent of insomnia as well as to depression secondary to sleep loss, is most useful in the initial stages of the evaluation. Some patients could be driven away by the feeling that their sleep disturbance is being given short shrift or that their insomnia is being conveniently explained away via psychiatric diagnosis. Keeping the question open allays these concerns, while also keeping the possibility of clinical depression on

the table, to be decided one way or the other in the course of most effectively re-
solving the sleep problem. (See Table 8.5 later in the chapter for a list of symptoms of depression that are assessed at the initial interview.)

Assessment of Anxiety

Just as depression can become entwined with poor sleep, anxiety disorders are
commonly associated with insomnia. Depending on the individual, anxiety can
be manifest primarily through somatic changes or through alterations of cognition. Most people respond with both physiological and cognitive changes in an escalating interaction: We think the worst, our bodies react accordingly, and then
we scare ourselves even more with our beating hearts. As to instigating insomnia,
the reaction of choice is almost immaterial: Both physiologically and cognitively
mediated anxiety interfere with the process of gradually "winding down" that
optimally induces and maintains sleep. However, to select a targeted treatment
strategy, the clinician should take the patient's manifestations of anxiety into
consideration.

Anxiety scales that are brief yet sensitive are available (5–6). In many cases,
the threshold for formal diagnosis of a mental disorder may not be met, yet the
patient's level of arousal is sufficiently elevated to lead to sleep problems. An
anxiety disorder label need not be provided to convey that psychological and
physiological intensity is contributing to these individuals' sleep disturbances.

Assessment of Cognitive Beliefs

As explored in detail later, the beliefs an individual holds about the determinants
and functions of sleep and the consequences of sleeplessness greatly affect the
course of a sleep disturbance and its response to treatment. These beliefs may not
announce themselves without prompting. They are often sufficiently ingrained in
the patient's mind as to be considered wholly unremarkable. In contrast, external
factors such as job stress or physical internal factors such as a presumed "chemical imbalance" may be seized and elaborated on. A survey of cognitive beliefs
can be administered before the clinical interview, providing a guide to attitudes
that should be revisited in depth (7).

Survey of Sleep Hygiene Practices

An overview of sleep hygiene practices is likewise helpful to have on hand when
allocating time during the initial interview (1). Some of these issues are so basic
as to easily get lost among the more compelling features of a patient's story. The

initial evaluation could be completed without the clinician's realizing that the light stays on after the patient finally dozes off or that the patient's "half a pack a day" of cigarettes is actually smoked during evening and nighttime hours. There is often a tendency to discount the contributions of sleep hygiene, on the part of both patients and clinicians, as being too straightforward to possibly account for the interesting case at hand. A survey of sleep hygiene practices can highlight these contributions and ensure that even the most mundane of factors is not overlooked.

Depiction of the Sleep Pattern with a Sleep Log

It is often valuable to obtain a graphic representation of the patient's sleep pattern, completed each day over a typical week. The patient should be instructed not to use the clock but rather to estimate features such as sleep latency and timing and duration of nocturnal awakenings. Considerable sleep disruption may be caused if the patient attempts to give an accurate portrayal of the timing of nocturnal events.

Surprisingly, patients may resist this relatively simple request. Their objections often take one of two forms: Either they protest that their pattern is always the same (e.g., "I usually get two or three hours of sleep and wake up around 4 A.M."), or they assert that there is simply no rhyme or reason to their sleep pattern (without appreciating that this very lack of a pattern, if confirmed by log, may itself suggest effective treatment strategies).

Patients in these cases often push to have treatment proceed on the basis of a synthesized pattern, drawn from memory, or more simply, on the experience of the previous night—it being as representative as any other. There are good reasons not to acquiesce in this request. The patient's history is often prone to error. This may result from insufficient attention to details, memory limitations, undue emphasis on more recent sleep experience, or exaggeration. Our sense of time is easily distorted around sleep, and we may tend to forget sleeping past 9 A.M. on weekends or dozing on the couch after work. These omissions and distortions are then compounded when we try to recall our experiences over several nights.

The sleep log offers, by contrast, a systematic portrayal of key features of the sleep pattern, as well as tallying medication, caffeine, and alcohol intake. While it records subjective experience (as opposed to the "objective monitoring" offered by means such as polysomnography or actigraphy), the act of logging renders this experience in a more neutral fashion than is typically obtained through interview. Rather than taking "too long to fall asleep," the patient simply records a bedtime of, for example, 10 P.M. and an estimated sleep onset time of 11:30 P.M. Rather than "oversleeping" on weekends, the log straightforwardly records a difference of, for example, two and a half hours noted between the average weekday and weekend times of arising. The week-long task of filling out a sleep log also signals to the patient that evaluation and treatment will likely have a time course of at least several weeks, or even a number of months, rather than just a few nights.

It is not uncommon for patients to be surprised by the results of their sleep logs. It is important to ascertain if the week documented on the log is representative. If it is atypical, the sleep history should be relied on more heavily, with allowances made for the biases discussed previously. The patient should also be supplied with additional logs for the coming weeks, even if these will now be reflecting interventions introduced during the session rather than baseline sleep.

An example of the graphical portion of the sleep log without the reports of medication use and other practices is rendered in Figure 8.1. It can be quickly seen that this patient takes more than two hours to fall asleep during the week. In contrast, on the weekend when bedtime is late, sleep onset is rapid. There is no trouble staying asleep and, in fact, sleeping in on weekends is significant. All of these features are readily grasped from the log, and the clinician gains considerable clarity by assimilating the details of this pattern.

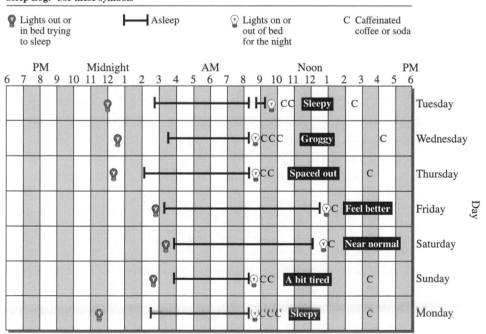

Figure 8.1   The Graphical Portion of a Typical Sleep Log Depicting the Sleep-Wake Pattern for a Week

Sleep Questionnaires

There are a number of instruments that survey a wide range of features of insomnia (11–21). Answered before the initial visit, the questions serve to harvest information for the clinician, sharpen the patient's focus on various details of the presenting problem, and give the patient a preview of the perhaps surprisingly wide scope of questions that will be considered. The clinician may wish to review the answers to these questions during the interview, thereby organizing the sleep history while at the same time assuring that unusual responses will be flagged and followed up.

THE SLEEP HISTORY

The interview is the crucial element in the evaluation of insomnia. Nothing is as effective in clarifying a complex clinical picture as the processes of hypothesis generation and hypothesis testing that can unfold during a face-to-face encounter. The clinician will probe for and follow up on suggestive leads that arise, and the various lines of questioning may stimulate the patient toward new insights.

A patient's sleep problem is more thoroughly comprehended if the evolution of the problem is understood. We have emphasized a simple schema that takes into account factors that may predispose an individual to insomnia, triggering conditions at the onset of the problem, and features that sustain the sleep disorder once it has begun (see Table 8.4 and Figure 8.2). By the time many cases of chronic insomnia present to clinical attention, their triggering events are already in the remote past and reduced in significance. As Figure 8.2 depicts, it is the perpetuating factors that are often the most salient features to assess and address when faced with chronic insomnia.

Predisposing factors include personality traits, basal physiological arousal level, and a host of other circumstances that render an individual prone to insomnia. The inability to regulate anxiety, for example, is a characteristic that creates the potential for sleep disturbance when the individual feels threatened. Most people react to a perceived threat with anxiety, but the magnitude of that reaction and the time course of subsequent settling down vary among individuals. If sufficient anxiety and agitation carry over into the habitual sleep period, insomnia is more likely to ensue.

Precipitating events, such as a critical job assignment, an upcoming wedding, or the loss of a loved one, are of sufficient magnitude that they overwhelm coping capacity. These events loom before us or cast shadows on our lives for weeks, months, or even years, demanding to be acknowledged. Oftentimes, we are more

Table 8.4   A Model of Insomnia for Categorizing Case Material

- Predisposing Factors: Features present before onset of insomnia that lower the threshold for developing insomnia. These features may precipitate the insomnia if they are sufficiently intense.

  –Physiological hyperarousal—high resting metabolic rate, taking steroids, caffeine consumption, strong time of day preference (e.g., evening-type and morning-type individuals)

  –Psychological traits—internalization of conflict such as highly sensitive or reactive to emotional arousal, depression-prone, ruminative tendency

- Precipitating Factors: Events that trigger the insomnia.

  –Stress—new job, having a baby, moving

  –Psychological threat or damage—anticipation of a challenge, loss of a loved one, lowered self-esteem, concern over medical illness

  –Change of habits—assigned to the night shift, having a new bed-partner

- Perpetuating Factors: Conditions and habits that accrue as the insomnia becomes chronic and help sustain the sleep disturbance. Frequently, the individual changes habitual practices in an attempt to cope with the sleep problem and inadvertently prolongs the problem.

  –Sleep schedule—napping, increased time in bed, staying in bed resting

  –Habits—increased caffeine consumption, reducing exercise, increased alcohol consumption

  –Cognitive—worrying about sleeplessness, catastrophic thinking, unrealistic expectations of sleep

Note: Adapted from "Assessment of Insomnia," by A. J. Spielman, 1986, *Clinical Psychology Reviews* 6, pp. 11–25, and "A Behavior Perspective on Insomnia Treatment," by A. J. Spielman, L. Caruso, and P. Glovinsky, 1987, *Psychiatric Clinics of North America* 10(4), pp. 541–553.

successful at keeping them "out of mind" during the day, when we can take refuge in daily routine. At night, with no other competing distractions, their full power to disrupt sleep becomes apparent. However, the greater the predisposition to insomnia, the less intense a triggering event needs to be to initiate a sleep problem.

In cases where the patient is able to precisely date the start of the sleep disturbance, the clinician has a special opportunity: In addition to a greater likelihood of identifying the triggering factors responsible for the appearance of the insomnia, clear demarcation of the onset of the problem allows for comparison between retrospective and prospective views. Historical review of what sleep quality, bedtimes, sleep hygiene, and the fabric of life were like before the appearance of the insomnia can help both the clinician and patient discern what key features might have come into play to precipitate the disturbance.

Once insomnia is established, it sets in motion a number of changes that may become perpetuating factors. The individual will make adaptations to accommodate

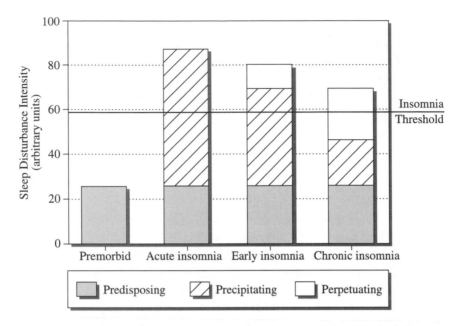

Figure 8.2   A Model of the Development of Insomnia. It is proposed that predisposing, precipitating, and perpetuating factors emerge at different times and with differing intensity over the course of insomnia (adapted from 22–24).

the sleep disturbance, such as staying in bed later trying to catch up on sleep, reducing social activities and exercise because of lack of energy, or drinking more coffee for a boost. These changes in habit may ultimately be counterproductive, sustaining the insomnia even as they bring short-term relief. For example, weekend oversleeping may bring immediate benefit in that it pays off a "sleep debt" accumulated across the week. However, it can begin to delay the timing of circadian rhythms such as the body temperature cycle and hormone release, making sleep at the individual's targeted weekday bedtime less likely.

Changes in thinking are common once insomnia takes hold, and they can also perpetuate the problem. Fretful apprehension during the evening of the dreaded night to come, worrying about the ability to perform during the day, a sense of vulnerability becoming incorporated into self-image—these cognitive changes can all effectively maintain an insomnia. Some individuals focus so intensely on their sleep disturbance, whether on causes or possible cures, that the increased thinking about sleep itself becomes part of the problem. Long after the individual has dealt with the triggering event, the accrual of perpetuating factors, represented by both behavioral and cognitive changes, may be enough to sustain perturbed sleep.

In addition to the historical perspective emphasized by focusing on predisposing, precipitating, and perpetuating factors, the clinician needs to survey a number of domains to ensure that a comprehensive evaluation is performed. A number of valuable approaches have been recommended (25, 26). We follow an outline organized as a semistructured interview (1).

Complaint

The patient's description of the presenting complaint points to what part of the night is most troubling and how frequently the problem occurs (see Table 8.1). The complaint can be narrowly focused or diffused, fixed, or fluid. Often, descriptions are offered at the outset of the interview as to the frequency, intensity, and consequences of the problem that are upgraded, discounted, or otherwise modified as the details are filled in. The clinician should encourage the patient to go beyond capsule descriptions when presenting the problem and instead try to convey its landmark features, whether commonplace or atypical, and its most distressing aspects.

Sleep-Wake Pattern

Near the beginning of the interview, a snapshot of the current sleep schedule during the weekdays, on weekends, and on extended holidays provides a context for all of the following case material. A completed sleep log provides key information on:

1. Type, dosage, frequency, and timing of sleep medication administration
2. Time and activities surrounding when the patient first gets into bed
3. Time the patient turns lights out and starts to try to fall asleep
4. Estimated sleep latency
5. Frequency, timing, duration, cause, and behavioral consequences of nocturnal awakenings
6. Time of final wake-up
7. Time out of bed
8. Estimate of total sleep time
9. Frequency, timing, and duration of napping or rest periods
10. Quality of sleep
11. Daytime consequences such as fatigue level or cognitive alertness

This list is deceptively straightforward. In reality, the information often emerges in a branching structure. For example, the sleep pattern may be radically different depending on whether the patient takes a sleep medication. In this case, all the information should be collected twice—both when on and off medication. The cognitive and behavioral consequences of this dichotomy require exploration. For example, it may serve to reinforce the patient's belief that good sleep requires medication. Similarly, the distinctive properties of "good" versus "bad" nights may require double entries. To make matters even more interesting, there may be "good" and "bad" nights on medication and so on. The clinician must be active and flexible to obtain a comprehensive picture of the sleep pattern.

In addition to the essential information on this list, the clinician directs the inquiry down particular paths that cannot be specified ahead of time. Commonly, it is useful to know what circumstances improve or degrade sleep, responses to treatments that have been tried in the past, and how the individual sleeps away from the habitual sleeping environment. Although it is important that the details of the sleep pattern be systematically pursued, we suggest that other features of sleep hygiene be surveyed later (see later section on sleep hygiene). The more time spent on the sleep schedule, the less time is available for the exploration of the patient's inner world.

Sleep-Related Cognitions

While worries have been implicated as exacerbating factors in a broad range of medical conditions, they are particularly effective when it comes to engendering insomnia. A hypochondriac's chronic worrying about illness certainly affects his or her quality of life, but it is not expected to bring on the dreaded disease itself. Yet this is exactly what happens when we worry too much about sleep. The apprehension of a poor night's sleep may be enough to ruin the night. A vicious cycle is set up where the experience of insomnia serves to justify dread of another poor night, which in turn becomes a self-fulfilling prophecy.

The clinician should be aware of the many other ways in which worries over sleep can impact the course of sleep itself, as well as the insomniac's self-image. Thoughts such as "Insomnia is ruining my life," "I can't function because of sleeplessness," or "Without eight hours of sleep, I get physically sick" need to be elicited and addressed to achieve the level of calm prerequisite to satisfactory sleep.

Obsessional thinking is a very effective means of forestalling sleep. The mind remains on alert, rehearsing responses to real or imagined crises. It doesn't matter that not much is likely to be accomplished at, for example, 12:30 A.M. concerning office politics or that new muffler for the car. It doesn't matter that the state of the world, as just reported on the late news show, will remain unaffected by an individual's unrelenting focus. The only reliable effect of such cognitive hyperarousal is on sleep, which is either delayed until exhaustion finally wins out or else peppered with interruptions.

Sometimes, patients do not have any particularly distressing thoughts in mind but complain instead that their minds flit from one mundane thought to another without cease. In these cases, it is the mode of cognitive processing itself that is interfering with sleep. Patients lament "I can't turn my mind off." They perceive a disconcerting split among their exhausted selves, longing for sleep, and their unruly minds, speeding along unrestrained. This split can lead to a sense of help-lessness. The poor sleeper may grow to live in fear of his or her own mind, wait-ing for it to erupt at that most inopportune time—when the light goes off.

The clinician should spend some time learning how the insomnia appears to the insomniac. Are anticipation of a poor night's sleep and its resultant self-fulfilling prophecy salient features? What are the patient's ideas about the causes of the in-somnia and the consequences of poor sleep? An individual who attributes poor sleep to "job stress" may feel like a passive victim and pessimistic that any efforts will improve sleep as long as this stress must be endured. The consequences of making a mistake at work because of diminished concentration just serve to raise the stakes over getting a good night's sleep.

In addition to identifying beliefs that may be contributing to the sleep distur-bance, the clinician should gain an appreciation for the form in which thoughts are being processed and the affect that accompanies this cogitation. Is the patient obsessively fixed on some problem or unable to focus on any one thought? During periods of sleeplessness, is the emotional tone one of anger, agitation, resigna-tion, or detachment? Occasionally, patients are encountered who enjoy their noc-turnal reveries because there may be no other occasion for such "daydreaming." Nocturnal awakenings may persist until another venue for unstructured thought is provided.

Psychological and Social Determinants

Elucidating the psychological underpinnings of insomnia is often essential for effective treatment. The common role of depression and anxiety in sleep prob-lems has been mentioned previously. The more explicit forms of depression are generally discernable by assessment scales and inquiry into affective, biological, and cognitive features. In less obvious cases, it takes considerable clinical skill to elicit the inner experience of a damaged self or latent guilt that makes sense of insomnia. If the clinician suspects the presence of depression or self-report scales are suggestive, the range of symptoms associated with depression should be assessed (see Table 8.5).

The association of sleep with darkness, quiet, comfort, and either solitude or a single bed partner is a fairly recent development and still not the norm in many societies. In Western countries, parents with young children may get just

Table 8.5 Features of Depression

- Mood
  –Sadness, crying, inability to enjoy oneself, irritability, reduced motivation, diurnal mood variation (worse in the morning)
- Cognitive
  –Reduced attention and concentration, reduced speed of processing, preoccupations, guilt, hopelessness, helplessness, worthlessness, catastrophic thinking
- Physiological
  –Reduced (or increased) appetite, diminished sex drive, poor sleep, early morning awakening, psychomotor agitation or lethargy, increased fatigue
- Other
  –Depressed facies; social withdrawal; suicidal thoughts, intentions, plans, and attempts

a suggestion of the social aspects of sleep that prevail elsewhere at present and that prevailed everywhere in the past. Historically, the sleep unit may have been a family or an extended clan, with members of varying ages on different schedules, catching sleep as they could amid conversations and other activities and with visits from both domestic pets and intruding pests.

The social context of sleeping behavior may have changed in industrial and postindustrial societies, but social inputs still markedly affect sleep in these societies. Shorter workdays and labor-saving appliances have opened up free time in the evening to watch television, doze on the couch, go out carousing, be with the family, go to the bowling alley, or work a second job. Each choice brings different ramifications for sleep.

Those who think to preserve a period of "winding down" before sleep, relatively free from social influences, are facing an uphill battle. The telephone rings, with friends, telemarketers, or committee organizers on the other end, each capable of fostering hyperarousal. The sitcom ends, and the nightly news headlines shatter quietude before you can reach for the remote. Internet chat rooms and instant messaging allow socializing to occur, with opportunities for emotional stimulation, even when you have chosen a quiet night at home.

People with chronic sleep difficulties vary in their approaches to meeting the threat that social factors pose for their sleep. Some insomniacs become very protective of their sleep, to the point that they forego invitations to evening social events. Others may follow their night-owl tendencies, reasoning that they are going to be up anyway. Some ask friends not to call late at night, or they set up an answering machine to pick up calls without ringing, while others remain permeable to these intrusions. Some have reached an agreement with family members to taper potentially overly stimulating interactions as the night approaches, while others seem to always end up dealing with thorny issues, or arguing outright, just before bedtime. Appreciation of the social context of the patient's sleep disorder, as well as the patient's responses to social stimuli, is especially helpful in planning treatment strategies—because these treatments will themselves be implemented within that same social context.

Sleep Hygiene

Many activities of everyday living do not facilitate good sleep. It is well known, for example, that excess caffeine may interfere with sleep. Other habits, less well appreciated, may also contribute to insomnia (see Table 8.6). Addressing these practices is commonly a part of the overall treatment plan. It is important to note

Table 8.6   Sleep Hygiene: Practices and Habits That Interfere with Sleep

Daytime and Evening Habits
1. Caffeine consumption, especially later than the morning
2. Smoking
3. Alcohol consumption
4. Napping, nodding, and dozing
5. Lying down to relax or meditate in the evening
6. In a trance, semi-awake in the evening
7. Exercising in the late evening
8. Worry about sleeplessness
9. Getting home too late to wind down
10. Insufficient wind-down in evening
11. Preparations for bed are arousing
12. No regular presleep ritual
13. Distressing "pillow talk"
14. Late evening meal (acid reflux), fluid near bedtime (nocturnal urination)
15. In-bed engaging in behaviors that are not compatible with sleep (e.g., talking on the phone, reconciling checkbook)

Nighttime Habits
1. Irregular sleep-wake schedule
2. Spending too much time in bed
3. Falling asleep to the TV/radio (sleep timer)
4. Trying too hard to sleep
5. Snoring bed-partner
6. Watching the clock during the night
7. Tossing and turning in the bed during long awakenings

Morning Habits
1. Lingering in bed awake in the morning
2. Extra sleep on the weekends
3. Bedroom disturbances (e.g., noise, sunlight, and pets)
4. Outdoor light exposure soon after awakening in the morning may result in early morning awakening due to a phase advance in circadian rhythms

Note: Adapted from "The Clinical Evaluate as Guide to Understanding the Nature of Insomnia: The CCNY Semi Structured Interview for Insomnia," by A. J. Spielman and M. A. Anderson, 1999, in S. Chokroverty, ed. *Sleep Disorders Medicine* (2nd Edition), Boston, MA: Butterworth-Heinemann, pp. 385–426.

that many patients have followed the "sleep hygiene tips for good sleep" suggested in the media to no avail. Chronic insomniacs are often scornful of these tips, having "proven" through trial and error that the tips have little bearing on their own case. The experienced clinician will not be deflected from targeting these practices when prescribing treatment. The patient must become convinced that contributing factors act in concert, no one factor is necessarily responsible for the sleep disturbance, and the potential contribution of these factors cannot be discounted haphazardly. Effective treatment instead depends on a systematic, comprehensive approach, allowing sufficient time for the effects of various interventions to make themselves apparent over the "noise" of expected night-to-night variations in sleep quality.

To facilitate the interview, the individual sleep hygiene items in Table 8.6 are organized into groups according to when they occur in the day.

Physiological Hyperarousal

Abundant anecdotal evidence, as well as scientific studies, has confirmed that heightened physiological arousal is present in individuals with sleeping problems and that increased arousal inhibits sleep (27–32). While techniques are available to measure indexes such as heart rate, body temperature, and muscle tension, thresholds that are considered to invariably trigger insomnia have not been established. Therefore, in the therapeutic realm of biofeedback, relative changes rather than absolute levels have been used as targets of intervention. Assessment of basal metabolic rate, which has normative data, is beyond the scope of clinical practice.

There is currently no suitable assessment instrument for quantifying physiological arousal in the clinical setting. The state of the art is currently limited to subjective report (see Table 8.7). This is an area in great need of development.

Table 8.7   Domains of Clinical Inquiry for Physiological Arousal

Muscle tension: neck tightness, tension headaches
Agitation: motor restlessness, rapid speech
Reactivity: increased startle response, heightened vigilance
Cardiac: increased heart rate, pounding in chest
Anxiety: air hunger, cold and clammy hands
Sleep: unable to nap, nocturnal awakenings are abrupt

Note: See also "Daytime Alertness in Patients with Primary Insomnia," by Q. Regestein and J. Dambrosia, 1993, *American Journal of Psychiatry* 150, p. 10.

Circadian Rhythms

The circadian system promotes sleep as well as wakefulness. Knowing the phase position of endogenous rhythms such as the temperature cycle can be of great help in understanding why a particular sleep pattern is manifest. Exotic experimental protocols with sophisticated data analysis techniques are capable of determining the relationship of the underlying circadian phase to an overt sleep-wake schedule. A delay in rhythms (for example, peak and trough of the core body temperature rhythm occurring later in the day) is associated with delayed sleep phase syndrome, while an advance in rhythms is associated with advanced sleep phase syndrome or early morning awakening insomnia. However, as with the assessment of physiological arousal, the clinical setting relies on indirect reports to estimate the position of the circadian system. Scale scores (33) and clinical features, such as the timing of the afternoon dip in alertness, ability to sleep late on weekends, and the preferred timing of sleep when there are no schedule constraints, reflect the timing of the sleep propensity rhythm.

Knowing the phase position of the circadian system is helpful in designing an initial sleep schedule that is in accord with the underlying rhythm. An individual who is going to bed at 11 P.M. but consistently unable to sleep until 1 A.M., who has great difficulty rising at 7 A.M. for work and who can easily sleep late into the morning on weekends, is manifesting a delayed sleep phase. Along with other treatment measures such as timed exposure to bright light, an initial sleep schedule might be designed that more closely matches the current propensity for sleep, with the aim of gradually advancing it to the desired bedtimes. This strategy would immediately address the frustration engendered by lying in bed for hours unable to sleep.

Sleep-Related Disorders

Restless Legs Syndrome (RLS)

The patient's description is necessary and sufficient for the diagnosis of restless legs syndrome. Discomfort in the thigh or calf is most common. Descriptions include "like something crawling on [or under] my skin," "a charged feeling," "a need to move my legs," "they jump on their own," and "it's hard to describe." These uncomfortable sensations occur almost exclusively in the evening when at rest. Relief can be achieved—often only fleetingly—by stretching, kneading, and moving the legs. In some cases, the feeling may occur during the day or within nocturnal awakenings. Frequency varies from virtually every night to only rarely. The vast majority of individuals with RLS also have periodic limb movement disorder, described in the next section.

Periodic Limb Movement Disorder

In contrast to the obvious discomfort of restless legs syndrome during wakefulness, patients are rarely aware of periodic limb movements (PLMs) during sleep, although they may complain of one of its potential consequences—daytime sleepiness. The bed partner may bear the brunt of the disorder by being kicked. Awakened from sleep, the bed partner may be able to observe the limb movements and thereby provide the essential description of the problem. A polysomnogram (PSG) recording can document the number and pattern of the movements and any associated arousals. It is unclear if or to what extent PLMs without associated arousals are clinically significant. In a patient who is somewhat sleep deprived before a PSG, for example, there may be no arousals associated with PLMs because of the raised arousal threshold due to sleep loss. On other nights when no sleep debt is present, there may be many arousals in conjunction with the PLMs.

PLMs range from a subtle writhing of the foot to distinct rapid jerks. PLMs are usually confined to the lower limbs. However, the arms and shoulders may be involved in rare cases. The movements come at relatively equal intervals, commonly between 20 and 40 seconds.

Sleep-Disordered Breathing

Breathing is vulnerable during sleep, and respiratory disturbance may produce arousals or full awakenings. The vast majority of patients with sleep-disordered breathing present with sleepiness. However, awakenings from disordered breathing events may be followed by trouble falling back to sleep. Therefore, sleep apnea is part of the differential diagnosis of insomnia. Disruptive snoring is a cardinal symptom of obstructive sleep apnea—although it is now recognized that increased upper airway resistance can lead to frequent transient arousals even in the absence of overt snoring. In addition, no obvious snoring may accompany central sleep apnea, secondary to pulmonary, cardiac, or neurological disease.

OBJECTIVE TESTS AND PROCEDURES FOR THE ASSESSMENT OF INSOMNIA

Overnight Sleep Study—The Polysomnogram (PSG) Recording

Objective assessment of the patient's sleep physiology by an overnight sleep study may play an important role in the evaluation of insomnia. If the clinician suspects, for example, that another primary sleep disorder might be producing the insomnia complaint, a PSG recording will be recommended. Complaints of snoring, pauses in breathing, uncomfortable leg sensations, kicking, or excessive restlessness at night may signal to the clinician that a sleep study is indicated to assess sleep apnea or periodic limb movement disorder. In other cases, a PSG study may be necessary when insomnia is unresponsive to behavioral or pharmacological treatments.

Individuals who complain of little or no sleep will benefit from a PSG recording that objectively documents substantial sleep and confirms the diagnosis of sleep state misperception. These patients may be reassured that they are objectively getting more sleep than they appreciate. We recommend that, before scheduling a PSG, these patients call an answering machine that has a time stamp, every hour on the hour, during their time spent in bed not sleeping. Some patients may make few, if any, calls during the night and thus gain an awareness that they must be sleeping. This would obviate the need for a PSG.

Physical Exam

A host of medical conditions may be responsible for insomnia. Therefore, a physical exam in conjunction with a medical history may be useful. However, in most cases of insomnia, there are few indications of a relevant medical condition and high suspicion of the most common behavioral and psychological causes of sleep disturbance. In these cases, we recommend proceeding with treatment trials based on current understanding. If the insomnia proves to be recalcitrant to treatment, physical examination, referral to other experts, or performing a PSG, as well as other ways of reevaluating the problem, remain options.

Actigraphy

Behavioral quiescence is a defining characteristic of sleep, and new technology, known as actigraphy, is available to measure ambulatory activity over long periods of time (34). Although actigraphy has face validity, there is certainly some discrepancy between this new method and the well-established standard of polysomnographic recording. Lying still while awake and trying to sleep, for example, will be incorrectly categorized as sleep by actigraphy. Nevertheless, in conjunction with a sleep log, actigraphy can detail the sleep and waking pattern over many days or weeks with minimal cost in the habitual sleeping environment.

Screening Laboratory Tests: Blood

Although not a standard component of the evaluation of insomnia, the levels of particular blood constituents may confirm clinical suspicion. If hyperthyroidism

Table 8.8   Signs and Symptoms of Hyperthyroidism

Heat intolerance, warm moist skin
Heart palpitations, chest pain, dyspnea on exertion
Nausea, vomiting, increased defecation
Polyuria, nocturia, decreased libido
Weakness, distal tremor
Fatigue, nervousness, depression, insomnia

(see Table 8.8) or menopause, for example, is suspected of playing a role in the sleep disturbance, blood levels of thyroid stimulating hormone and estrogen, respectively, are needed to evaluate these hypotheses. However, this screening is suggested only when there is independent evidence for an endocrine abnormality. In patients with possible periodic limb movement disorder, iron, ferritin, and blood levels of other factors may assist in diagnosis and treatment. Similarly, prostate-specific antigens (PSA) levels may be helpful in male patients who complain of frequent urination at night to rule out prostate disease.

Trial Treatment as Evaluation

As discussed previously, patients with restless legs syndrome (RLS) complain of "pins and needles" or "creeping or crawling" sensations in their legs during the evening when at rest, which can be relieved only by moving, stretching, or crossing their legs. The majority of patients with RLS also have periodic limb movement (PLM) disorder, a rhythmic dorsiflexion of the toe or flexion of the leg that typically occurs about once every 20 to 40 seconds. Dopaminergic agents are often the recommended treatment for RLS and associated PLMs. While a sleep study is the only definitive way of diagnosing PLM disorder, if there is a clinical response to the administration of dopaminergic agents such as Mirapex or Sinemet, there is increased diagnostic certainty.

CONCLUSION

Clinicians and patients hoping to effectively evaluate insomnia can be stymied both by the disorder's straightforward surface appearance and the complexity that churns just below that surface. In the first case, the inquiry may quickly run out of leads as the handful of "usual suspects" are discounted; in the second, it may get lost in a crowd of possibilities. We advocate balancing a systemic approach based on several decades of research into factors present in large subgroups of insomniacs, with respect for the role that idiosyncrasies play in a particular case and development of an intuitive sense about these individual differences. A comprehensive evaluation makes varying use of psychometric scales, structured questionnaires, sleep logs, and objective tests. It also reserves time for a collaborative, reciprocal inquiry into the nature of the problem, with both clinician and patient offering ideas for consideration.

Consonant with exploration in any new field, the broader and more trustworthy behavioral outlines of insomnia took priority in early clinical descriptions of the problem and in formulating prescriptions. We have made much progress by focusing on the links between particular behaviors occurring across waking hours and their resultant effects on sleep. Our patients are sleeping better as a result. However, much work remains to be done, and to a large extent, the more difficult tasks lie ahead because they involve a greater appreciation of the patient's inner world. Dream-related insights notwithstanding, the mind has achieved most of its greatness during waking hours. We should, therefore, perhaps not be too surprised that it has its wiles when it comes to staying awake.

REFERENCES

1. Spielman, A. J. and M. A. Anderson. The clinical evaluate as guide to understanding the nature of insomnia: The CCNY semi-structured interview for insomnia. In S. Chokroverty, ed. *Sleep Disorders Medicine* (2nd Edition). Boston, MA: Butterworth-Heinemann. 1999: 385 426.

2. American Sleep Disorders Association. *International Classification of Sleep Disorders, revised: Diagnostic and Coding Manual.* Rochester, MN: American Sleep Disorders Association. 1997.

3. Beck, A. T., C. H. Ward, M. Mendelson, J. E. Mock, and J. K. Erbaugh. An inventory for measuring depression. *Archive of General Psychiatry* 4: 561–571, 1961.

4. Benca, R. M. Mood disorders. In M. H. Kryger, T. Roth, and W. C. Dement, eds. *Principles and Practice of Sleep Medicine* (3rd Edition). Philadelphia, PA: W.B. Saunders Company. 2000: 1140–1157.

5. Bonnet, M. H. and D. L. Arand. 24-hour metabolic rate in insomniacs and matched normal sleepers. *Sleep* 19: 581–588, 1995.

6. Bootzin, R. R. and S. P. Rider. Behavioral techniques and biofeedback for insomnia. In M. R. Pressman and W. C. Orr, eds. *Understanding Sleep: The Evaluation and Treatment of Sleep Disorders.* Washington, DC: American Psychological Association. 1997: 315–338.

7. Brodman, K., A. J. Erdmann Jr., I. Lorge, and H. G. Wolff. The Cornell Medical Index: An adjunct to medical interview. *Journal of the American Medical Association* 140: 530–534, 1949.

8. Lacks, P. *Behavioral Treatment of Persistent Insomnia.* New York, NY: Pergamon Press. 1987.

9. Hauri, P. and S. Linde. *No More Sleepless Nights.* New York, NY: John Wiley. 1990.

10. Metrodesign Associates/Charles Pollak, MD, 90 Clinton Street, Homer, NY. 1989.

11. Spielman, A. J. and P. B. Glovinsky. The evaluation and differential diagnosis of insomnia. In M. Pressman and W. Orr, eds. *Sleep and Biological Rhythms in Health and Sickness.* Washington, DC: American Psychological Association. 1997: 125–160.

12. Spielman, A. J., Y. Chien-Ming, and P. Glovinsky. Assessment techniques for insomnia. In M. H. Kryger, T. Roth, and W. C. Dement, eds. *Principles and Practice of Sleep Medicine* (3rd Edition). Philadelphia, PA: W.B. Saunders Company. 2000: 1239–1250.

13. Buysse, D. J., C. F. Reynolds, T. H. Monk, S. R. Berman, and D. J. Kupfer. The Pittsburgh Sleep Quality Index: A new instrument for psychiatric practice and research. *Psychiatry Research* 28: 193–213, 1989.

14. Miles, L. Sleep questionnaire and assessment of wakefulness (SQAW) In C. Guilleminault, ed. *Sleeping and Waking Disorders: Indications and Techniques.* Menlo Park, CA: Addison-Wesley. 1982: 383–413.

15. Douglass, A., R. Bornstein, G. Nino-Murcia, and S. Keenan. Creation of the "ASDC Sleep Questionnaire" *Sleep Research* 15: 117, 1986.

16. Ellis, B. W., M. W. Johns, R. Lancaster, P. Raptopoulos, N. Angelopoulos, and R. G. Priest. The St. Mary's Hospital Sleep Questionnaire. *Sleep* 4(1): 93–97, 1981.

17. Domino, G., G. Blair, and A. Bridges. Subjective assessment of sleep by sleep questionnaire. *Perceptual and Motor Skills* 59(1): 163–170, 1984.

18. Webb, W. B., M. Bonnet, and G. Blume. A postsleep inventory. *Perceptual and Motor Skills* 43: 987–993, 1976.

19. Zammit, G. K. Subjective ratings of the characteristics and sequelae of good and poor sleep in normals. *Journal of Clinical Psychology* 44(2): 123–130, 1988.

20. Akerstedt, T., K. Hume, D. Minors, and J. Waterhouse. The subjective meaning of good sleep, an intra-individual approach using the Karolinska Sleep Diary. *Perceptual and Motor Skills* 79: 287–296, 1994.

21. Johns, M. W., T. J. Gay, M. D. Goodyear, and J. P. Masterson. Sleep habits of healthy young adults: Use of a sleep questionnaire. *British Journal of Prevention and Social Medicine* 25: 236–241, 1971.

22. Spielman, A. J. Assessment of insomnia. *Clinical Psychology Reviews* 6: 11–25, 1986.

23. Spielman, A. J., L. Caruso, and P. Glovinsky. A behavior perspective on insomnia treatment. *Psychiatric Clinics of North America* 10(4): 541–553, 1987.

24. Spielman, A. J. and P. Glovinsky. The varied nature of insomnia. In P. Hauri, ed. *Case Studies in Insomnia.* New York, NY: Plenum Publishing Company. 1991: 1–15.

25. Lacks, P. *Behavioral Treatment for Persistent Insomnia.* New York, NY: Pergamon Press. 1987.

26. Morin, C. M. *Insomnia: Psychological Assessment and Management.* New York, NY: Guilford Press. 1993.

27. Monroe, L. J. Psychological and physiological differences between good and poor sleepers. *Journal of Abnormal Psychology* 72(3): 255–264, 1967.

28. Bonnet, M. H. and D. L. Arand. The consequences of a week of insomnia. *Sleep* 19(6): 453–461, 1996.

29. Bonnet, M. H. and D. L. Arand. Physiological activation in patients with sleep state misperception. *Psychosomatic Medicine* 59(5): 533–540, 1997.

30. Bonnet, M. H. and D. L. Arand. 24-hour metabolic rate in insomniacs and matched normal sleepers. *Sleep* 18(7): 581–588, 1995.

31. Regestein, Q. and J. Dambrosia. Daytime alertness in patients with primary insomnia. *American Journal of Psychiatry* 150: 10, 1993.

32. Pavlova, M., O. Berg, R. Gleason, F. Walker, S. Roberts, and Q. Regestein. Self-reported hyperarousal traits among insomnia patients. *Journal of Psychosomatic Research* 51(2): 435–441, 2001.

33. Horne, J. A. and O. Ostberg. A self assessment questionnaire to determine morningness—eveningness in human circadian rhythms. *International Journal of Chronobiology* 4: 97–110, 1976.

34. Ancoli-Israel, S. Actigraphy. In M. H. Kryger, T. Roth, and W. C. Dement, eds. *Principles and Practice of Sleep Medicine* (3rd Edition). Philadelphia, PA: W.B. Saunders Company. 2000: 1295–1301.

Chapter 9

PRIMARY INSOMNIA: DIAGNOSTIC ISSUES, TREATMENT, AND FUTURE DIRECTIONS

MICHAEL T. SMITH, LEISHA J. SMITH, SARA NOWAKOWSKI, AND MICHAEL L. PERLIS

Insomnia is undoubtedly one of the more common maladies of modern life. Epidemiological surveys estimate that the point prevalence of any insomnia complaint in adults ranges from approximately 30% to 50% (1). Women and older adults (2–3) are approximately 1.3 to 1.5 times more likely to report symptoms (4–5). Only a few large-scale surveys, however, have used rigorous definitions of insomnia. In the studies that have incorporated more stringent criteria, approximately 10% to 15% of adults report disturbed sleep as a serious and persistent problem (4). For example, Ohanyon reported that 11.1% of the general population described difficulty initiating/maintaining sleep (or nonrestorative sleep) for at least three nights a week with concomitant daytime consequences for at least one month (2). Because insomnia research has lacked consistent standards defining the disorder and because the diagnosis of primary insomnia requires the careful evaluation of comorbid medical and psychiatric disorders, prevalence estimates continue to be a source of confusion and debate.

Despite this debate, it is clear that insomnia is a highly prevalent and serious problem, which is often ignored at the clinical level. Most often, insomnia is minimized as an orphan symptom of other disorders. Little attention is given to the aggressive management and monitoring of insomnia as an active symptom—one that has detrimental ramifications for health in general or on the course of the parent disorder in particular (6). Even less attention is given to the thorough evaluation and treatment of primary insomnia itself. This is unfortunate for two reasons. First, several longitudinal studies have found insomnia to be a substantial risk factor for psychiatric (7–9) and medical morbidity (10–12). Second, cognitive-behavioral therapies (CBTs) for primary insomnia are substantially effective (have moderate to large effect sizes; 13–15), with CBT showing effects comparable to medical interventions in the short term (16) and substantially better durability over time (17, 18).

Given that CBT for insomnia is fast becoming the standard of practice for sleep medicine, it is now time to address the issue that most patients with primary insomnia will not receive this form of treatment. This is likely true because most general practice clinicians do not recognize that insomnia may exist as a primary disorder and/or as an independent comorbid symptom that requires specialized evaluation and treatment. Most clinicians conceive of insomnia solely as a symptom of other diseases. Along with this diagnostic bias comes the assumption that "if the parent disorder is successfully treated, the insomnia symptoms will remit" (19). This assumption, however, may be challenged on at least two grounds. First, the diagnosis of secondary insomnia is often hastily made and based solely on whether there is a concomitant medical or psychiatric diagnosis (19). Second, very few data support the concept that remission of the primary medical/psychiatric disorder actually results in the cessation of sleep initiation and/or maintenance problems. This latter problem has become more evident in recent years, with the clear and ubiquitous problem of persistent insomnia in patients with major depression who are successfully treated with selective serotonin reuptake inhibitors (SSRIs; 20–24).

Leaving aside whether the majority of insomnia is properly secondary, there is now a nascent literature showing that patients with pain (25–27), cancer (28–29), and psychiatric disorders (26, 30) respond well to CBT treatment for insomnia. These studies suggest that even in cases where the insomnia is clearly precipitated by other factors, the sleep initiation and/or maintenance problems may exist (or persist) as independent comorbid symptoms. This may be so because the maintaining factors that are thought to contribute to the persistence and severity of primary insomnia can become of greater relevance for the persistence of insomnia symptoms in medically or psychiatrically ill patients than the precipitating or continuing primary conditions (31). If this is the case, an argument can be made that CBT should always be considered for the treatment of *chronic insomnia,* regardless of whether the condition is identified as primary or secondary. The key determination being whether there is evidence of maintaining factors, such as conditioned arousal, irregular sleep wake times, maladaptive beliefs about sleep, etc, which perpetuate the symptom and are amenable to cognitive-behavioral intervention.

In this chapter, we provide an overview of how chronic insomnia is assessed and treated. We hope that this overview (and all of this textbook) will stimulate more clinicians to develop skills within the area of behavioral sleep medicine. It is also our hope that our coverage of alternative methods for standard practices, information on a broad range of interventions, and a discussion of possible directions for research will also prove of interest to expert clinicians.

DEFINITIONS OF INSOMNIA

The World Health Organization defines *insomnia* as a problem initiating and/or maintaining sleep or the complaint of nonrestorative sleep that occurs on at least three nights a week and is associated with daytime distress or impairment (32).

Primary Insomnia

The term *primary insomnia,* which is adopted by the American Psychiatric Association's diagnostic nomenclature (33), is used to distinguish insomnia that is considered to be a distinct diagnostic entity from insomnia that is a secondary symptom of an underlying medical and/or psychiatric condition. The American Psychiatric Association specifies a duration criteria of one month and stipulates that the diagnosis be made when the predominant complaint is difficulty initiating or maintaining sleep or nonrestorative sleep. In either case, the complaint must be associated with significant distress and daytime impairment and not due to other medical, psychiatric, or sleep disorders.

Psychophysiologic Insomnia

In the American Academy of Sleep Medicine's nosology (the *International Classification of Sleep Disorders-Revised* [ICSD-R]), primary insomnia is referred to as *psychophysiologic insomnia.* The ICSD-R definition is more directly tied to the etiologic underpinnings of the disorder. While we do not use this phrase throughout this chapter, it has the advantage of describing the disorder in terms that suggest how insomnia is initiated and maintained. *Psychophysiologic insomnia* is described as "a disorder of somatized tension and learned sleep-preventing associations that results in a complaint of insomnia and associated decreased functioning during wakefulness." (34) *Somatized tension* refers to either the patient's subjective sense of, or objective measures of, somatic hyperarousal while attempting to sleep. Somatic arousal is characterized by peripheral nervous system activity, which is commonly marked by increased muscle tension, rapid heart rate, sweating, and so on. *Learned sleep-preventing associations* refers to the pattern of presleep arousal that appears to be classically conditioned to the bedroom environment, where intrusive presleep cognitions, racing thoughts, and rumination are often taken as indicators of presleep arousal.

Interestingly, none of the nosologies formally embrace the older descriptive clinical characterizations of insomnia in terms of initial, middle, and terminal (late) insomnia. Trouble falling asleep is often referred to as *initial, early,* or *sleep-onset* insomnia. Trouble with frequent or prolonged awakenings is often labeled *middle* or *sleep maintenance* insomnia. Waking up earlier than desired and being unable to fall back asleep is referred to as *late, terminal,* or *early morning awakening* insomnia. Waking up feeling unrefreshed is commonly referred to as *nonrestorative* sleep. Patients often report some combination of these descriptions, which is generally referred to as *mixed* insomnia. For the purpose of this chapter, although we consider the International Classification system to provide a more precise definition of the disorder, we use the term *primary insomnia* because it is the most widely embraced term in clinical practice in the United States. We adopt the more descriptive terminology when a more specific characterization of the presenting complaint is required.

Apart from presenting a specific definition of the disorder/disease entity, there is the need to qualify the duration and severity of the defined illness. Typically, duration is framed dichotomously in terms of acute and chronic stages. Severity can be construed in one of two ways. In one case, standards are set for what constitutes significant deviance from population norms with respect to frequency and intensity of presenting symptoms. In the other case, standards are set by setting the bar for pathologic at a level that is modal for patients who are help-seeking.

Duration of Illness

Insomnia lasting less than one month is generally considered acute and is often associated with clearly defined precipitants such as stress, acute pain, or substance abuse. Insomnia is characterized as being chronic when symptoms persist unabated for a duration of at least one month and, more typically, for durations of six months or greater. These cutoffs are relatively arbitrary and correspond to traditional medical definitions of what constitutes short and long periods of time. There are currently no studies that use risk models to evaluate the natural course of insomnia. Thus, there is no way of definitively defining *chronicity* in terms related to when the disorder becomes severe, persistent, and (for want of a better expression) self-perpetuating. One clinical cue for differentiating between acute and chronic insomnia resides in the way patients characterize their complaints. When patients stop causally linking their insomnia to its precipitant and instead indicate that their sleep problems seem "to have a life of their own," this change in presentation may:

1. Serve to define the *cut point* between the acute and chronic phases of the disorder
2. Suggest when CBT may be indicated

Severity of Illness

Intensity

Although there are no formal diagnostic criteria, most investigators consider 30 or more minutes to fall asleep and/or 30 or more minutes of wakefulness after sleep onset to represent the threshold between normal and abnormal sleep. Recent work by Lichstein and colleagues suggests that this criteria should be set at "more than 30 minutes" because this definition is better related to the occurrence of complaint in population studies (35). With respect to how much sleep, many investigators are reluctant to fix a value for this parameter. Of the investigators that are inclined to set minimums, most specify that the amount of sleep obtained on a regular basis be equal to or less than either 6.0 or 6.5 hours per night. The reluctance to establish total sleep time parameters is due, in part, to the difficulty in establishing precisely what is considered abnormal. Representing what is pathological with a single number is too confounded by factors such as age, prior sleep, and the individual's basal level of sleep need. The lack of an established total sleep time cutoff is also related to the possibility that profound sleep initiation or maintenance problems may occur in the absence of sleep loss. This is an important distinction, because it is often assumed that insomnia is synonymous with sleep deprivation. While it is certainly true that the daytime symptoms associated with insomnia might be explained, in part, by partial chronic sleep deprivation, daytime symptoms need not be ascribable only to lack of sleep. For example, it has been shown that patients with insomnia reliably exhibit sleep micro-architectural disturbances such as enhanced high-frequency activity during non-rapid eye movement (NREM) sleep (36–40). This type of activity, which appears to be independent from sleep continuity and architecture parameters, has been shown to be correlated with patient perceptions about their sleep quality and quantity (36, 41, 42).

Frequency

There is also no fixed benchmark for frequency of symptoms. Most clinical researchers, in this case, require that subjects experience problems on three or more nights per week, but this may have more to do with increasing the odds of studying the occurrence of the disorder in laboratory than an inherent belief that less than three nights per week is normal.

Commonalities and Problems with Current Definitions

All of these definitions show a degree of consistency, both in terms of what is and is not delineated. Common to all is that:

1. Insomnia is defined as a subjective complaint.
2. Patients must report compromised daytime functioning.
3. There are no specific criteria for how much wakefulness is considered pathologic (before desired sleep onset or during the night).
4. There are no criteria for how little total sleep must be obtained to fall outside the normal range.

The latter two of these issues have already been explicated (lack of quantitative criteria for sleep latency [SL], wake time after sleep onset [WASO], and total sleep time [TST]). The former two require further discussion.

Insomnia as a Subjective Complaint

Defining insomnia as a subjective complaint without requiring objective verification of signs and symptoms has advantages and disadvantages. The advantage of having subjective criteria is that it recognizes the primacy of the patient's experience of distress or disease. That is, ultimately, patients seek, comply with, and discontinue treatment based on their perception of wellness. The disadvantage is that such measures, when used alone, do not allow for a complete characterization of either the patient's condition or the disorder in general.

Insomnia and Daytime Impairment

Daytime complaints are required for diagnosis because, in the absence of such complaints, it is possible that the phenomena of short sleep may be misidentified as insomnia. Frequent complaints associated with insomnia include fatigue, irritability, problems with attention, and concentration and distress directly related to the inability to initiate and/or maintain sleep.

DIAGNOSTIC PROCESS

The clinical diagnosis of primary insomnia, like any disease or disorder, requires that the patient undergo a thorough evaluation. Typically, this process has two steps. First, an intake evaluation is conducted to characterize the history of the presenting complaint and to gather demographic, medical, and psychiatric information. The evaluation usually requires that subjects complete a variety of questionnaires and a face-to-face interview. Although each clinic varies as to what instruments are used, a typical battery is illustrated in Table 9.1. Second, most clinicians prospectively monitor the patient's sleep for one to two weeks. During this period, sleep-wake diaries are completed before bed and immediately on awakening. These data are used to better characterize the form, frequency, and severity of the sleep complaint. Diaries may also be used to assess the factors that might moderate the incidence or severity of the presenting complaint (e.g., presence or absence of bed partner, napping, medication use, food allergies, alcohol use). The combination of the intake interview and sleep diary data allows for the establishment of a final diagnosis and formation of a treatment

Table 9.1   Typical Set of Questionnaires Administered at Intake

Instrument	Purpose(s)
A general information questionnaire	Obtain demographic and psychosocial information.
A medical history survey	Obtain a list of the patient's past and present medical problems.
A medical symptoms checklist	Assess for current medical symptoms and aid in evaluating the possibility of occult medical disorders.
Beck Depression Inventory (BDI) Hamilton Rating Scale for Depression (HRSD)	Identify and quantify depressive symptoms and aid in the assessment of depression as a diagnosis.
Beck Anxiety Inventory (BAI) State-Trait Anxiety Inventory (STAI) Penn State Worry Questionnaire	Identify and quantify anxiety symptoms and aid in the assessment of anxiety disorders.
A general checklist of sleep disorders symptoms Pittsburgh Sleep Quality Index (PSQI) Insomnia Severity Index (ISI) Rochester Sleep Continuity Inventory (RSQI) Epworth Sleepiness Scale Multi-Dimensional Fatigue Inventory Beliefs and Attitudes about Sleep Scale	Assess for occult intrinsic sleep disorders. Quantify sleep disturbance (general). Profile insomnia complaint. Quantify severity of insomnia complaint. Quantify sleepiness and fatigue. Assess sleep-related worry and misinformation.

plan. For more information on the assessment of insomnia, see Chapter 8 (Spiel man et al.).

Differential Diagnosis

The inability to fall asleep (initial insomnia), stay asleep (middle insomnia), or the tendency to awaken early in the morning (terminal insomnia) may be related to a variety of factors, including primary medical or psychiatric conditions. Table 9.2 contains an abridged list for each of these categories.

Table 9.2   List of Contributing Factors for Each Type of Insomnia

Common Factors That Contribute to Insomnia

Medical illness:

Chronic and acute pain conditions (e.g., arthritis, fibromyalgia, back pain, headaches), chronic obstructive pulmonary disease, asthma, diabetes, cardiac conditions, head injuries, hyperthyroidism, gastroesophageal reflux disease, seizure disorder, Parkinson's disease, Alzheimer's disease, kidney disease, and so on

Psychiatric illness:

Major depression, generalized anxiety disorder, posttraumatic stress disorder, panic disorder, bipolar disorder, dementia, schizophrenia

Acute medication effects:

Alcohol, amphetamines, caffeine, reserpine, clonidine, SSRI antidepressants, steroids, L-dopa, theophyline, nicotine, nifedipine, Beta agonists (albuterol), and so on

Withdrawal medication effects:

Benzodiazepines, barbiturates, alcohol

Other sleep disorders:

Obstructive sleep apnea, narcolepsy, nocturnal myoclonus (periodic limb movement disorder), restless legs syndrome, phase advance sleep disorder, phase delay sleep disorder, sleep state misperception disorder, nightmare disorder, parasomnias, and so on

Poor sleep environment:

Noise, ambient temperature, light, sleeping surface, bed partner, family pets, and so on

Poor sleep habits:

Extended time in bed, naps, irregular schedule

Situational factors:

Life stress, bereavement, unfamiliar sleep environment, jet lag, shift work

Note: Adapted from "The Diagnosis of Primary Insomnia and Treatment Alternatives," by M. L. Perlis and S. Youngstead, 2000, *Comprehensive Therapy* 26, pp. 298–306.

In routine practice, it is tempting to assume that medical and psychiatric considerations are not important. After all, most patients must be referred for behavioral sleep medicine treatment; therefore, they have, in effect, been pre-screened. Even when the patient has been referred, a careful clinical history and review of the patient's medical and psychiatric record are required to determine how these factors may or may not account for their symptoms. It cannot be assumed that because the patient was referred as an insomniac, he or she actually has chronic or primary insomnia. The critical judgment required is whether there is an occult psychiatric or medical disorder responsible for precipitating or (more importantly) maintaining the insomnia. To do this, the symptoms that correspond to the traditional rule outs must be assessed, which may not have been considered by the referring clinician. Consider these two examples:

1. A family practice physician refers a patient for treatment for insomnia. On interview, it becomes clear that the insomnia is acute and is better characterized as total sleeplessness. This, along with other positive signs for bipolar disorder or schizophrenia, might suggest that this patient is in a prodromal phase for one of these disorders and would best be served by being referred for a full psychiatric evaluation.

2. A psychiatric social worker refers a patient for treatment for insomnia. On interview, it becomes clear that the insomnia developed within the last three to five months. There is no clear precipitating event, but the patient reports that she has been experiencing fatigue, irritability, problems with memory, and decreased libido. On a symptom checklist, she endorses several more somatic concerns including cold intolerance, brittle and dry hair and skin, hair loss, abnormal menstrual cycles, and muscle aches and cramps. This set of signs and symptoms, while suggestive of depression, is also entirely consistent with hypothyroidism. Accordingly, the patient may be best served by first having a physical to rule out organic factors that may be directly contributing to the insomnia.

As clear as these examples are, making the distinction between primary and secondary insomnia can be challenging. In clinical practice, there is often considerable overlap of symptoms. In the case of diagnosed illness, another critical decision must be made: If the patient has one or more diagnosed medical or psychiatric conditions, are those conditions likely to be maintaining the insomnia? To address this question, the clinician must determine if the underlying condition is adequately treated, stable, and/or truly in remission. If the answer is no, it may be prudent to delay the CBT treatment for insomnia. If, on the other hand, the data provided by the patient and the collaborating clinicians suggest that the other disease entities are indeed adequately treated and stable and there is evidence that there are cognitive behavioral factors maintaining the insomnia, a trial of CBT is warranted.

Establishing that the patient's insomnia is not maintained by medical or psychiatric illness constitutes one-half of the differential diagnosis process. The other half of the process requires the determination of whether the insomnia is a symptom of one of the other intrinsic sleep disorders or is primary along this dimension as well. This process is complicated, in part, because insomnia is both a formal and vernacular term. For example, many patients with obstructive sleep apnea (OSA) report at intake that they have insomnia. On interview, it usually becomes clear that this is more of an attribution than a clear statement of the facts. OSA patients are profoundly sleepy during the day and often attribute this to insomnia. What is meant by insomnia, however, has nothing to do with the inability to fall asleep and stay asleep. Instead, OSA patients infer that their sleep must be nonrestorative for them to feel so sleepy during the day. Because their sleep is nonrestorative, they characterize it as insomnia. Interestingly, our current classification systems also allow for the complaint of nonrestorative sleep to be synonymous with insomnia. Most would agree, however, that:

1. Sleep initiation and/or maintenance problems are required for the diagnosis of insomnia.
2. The complaint of nonrestorative sleep better represents and/or corresponds to complaint of impaired daytime function.

Once it is determined whether the patient has difficulty initiating or maintaining sleep and/or significant problems with excessive daytime sleepiness, it is possible to differentiate between the two major classes of intrinsic sleep disorders: those associated with problems initiating and maintaining sleep (DIMS) and those associated with problems of excessive daytime sleepiness (DOES). Figure 9.1 provides a schematic that characterizes the differential diagnostic process and illustrates how the decision tree incorporates circadian rhythm disorders and periodic leg movements of sleep as they occur in association with the complaint of insomnia. Table 9.3 contains a complete list of intrinsic, circadian, and extrinsic sleep disorders as they are defined by the ICSD nosology (34).

Detailed Information on the Major Diagnostic "Rule Outs" for Primary Insomnia

Medical Conditions

Common medical illnesses that should be considered in ruling out the diagnosis of primary insomnia include insomnias secondary to inadequately treated, unstable,

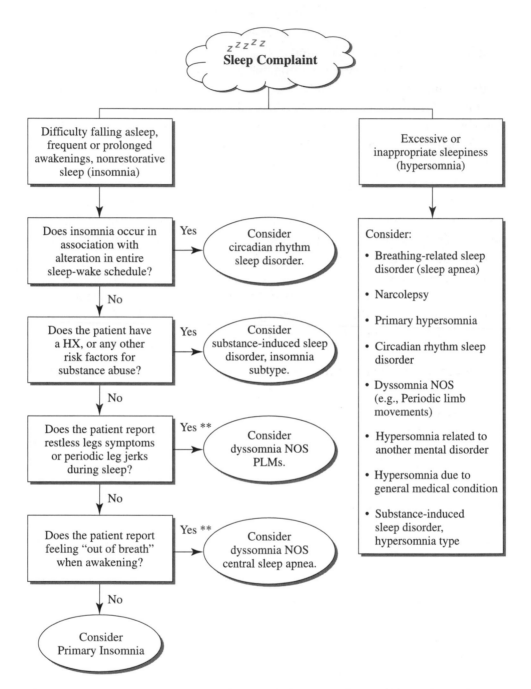

**Figure 9.1 A Schematic of the Differential Diagnosis Process for Primary Insomnia. ****Note that the two last-choice boxes are flagged because there are no reliable signs and symptoms that can be obtained on clinical interview to detect occult CSA or PLMs. Adapted with permission from "The Evaluation and Treatment of Insomnia," by D. J. Buysse and M. L. Perlis, March 1996, *Journal of Practical Psychiatry and Behavioral Health,* pp. 80–93.

Table 9.3   List of ICSD Sleep Disorders

Dyssomnias		
Intrinsic Sleep Disorders	Circadian Rhythm Sleep Disorders	Extrinsic Sleep Disorders
Psychophysiological insomnia	Time zone change (jet lag) syndrome	Inadequate sleep hygiene
Sleep state misperception		Environmental sleep disorder
Idiopathic insomnia	Shift work sleep disorder	Altitude insomnia
Narcolepsy	Irregular sleep-wake pattern	Adjustment sleep disorder
Recurrent hypersomnia	Delayed sleep phase syndrome	Insufficient sleep syndrome
Idiopathic hypersomnia	Advanced sleep phase syndrome	Limit setting sleep disorder
Posttraumatic hypersomnia	Non-24-hour sleep-wake disorder	Sleep-onset association disorder
Obstructive sleep apnea syndrome	Circadian rhythm sleep disorder NOS	Food allergy insomnia
Central sleep apnea syndrome		Nocturnal eating (drinking) syndrome
Central alveolar hypo-ventilation syndrome		Hypnotic-dependent sleep disorder
Periodic limb movement disorder		Stimulant-dependent sleep disorder
Restless legs syndrome		Alcohol-dependent sleep disorder
Intrinsic sleep disorder NOS		Toxin-induced sleep disorder
		Extrinsic sleep disorder NOS

Note: Adapted from "The Diagnosis of Primary Insomnia and Treatment Alternatives," by M. L. Perlis and S. Youngstead, 2000, *Comprehensive Therapy* 26, pp. 298–306.

and/or recurrent chronic pain, cardiopulmonary diseases (e.g., chronic obstructive pulmonary disease), gastrointestinal disorders (e.g., gastroesophageal reflux disease), renal disease, neuroendocrine disorders (e.g., hyperthyroidism or hypothyroidism, estrogen deficiency), and neurologic conditions (e.g., dementia). In these instances, it would be prudent to assume that the first step in treatment is the appropriate medical or psychiatric intervention. If the insomnia persists, CBT may be indicated in conjunction with ongoing medical/psychiatric treatment.

Little empirical work has been done on:

1. Whether unique sleep continuity profiles map onto any one set of medical disorders
2. Reciprocal interaction effects (the possibility that poor sleep may be precipitated by the medical disorder but then may serve to exacerbate it)
3. The possibility that effective insomnia treatment may positively impact on the parent or primary disorder

Psychiatric Disorders

Insomnia is a significant feature of the majority of Axis I psychiatric conditions, particularly affective and anxiety disorders. Conversely, many patients with primary insomnia exhibit at least subsyndromal levels of psychiatric symptomatology (43). There is also a fair amount of evidence that the two classes of disorders may interact. For example, primary insomnia may be a risk factor for new onset and/or recurrent major depression (see Figure 9.2; 23, 32, 41, 44, 49, 94, 104) and may be a prodromal symptom of both (45).

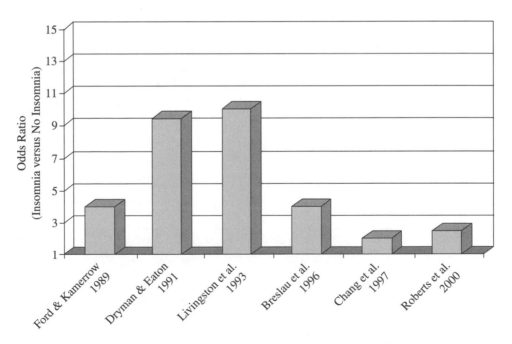

Figure 9.2   The Behavioral Model of Insomnia

In clinical practice, it is often difficult to distinguish the primacy or directionality of the relationship, that is, whether the insomnia represents a subsyndromal form or a residual symptom of a psychiatric disorder or whether the insomnia is primary and the psychiatric symptomatology (e.g., mood disturbance, attention and concentration difficulties) is secondary to sleep loss. While such distinctions may seem academic, identifying which disorder is primary is likely to have important treatment implications. As with medical illness, when the psychiatric illness is deemed primary (and is untreated or unstable), pharmacologic and/or nonpharmacologic strategies that specifically target the psychiatric illness should be the first line of treatment. Alternatively, if the insomnia is identified as primary, pharmacologic and/or nonpharmacologic strategies that specifically target the insomnia should be the first line of treatment. In either case, both forms of symptoms should be monitored to allow a change in treatment strategy as the clinical situation warrants.

Intrinsic Sleep Disorders

The primary rule outs in this domain are sleep apnea, narcolepsy, periodic limb movement disorder, and restless legs syndrome. Each of these disorders may have insomnia as a chief complaint. During the screening process, it is important to distinguish between the complaint of fatigue and excessive daytime sleepiness (EDS). Often, patients use the terms *fatigue* and *sleepiness* interchangeably. *Fatigue* refers to physical and/or mental weariness; the patient clearly indicates that his or her performance is compromised and attributes this to being worn out. *Sleepiness,* on the other hand, may or may not include fatigue but is characterized by patients clearly indicating that they are fighting to stay awake or that they cannot resist falling asleep. Patients with primary insomnia often report fatigue and anergia but less frequently complain of or demonstrate EDS. As indicated throughout this chapter, EDS is more characteristic of other intrinsic sleep disorders such as obstructive sleep apnea, periodic limb movement disorder, and narcolepsy. It should also be noted, however, that daytime sleepiness may be associated with insufficient sleep syndrome. Insufficient sleep syndrome is essentially involuntary or voluntary sleep deprivation in the absence of insomnia symptoms. It has been estimated that 2% of the general population experience significant daytime sleepiness due to failing to get enough sleep for reasons such as work schedule or leisure activities (46).

In the absence of a formal assessment using polysomnographic procedures such as the Multiple Sleep Latency Test (MSLT; 47), brief self-report measures such as the Epworth Sleepiness Scale (48) can serve as a rough guideline to differentiate between disorders of excessive daytime somnolence (DOES) or disorders of initiation and maintenance of sleep (DIMS). When daytime sleepiness is the key complaint, referral for nocturnal polysomnographic assessment is indicated.

Circadian Rhythm Disorders

When the presenting complaint is an extreme and pure sleep onset or early morning awakening problem, the possibility of a chronobiologic disorder should be considered. In general, chronobiologic sleep disorders result when the circadian sleep-wake cycle becomes out of phase with the desired sleep period. Such patients have normal sleep when they adjust their sleep window to match their chronobiologic clocks. The two most common circadian problems are phase delay and phase advance. Phase delays are more common during adolescence and usually involve a sleep onset complaint of two hours or more, with difficulty rousing in the morning. An individual with phase advance syndrome normally presents with the complaint of sleepiness in the early evening and significant early morning awakenings of two hours or more. Persons with phase disorders often report normal sleep on weekends when they naturally shift their sleep pattern to match their circadian rhythm because of lack of work-related constraints. Classification of sleep disorders is not necessarily mutually exclusive, and many disorders may exist and coexist on a continuum. Thus, it is possible that individuals meeting criteria for psychophysiologic insomnia may also have circadian factors that contribute to their sleep disturbance. While there are a number of diagnostic tests such as assessing dim light melatonin onset and measuring core body temperature, which provide markers of the circadian disturbance, such tests are primarily used in research settings and are currently impractical and typically not necessary in the clinical setting.

Extrinsic Sleep Disorders

Another important differential diagnostic category to rule out is external factors that interfere with sleep processes. Among the most common extrinsic sleep disorders are dyssomnias associated with medication, drug, or alcohol use. As shown in Table 9.2, insomnia is often associated with medications, either as an acute side effect or as part of a withdrawal syndrome. The behavioral sleep medicine specialist should consider the possible side effect profiles of any medication taken by the patient, including over-the-counter remedies, such as allergy medications and analgesics, which frequently contain sympathomimetics or caffeine. Although it may not be possible to discontinue medications deemed to be aggravating the insomnia, the timing, dosing, or decision to switch to an alternative medication may be a feasible option to discuss with the patient's physician.

A common problem seen in patients discontinuing chronic use of sedative hypnotics is rebound insomnia. Such effects may be directly related to the withdrawal process. Unfortunately, many patients find it difficult to stop taking sedative hypnotics, because the resumption of insomnia on discontinuation is often believed to indicate a relapse, rather than a transient effect of medication withdrawal. The attribution of relapse often prompts a vicious cycle of continued medication use.

In addition to evaluating medication usage, a thorough history of substance use and abuse should be a routine part of the evaluation of insomnia. While stimulant use such as cocaine and methamphetamines is often recognized by patients as aggravating insomnia, many are unaware of alcohol's detrimental effects on sleep continuity and architecture. In fact, alcohol is often used by the patient to promote sleep (4), but it can contribute to sleep maintenance insomnia with moderate to heavy consumption.

Lifestyle and environmental factors, such as noise, lighting, diet, timing of exercise, and so on, are also common extrinsic causes of insomnia. When they are deemed the primary cause of insomnia, such factors are used to make the diagnosis of inadequate sleep hygiene in the ICSD classification scheme, or dyssomnia-NOS in the American Psychiatric Association classification (*DSM*). However, many patients with primary insomnia engage in a number of maladaptive sleep hygiene practices, such as smoking cigarettes before going to bed, napping excessively, and/or failing to sound- and light-attenuate their sleep environment.

Assessment and Measurement

Self-Report Assessment

As indicated in Table 9.1, behavioral sleep medicine specialists often use a number of retrospective assessment tools to gather more precise diagnostic information. In addition, behavioral sleep medicine specialists use daily sleep diaries (49) to prospectively monitor sleep complaints. Prospective assessment is important for:

1. Evaluating the severity of insomnia complaints on a day-to-day basis
2. Identifying the behaviors that maintain the insomnia
3. Determining to what extent circadian dysrhythmia is present
4. Gathering the data needed to measure and guide treatment response

The sleep component of sleep-wake diaries is typically completed after waking and obtains information on time to bed, wake time, sleep latency (SL), frequency of nightly awakenings (FNA), wake time after sleep onset (WASO), total sleep time (TST), early morning awakenings (EMA), medication/substances taken before bed, and subjective assessments of sleep quality. The daytime measures, which are completed before going to bed, include nap frequency and duration, fatigue ratings, stimulant consumption, and medication usage. For additional information on sleep diaries, see Chapter 2 in this text (Smith et al.).

Objective Assessment

In current clinical practice, the diagnosis of primary insomnia does not require an in-laboratory, polysomnographic (PSG) study to substantiate the diagnosis for three primary reasons. First, there is enough of a general correspondence between the subjective complaint and objective measures that PSG assessment is not required to verify the sleep continuity disturbance. Second, traditional polysomnography does not reveal, or allow for the quantification of, the underlying sleep pathophysiologies that presumably give rise to the patient's complaints. Third, and most pragmatically, third-party payers will not reimburse for sleep studies on patients with likely primary insomnia. Sleep studies are, however, indicated if the patient demonstrates symptoms consistent with other intrinsic sleep disorders and/or fails to respond to treatment.

When assessed with polysomnography, patients with primary insomnia reliably exhibit increased sleep latency, increased frequency of nightly awakenings, increased wake after sleep onset time, and decreased total sleep relative to good sleeper controls. PSG findings, however, do not correspond in a one-to-one fashion to patient perceptions of sleep continuity. Patients with insomnia routinely report more severe sleep disturbance than is evident on traditional PSG measures (50–52). Some have argued that this discrepancy might be explained by the findings that patients with primary insomnia show a greater degree of psychopathology, including tendencies to somatize internal conflicts and exaggerate symptoms (53–55). Others have argued that the subjective-objective discrepancy findings reflect a cardinal feature of the disorder, that is, the persistence of sensory and information processing into NREM sleep. The continuance of such processes into PSG-defined sleep is thought to be the basis for patient difficulties distinguishing between wakefulness and sleep (56). The extent to which one or both of these factors contribute to the discrepancies between subjective and objective measures of sleep in insomnia continues to be a matter of ongoing debate. (For additional information on these issues, see the following section on the cognitive-behavioral perspective on insomnia.)

When polysomnography is not feasible, the use of alternative, less costly objective devices can be particularly helpful when the clinician suspects a high degree of sleep state misperception. *Sleep state misperception* is a term (as well as a disorder) used to describe the common finding among patients with insomnia that there is a discrepancy between a patient's subjective impression of sleep parameters and what is measured via objective recording methods. At the level of

self-report, extreme values (gathered retrospectively or prospectively) may sug
gest that this is a component of the disorder (e.g., sleep latencies of greater than
two hours, wake after sleep onset of greater than two hours, or a total sleep time
of equal to or less than four hours). In the absence of a PSG study, actigraphs
may be used to obtain corroborating prospective data. Actigraphs are wristwatch-like devices that use sophisticated movement detectors to estimate the traditional sleep continuity parameters (e.g., SL, WASO, FNA, and TST). This
information may, in turn, be compared to the self-report data to assess the degree
to which sleep state misperception is occurring. The extent to which subjec-
tive/objective discrepancies can be resolved using actigraphy has not yet been
subjected to adequate empirical validation. In our clinical practice, however, we
have found that actigraphy can be used to assess for sleep state misperception.
For additional information on actigraphy, see Chapter 2 in this text (Smith et al.).

THE COGNITIVE-BEHAVIORAL PERSPECTIVE ON INSOMNIA

Behavioral Perspective

Since the late 1980s, insomnia has largely been conceptualized from within a behavioral framework. The original model was proposed by Spielman and colleagues,
and it continues to be the leading theory for both sleep medicine and the subspecialty area of behavioral sleep medicine (57). As illustrated in Figure 9.3, the behavioral model posits that insomnia occurs acutely in relation to both predisposing
(trait) and precipitating (state) factors and occurs chronically in relation to perpetuating or maintaining factors. Thus, an individual may be prone to insomnia due
to trait characteristics, experience acute episodes because of precipitating events,
and have chronic insomnia because of a variety of perpetuating factors. With respect to trait factors, personality characteristics (56, 58), physiologic arousal (56,
58), and genetic predisposition (59) are each thought to predispose the individual
to acute episodes of insomnia. Typical precipitating events (which represent stressors within the larger stress diathesis model of disease) include situational stress
(60), acute injury or pain, bereavement, and so on. Perpetuating factors, as the
term implies, maintain the chronic form of the disorder even after the precipitating
events have either been stabilized or resolved. Perpetuating factors are any of a variety of maladaptive, compensatory strategies in which the patient engages in an
attempt to cope with insomnia symptoms. Typical examples of such factors are excessive daytime napping, extending sleep opportunity, keeping variable sleep-wake
schedules, using alcohol as a hypnotic, spending excessive time awake in bed, and
diminishing daily activity level due to fatigue. Central to the behavioral model of

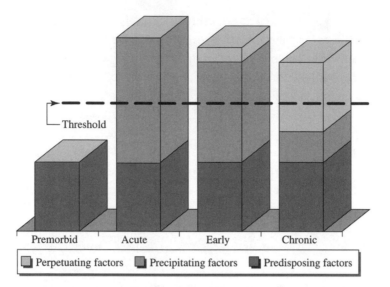

Figure 9.3   A Graphic Representation of Insomnia as a Risk Factor for Depression. Adapted with permission from "The Varied Nature of Insomnia" by A. J. Spielamn and P. Glovinsky, in P. J. Hauri (Ed.), *Case Studies in Insomnia* (pp. 1–15). New York: Plunum Press, 1991.

chronic insomnia is the role of classical conditioning as the primary maintaining factor. It is hypothesized that, over time, insomnia becomes a conditioned response to the bed and bedroom environment (stimuli). This process presumably occurs via traditional principles of classical conditioning, due to repeated parings of the bed and bedroom (conditioned stimuli) with states of psychophysiologic hyperarousal (unconditioned stimuli) that are thought to interfere with the normal biologic processes of sleep initiation and maintenance.

Cognitive Perspective

A number of authors have stressed the importance of cognitive factors in primary insomnia (61–63). Given their emphasis on the role of cognition, they and others have developed the interventions that provide for the cognitive component of the more broad-based cognitive-behavioral approach. In this perspective, two related types of cognitions are thought to be operational: One set is related to patients' beliefs about their disorder; the other set is related to cognitive processes such as intrusive thoughts and worry.

Morin et al., for example, has found that patients with primary insomnia have a number of maladaptive beliefs about sleep, including unrealistic views about what constitutes adequate sleep and catastrophic beliefs about the consequences of insomnia. Such beliefs presumably contribute to insomnia via:

1. Increasing sleep-related performance anxiety
2. Prompting and promoting maladaptive compensatory behaviors

Support for the role of such factors derives from data showing that successful cognitive-behavioral treatment of insomnia is associated with a reduction in negative beliefs and attitudes about sleep (15, 64). While this is suggestive, more work is needed to demonstrate the insomnogenic potential of such cognitions because it is easy to imagine that successful therapy may change an individual's thoughts and beliefs but also that such changes may not be responsible for the treatment gains.

Hall et al. and Harvey and colleagues have focused more on cognitive process (versus content) issues. Central to this area is that patients with insomnia often complain that they are unable to sleep because of intrusive thoughts or excessive worry. These thoughts and images are characterized as being intrusive and may occur in isolation or as unwanted perseverative-type problem solving (worry). The content of the thoughts and worry may be centered on the kind of dysfunctional attitudes and beliefs described previously, but they are often more general in content. The ideation and imagery that occur as intrusive thoughts are often related to mundane daily activities and/or work or relationship issues. As with dysfunctional attitudes and beliefs, intrusive thoughts and perseverative thinking (from within the radical cognitive perspective) are thought to be responsible for the occurrence and severity of insomnia. The more moderate view is that these phenomena are, along with behavioral and conditioning factors, contributory.

Support for the cognitive perspective comes from a variety of studies that have found that patients with primary insomnia complain of higher levels of presleep rumination compared to normal controls (65–66). Investigations of presleep thought content have found that the presleep cognitions of patients with primary insomnia tend to be more negatively toned and that patients report increased general problem solving and thoughts pertaining to environmental stimuli at or around sleep onset (67–69).

Neurocognitive Perspective

In sharp contrast to the cognitive model, the neurocognitive perspective all but suggests that dysfunctional beliefs and worry are epiphenomena. It is posited that cognitive factors are likely to mediate the occurrence and severity of insomnia when the disorder is acute. When, however, the disorder is chronic, cognition occurs secondary to conditioned arousal. That is, patients with chronic insomnia are not awake because they are given to rumination and worry, but, rather, they ruminate because they are awake.

The neurocognitive perspective (56) is an extension of the traditional behavioral model. As laid out by Spielman and colleagues (57), the behavioral model allows for a compelling conceptualization as to how maladaptive behaviors lead to conditioned arousal and chronic insomnia. The Spielman model does not, however, spell out what the conditioned arousal is or why and how arousal interferes with sleep initiation and/or maintenance and/or the perception of sleep. These latter issues are explained in the neurocognitive model, which defines *arousal* as conditioned cortical arousal. This form of arousal may be observed in patients with primary insomnia as high-frequency EEG activity (14 to 45 Hz) at or around sleep onset and during NREM sleep (36–37). High-frequency EEG activity, it is hypothesized, allows for abnormal levels of sensory and information processing and long-term memory formation. Increased sensory processing is thought to interfere with the ability to initiate sleep (as measured by traditional PSG measures). Increased information processing during PSG-defined sleep is thought to interfere with the subject's ability to perceive PSG sleep as sleep. Increased long-term memory formation (attenuation of the normal mesograde amnesia of sleep) is thought to interfere with the patient's morning judgments about sleep quality and quantity.

Support for the neurocognitive perspective (70) comes from a variety of studies, which have found Beta EEG (14 to 45 Hz) to:

1. Be elevated in patients with insomnia (36–40)
2. Be positively associated with patient perceptions of sleep quality (41–42, 71)
3. Be positively associated with sleep state misperception (the degree of discrepancy between subjective and objective measures of sleep; 36, 72)
4. Vary with successful CBT treatment for insomnia (73)

There is also preliminary evidence that the occurrence of elevated NREM Beta activity is sensitive and specific to primary insomnia (versus insomnia secondary to major depressive disorder; 36) and data that suggest the long-term memory function at peri-sleep onset intervals is altered in patients with chronic insomnia (74).

COGNITIVE-BEHAVIORAL TREATMENT

The most common cognitive-behavioral therapies for primary insomnia are sleep hygiene education, stimulus control, sleep restriction, relaxation training, and cognitive therapy. For a detailed explanation of each of these therapies, see *Insomnia: Psychological Assessment and Management,* by Charles Morin (61). As for the clinical efficacy of the behavioral approach, there is clear evidence that the treatment modality is effective (13–14). When either stimulus control and/or sleep restriction is used, clinical gains at five weeks are comparable to, if not more effective than, those produced by benzodiazepine receptor agonist hypnotics (16–18). Unlike hypnotics, behavioral interventions have demonstrated long-term benefits after treatment is discontinued (up to two years; 17). Of all the available psychological treatments, stimulus control therapy is the most well validated and is considered the gold standard for the behavioral treatment of insomnia. In practice, most behavioral sleep medicine clinicians adopt a multicomponent approach, which usually contains at least stimulus control, sleep restriction, and sleep hygiene therapies.

Therapeutic Regimen

The cognitive-behavioral treatment of insomnia generally requires four to eight weeks' time with once a week face-to-face meetings with the clinical provider. Sessions range from 30 to 90 minutes depending on the stage of treatment and the degree of patient compliance. Intake sessions are usually 60 to 90 minutes in duration. During this session, the clinical history is obtained and the patient is instructed in the use of sleep diaries. No intervention is provided during the first week. This time frame is used to collect the baseline sleep-wake data that will guide treatment for the balance of therapy. The primary interventions (stimulus control and sleep restriction) are deployed over the course of the next one to two 60-minute sessions. Once these treatments are delivered, the patient enters into a phase of treatment where total sleep time is upwardly titrated over the course of the next two to five visits. These follow-up sessions require about 30 minutes unless additional interventions are being integrated into the treatment program. Adjunctive treatments include cognitive therapy, relaxation training, and relapse prevention.

First-Line Interventions

Stimulus Control Therapy

Stimulus control therapy (SCT) is recommended for both sleep initiation and maintenance problems. The therapy is generally considered as the first-line behavioral treatment for chronic primary insomnia because it has the most research support (75). Stimulus control instructions limit the amount of time patients spend awake in the bed/bedroom and are designed to decondition presleep arousal and reassociate the bed/bedroom environment with rapid, well-consolidated sleep. Typical instructions include:

1. Keep a fixed wake time seven days per week, irrespective of how much sleep you got during the night.
2. Avoid any behavior in the bed or bedroom other than sleep or sexual activity.
3. Sleep only in the bedroom.
4. Leave the bedroom when awake for approximately 15 to 20 minutes.
5. Return only when sleepy.

Some clinicians, in an effort to prevent clock watching behavior, encourage patients to leave the bedroom as soon as they feel clearly awake or experience annoyance and irritation over the fact that they're awake. The combination of these instructions reestablishes the bed and bedroom as strong cues for sleep and entrains the circadian sleep-wake cycle to the desired phase.

Sleep Restriction

Sleep restriction therapy (SRT) is recommended for both sleep initiation and maintenance problems. The therapy requires patients to limit the amount of time they spend in bed to an amount equal to their average total sleep time (determined from baseline sleep diary data). To accomplish this, the clinician works with the patient to:

1. Establish a fixed wake time
2. Decrease sleep opportunity by limiting subjects' time in bed (TIB) to an amount that equals their average total sleep time (TST) as ascertained by baseline sleep diary measures

Once a target amount of time in bed is set, the patient's bedtime is delayed to later in the night so that the TIB and average TST are the same. Initially, this intervention results in a reduction in total sleep time, such that patients get less total sleep than they are accustomed to. This controlled form of sleep loss usually corresponds to a decrease in sleep latency and wake after sleep onset time. Thus, during the acute phase of treatment, patients get less sleep but sleep in a more consolidated fashion (i.e., they fall asleep more quickly and stay asleep for longer periods of time). The increase in consolidated sleep is formally represented as sleep efficiency (TST/TIB).

The patient's sleep efficiency is monitored on a weekly basis. If the patient's average weekly sleep efficiency reaches 85% to 90% (depending on age), the patient's sleep opportunity is incrementally increased by 15 minutes. The increase in sleep opportunity is accomplished by having the patient retire 15 minutes earlier for the next week of treatment. The upward titration process is usually continued for about four weeks, thus allowing for an increase of about one hour in sleep opportunity. When the patient does not reach the 85% to 90% benchmark, some clinicians reduce the total sleep opportunity to the previous set point, others maintain the subject's total sleep opportunity until adequate sleep efficiency is observed, while still others combine these approaches. With respect to the last possibility, the clinician may maintain total sleep opportunity for two to three weeks and then downwardly titrate the TIB when there is clear evidence that patients cannot sustain their clinical gains.

This therapy is thought to be effective for two reasons. First, it prevents patients from coping with their insomnia by extending sleep opportunity. This strategy, while increasing the opportunity to get more sleep, produces a form of sleep that is shallow and fragmented. Second, the initial sleep loss that occurs with SRT is thought to increase the pressure for sleep, which in turn produces quicker sleep latencies, less wake after sleep onset, and more efficient sleep.

Three points merit further comment. First, total time in bed is manipulated by phase delaying the patient's sleep period. This, along with keeping a fixed wake time, results in sleep restriction. It is plausible, however, that total time in bed could be altered by having the subject wake up at an earlier time. This approach is not adopted because fixing wake up time at an early hour:

1. Does not capitalize on the fact that extending wakefulness is easier to tolerate than curtailing sleep
2. Delays the initial increase in time awake before sleep for 24 hours (and thus delays the clinical effect)
3. May reinforce the tendency for early morning awakenings
4. Undermines the opportunity to pair sleep with the bed/bedroom

Second, it should be noted that SRT has a couple of paradoxical aspects to it. One paradox is that patients who report being unable to sleep are in essence being told to sleep less. The other paradox occurs over the course of treatment. With therapy, patients find that it is difficult to stay awake until the prescribed hour. This, if not paradoxical, is at least ironic for the patient who initially presents with sleep onset difficulties. Finally, it should be noted that sleep restriction may

be contraindicated in patients with histories of mania or seizure disorder because it may aggravate these conditions.

Adjunctive Interventions

Sleep Hygiene Education

Sleep hygiene education is recommended, along with SRT and SCT, for both
sleep initiation and maintenance problems. It may also have some value as a
means toward increasing total sleep time. Sleep hygiene education addresses a
variety of behaviors that may influence sleep quality and quantity. The intervention most often involves providing the patient with a handout and then reviewing the items and the rationales for them. Table 9.4 contains a set of sleep
hygiene instructions. In this formulation, several aspects of other therapies are
adopted. For example, items 1, 2, 12, 13, and 15 are traditionally considered part
of stimulus control and/or sleep restriction therapy.

Sleep hygiene education is most helpful when tailored to a behavioral analysis
of the patient's sleep-wake behaviors. The tailoring process allows clinicians to:

1. Demonstrate the extent to which they comprehend the patient's individual
   circumstances (increases the therapeutic alliance)
2. Explain important background about factors that influence sleep
3. Modify the sleep hygiene guidelines to increase compliance while continuing to encourage sleep promoting behaviors

   Rigid prescription of sleep hygiene guidelines can be short-sighted, over
   simplistic, and may jeopardize the therapeutic alliance/relationship. For
   example:

   —The admonishment to avoid caffeinated products may be, in general, too
   simply construed. Caffeinated beverages may be used to combat daytime
   fatigue (especially during acute therapy) and, if the withdrawal is timed
   correctly, may actually enhance the subject's ability to fall asleep.

   —Similarly, the prohibition against napping may be impractical and un-
   necessary. Elderly subjects or subjects with extreme work performance
   demands may indeed need to compensate for sleep loss. A more considerate approach to napping may entail taking into account the time of the
   nap, the duration of the nap, and how nocturnal sleep is handled on days
   when patients nap. Napping earlier in the day will allow for more homeostatic pressure for nocturnal sleep. Limiting the duration of the nap
   will allow for less of a discharge of the homeostat and enhance subjects'

Table 9.4   Sleep Hygiene Instructions

Sleep Hygiene Instructions

1. *Sleep only as much as you need to feel refreshed during the following day.* Restricting your time in bed helps to consolidate and deepen your sleep. Excessively long times in bed lead to fragmented and shallow sleep. Get up at your regular time the next day, no matter how little you slept.

2. *Get up at the same time each day, 7 days a week.* A regular wake time in the morning leads to regular times of sleep onset, and helps to set your biological clock.

3. *Exercise regularly.* Schedule exercise times so that they do not occur within 3 hours of when you intend to go to bed. Exercise makes it easier to initiate sleep and deepen sleep.

4. *Make sure your bedroom is comfortable and free from light and noise.* A comfortable, noise-free sleep environment will reduce the likelihood that you will wake up during the night. Noise that does not awaken you may also disturb the quality of your sleep. Carpeting, insulated curtains, and closing the door may help.

5. *Make sure that your bedroom is at a comfortable temperature during the night.* Excessively warm or cold sleep environments may disturb sleep.

6. *Eat regular meals and do not go to bed hungry.* Hunger may disturb sleep. A light snack at bedtime (especially carbohydrates) may help sleep, but avoid greasy or heavy foods.

7. *Avoid excessive liquids in the evening.* Reducing liquid intake will minimize the need for nighttime trips to the bathroom.

8. *Cut down on all caffeine products.* Caffeinated beverages and foods (coffee, tea, cola, chocolate) can cause difficulty falling asleep, awakenings during the night, and shallow sleep. Even caffeine early in the day can disrupt nighttime sleep.

9. *Avoid alcohol, especially in the evening.* Although alcohol helps tense people fall asleep more easily, it causes awakenings later in the night.

10. *Smoking may disturb sleep.* Nicotine is a stimulant. Try not to smoke during the night when you have trouble sleeping.

11. *Don't take your problems to bed.* Plan some time earlier in the evening for working on your problems or planning the next day's activities. Worrying may interfere with initiating sleep and produce shallow sleep.

12. *Train yourself to use the bedroom only for sleeping and sexual activity.* This will help condition your brain to see bed as the place for sleeping. Do not read, watch TV, or eat in bed.

13. *Do not try to fall asleep.* This only makes the problem worse. Instead, turn on the light, leave the bedroom, and do something different like reading a book. Don't engage in stimulating activity. Return to bed only when you are sleepy.

14. *Put the clock under the bed or turn it so that you can't see it.* Clock watching may lead to frustration, anger, and worry, which interfere with sleep.

15. *Avoid long naps.* Staying awake during the day helps you to fall asleep at night. Naps totaling more than 30 minutes increase your chances of having trouble sleeping at night.

Note: This list includes the usual practices described as *good sleep hygiene,* but it also includes some principles subsumed under *stimulus control therapy* (2, 12–13), *sleep restriction therapy* (1–2, 15), and *relaxation* (11, 13). Adapted from "The Diagnosis of Primary Insomnia and Treatment Alternatives," by M. L. Perlis and S. Youngstead. *Comprehensive Therapy* 26(4): 298–306, 2000.

sensation of feeling rested from the nap (by avoiding awakening from slow wave sleep). Going to bed later, when they nap during the day, may minimize the effects of the nap on nocturnal sleep.

Finally, it can be argued that one of the most important aspects of sleep hygiene education derives not so much from the tips provided, but from allowing clinicians the opportunity to demonstrate their knowledge. A thoughtful and elaborate review may enhance patients' confidence in their therapist and in the treatment regimen. Such enhanced confidence may, in turn, lead to greater adherence/compliance with the more difficult aspects of therapy.

Cognitive Therapy

Several forms of cognitive therapy for insomnia have been developed. Some have a didactic focus (61), others use paradoxical intention (76), others employ distraction and imagery (77), and still others use a form of cognitive restructuring (78). While the approaches differ in procedure, all are based on the observation that patients with insomnia have negative thoughts and beliefs about their condition and its consequences. Helping patients to challenge the veracity of these beliefs is thought to decrease the anxiety and arousal associated with insomnia. The cognitive restructuring approach is adapted from the procedure used for panic disorder (79–81).

Cognitive restructuring focuses on catastrophic thinking and the belief that poor sleep is likely to have devastating consequences. While psychoeducation may also address these kinds of issues, the more important ingredient of cognitive restructuring lies not in disabusing patients of erroneous information, but, rather, in having them discover that their estimates are inaccurate (a testament to the tendency to think in less than clear terms in the middle of the night). When undertaking this exercise with patients, it needs to be introduced in a considerate way, one that avoids any hint that the therapist is being pedantic, patronizing, or condescending.

The following are examples of catastrophic thinking that occurs when the patient is lying in bed trying to sleep. "If I don't get a good night's sleep:

- *I'll be in a bad mood tomorrow.* If my mood is poor tomorrow, I will—yet again—be short with my wife. If I'm irritable with my wife (again), she may start thinking about not putting up with this anymore. If she thinks about not putting up with this anymore, she'll consider leaving me . . ." [get divorced].
- *I won't be able to stay awake or concentrate when I'm driving to work.* If I don't stay awake or concentrate when I'm driving, I may get into an accident . . ." [wreck the car].

- *I won't be able to function tomorrow at work.* If I am not able to function at work, I may get a reprimand. If I get reprimanded . . ." [get fired].

The first step in the cognitive restructuring process is to have patients discuss and make a list of the kinds of negative things they think can happen when their sleep is poor. Usually, the list is constructed with the patient and placed on the cognitive therapist's ever present in-office chalkboard. Column one is the list of catastrophic events. The patient may need to be prompted to identify the underlying and most catastrophic thought. For example, the patient may say: "I worry about not being able to fall sleep," when what he or she is primarily worried about is the extreme version of this proposition: spending the entire night awake.

Once the list is compiled (5 to 10 things constitutes a reasonable list), patients are then asked how likely they think each of the events are, given a night of poor sleep. For instance, the therapist may ask, "When you are lying in bed imagining being so tired tomorrow that you might perform badly at work, *at that moment* how certain are you that your work will be 'substandard,' how certain are you that you'll be 'reprimanded'?" and so on. These data are represented in column two. Next, patients are asked how frequently their sleep is poor and for how many years they have been suffering from insomnia. This number is coded as the "number of days with insomnia" and is set to the side of the table (to be coded later in column 3). The final data needed from patients is an estimate of how frequently each of the catastrophic events has occurred. These are coded into the fourth column. The combination of these four sources of data are then used to show patients that there is a substantial mismatch between their degree of certainty and the number of times the negative events have actually transpired.

For example, the clinician might observe, "You have suffered from insomnia for five nights a week for the past three years. This means that you have had about 800 really bad nights. You also said that when you're thinking about what might happen if you don't fall asleep, you are 90% certain that on the next day you are going to perform so badly that you'll be reprimanded. If it happened 90% of the time and you've had 800 bad nights, then you should have been reprimanded about 700—lets say 500—times." These data are represented in the fifth column. The last column of data is then compared to the list in the fourth column so that the patient can see the mismatch between the number of instances that should have occurred and the number of instances that actually occurred. For an example of the chart described, see Table 9.5 on page 242.

Relaxation Training

Different relaxation techniques target different physiological systems. Progressive muscle relaxation is used to diminish skeletal muscle tension (82–86).

Table 9.5   An Example of a Typical Worksheet Used during Cognitive Restructuring for Insomnia

Number of Days with Insomnia *800*

1	2	3	4	5
Event	Certainty When Lying Awake and Unable to Sleep	Number of Days with Insomnia	Number of Event Occurrences	Number of Event Occurences Given Certainty
Get reprimanded	90%	800	5	620 (500)
Get fired				
Get divorced				
Wreck the car				
Be awake all night				

Diaphragmatic breathing is used to make respiration slower, deeper, and mechanically driven from the abdomen as opposed to the thorax. (It is interesting to note that this form of respiration resembles what occurs naturally at sleep onset.) Autogenic training focuses on increasing peripheral blood flow by having subjects imagine, in a systematic way, that each of their extremities feels warm. The use of imagery is often incorporated in each of these relaxation approaches.

Most practitioners select the optimal relaxation method based on the technique that is easiest for the patient to learn and most consistent with how the patient manifests arousal. Like cognitive techniques, learning to effectively use relaxation training often requires substantial practice. Many clinicians recommend that the patient rehearse the skill during the day in addition to practicing before sleep. When integrating into stimulus control instructions, if relaxation training causes some initial performance anxiety, it may be best to have the patient practice in a room other than the bedroom. It also should be borne in mind that some patients, especially those with a history of panic disorder, may experience a paradoxical response to relaxation techniques.

Phototherapy

While many may not consider phototherapy a behavioral intervention, the use of bright light is often important to integrate into the treatment regimen. This is especially true when circadian factors appear to substantially contribute to the insomnia complaint. There is substantial empirical evidence that bright light has sleep-promoting effects.

If the patient's insomnia has a phase delay component (i.e., the patient prefers to go to bed late and wake up late), bright light exposure in the morning for a period of 30 minutes or more may enable the patient to feel sleepy at an earlier time in the evening. If the patient's insomnia has a phase advance component (i.e., the patient prefers to go to bed early and wake up early), bright light exposure in the late evening/early night may enable the patient to stay awake until a later hour. Phototherapy is often accomplished via a light box, which typically generates white light or, more selectively, blue spectrum light at 5,000 to 10,000 lux. The dose is adjusted by altering the distance and duration of light exposure. It is generally assumed that phototherapy has no significant side effects, but this is not always the case. Mania may be triggered by bright light but rarely, if ever, in patients not previously diagnosed with bipolar mood disorder. Other side effects are insomnia, hypomania, agitation, visual blurring, eye strain, and headaches. Light boxes may not be recommended for individuals with certain eye conditions, including retinopathy secondary to diabetes. In some cases, equivalent or better phase-shifting properties may be accomplished by scheduling time outdoors by taking early morning walks, for example.

The sleep-promoting effects of bright light may occur via several mechanisms, including shifting the circadian system, enhancement of the amplitude of the circadian pacemaker, promoting wakefulness during the day and sleep at night, or indirectly, via its antidepressant effects.

Complicating Factors

A number of potential complicating factors require continuous monitoring and evaluation throughout the course of treatment, particularly if the patient fails to show expected clinical gains after two to four sessions of active treatment. The most common complicating factors are poor treatment compliance, issues related to comorbid psychiatric and medical disorders, and the simultaneous use of sedative hypnotics.

Treatment Compliance

The single most important complicating factor is poor treatment compliance. At the beginning of treatment, the clinician should proactively address the fact that the prescriptions may seem counterintuitive and that adhering to the treatment will be difficult. Providing the patient with a complete and thoughtful rationale for each aspect of the treatment, managing the patient's expectations, and encouraging an active self-management approach are essential. Providing the rationale for treatment is likely to gain compliance in at least two ways. First, the effort to explain therapy is less imperative and thereby makes the patient an active partner in the treatment process and less resistant or reactive to the prescriptions. Second, a fluid, interesting, and compelling explanation will support and enhance the patient's perception of the clinician as a competent authority.

With respect to expectation, patients should not anticipate that the results will be immediate. In fact, patients should be cautioned that their sleep problem is likely to briefly get worse before it gets better. Sometimes an appeal to the research literature, demonstrating that treatment gains are maintained and often continue to improve in the long term, may help maintain their motivation despite the short-term difficulty adjusting to the procedures.

With respect to active self management, it is important to remember that the treatment alternative is medication and that this requires very little in the way of lifestyle change. Thus, the clinician must spend a considerable amount of time working with the patient to make and stay with the investment.

Comorbity of Mental and Medical Disorders

Many patients with chronic insomnia report mild or subthreshold levels of depressive symptoms. When depressive symptoms become severe, they may interfere with the patient's ability and motivation to successfully follow the recommended protocol. If medical factors become exacerbated, expectations for clinical gains need to be tempered until there is stabilization. Throughout the course of treatment, both medical and psychiatric factors should be monitored and consideration given for the need for further evaluation and intervention.

Cognitive-Behavorial Therapy and Sedative Hypnotics

Not yet addressed is the possibility of using sedative hypnotics acutely, along with cognitive-behavioral treatment for insomnia (i.e., dual or combined therapy). This is a promising and underinvestigated area of inquiry. Initial studies were mixed (18, 87, 88), but promising work continues (89). The benefit of combined therapy is a more rapid reduction of symptoms. The risk of combining pharmacotherapy with behavioral treatment, however, is that once patients start using medications, they may be less inclined to adopt or tolerate the behavioral interventions. Work is ongoing to determine the most effective way to combine these two strategies to capitalize on the immediate reduction in symptoms afforded by sedative hypnotics and the long-term efficacy of cognitive-behavioral treatment (90).

Perhaps more important than the issue of combined therapy to the practice of CBT for insomnia is that many of the patients referred for cognitive-behavioral treatment have been taking sedative hypnotics for years and are very apprehensive about discontinuing treatment. Often, the initial phases of treatment involve collaboration with the referring physician to assist the patient in the weaning process. Use of sleep diaries to provide feedback about sleep continuity during the withdrawal process and education about rebound insomnia and the medication it-self are important for this kind of intervention. The chronic use of sedative hyp-notics often leaves the patient with as poor a sleep continuity profile as if no medications at all were being used. This is difficult for the patient to appreciate because of the rebound insomnia that occurs during the withdrawal period. As noted previously in this chapter, the natural assumption during the withdrawal from medication is "This is how I will sleep without medications from now on." In combination with a careful weaning process, sleep diaries may serve as the hard data to demonstrate to the patient that this assumption is not true.

Case Example

April 1, 2002

Demographic Information. (Identifying information has been altered to protect confidentiality.) Mrs. McMuffin is a 51-year-old married European American. She currently works in part-time private practice as an attorney. She is 5′5″ and weighs 150 lbs (body mass index = 25).

Chief Complaint

"I have had trouble falling asleep since high school. Now I have trouble with both falling asleep and staying asleep. It's been pretty bad lately, and I am afraid it will keep me from returning to working full time."

Sleep Continuity/Quality. In the past six months, Mrs. McMuffin reported trou-ble falling asleep with an average sleep latency ranging from 60 to 90 minutes on five or more nights per week. Although her sleep latency varies from night to night, she stated that she rarely falls asleep in less than 30 minutes. Mrs. McMuf-fin also reported sleep maintenance insomnia, stating that she wakes up three to four times per night for about 30 to 45 minutes total approximately three nights per week. She has trouble sleeping on both weekdays and weekends. She denied early morning awakenings and stated that she often has difficulty waking up on time and sleeps late into the morning. When attempting to fall asleep or return to sleep, Mrs. McMuffin ruminates and feels mentally alert ("can't turn my mind off"), despite being tired and fatigued during the day. She describes feeling ag-gravated when she is unable to sleep and worries that she will have trouble con-centrating at work. When sleeping in novel environments (work travel or vacations), Mrs. McMuffin reports her insomnia is reliably less severe. She de-nied waking up gasping for breath, loud snoring, or symptoms of periodic limb movements and restless legs syndrome at this time.

(continued)

Daytime Functioning/Symptoms. Mrs. McMuffin reportedly wakes up with a dry mouth and headaches one to two mornings per week. She stated that daytime fatigue and irritability (which is ascribed to her insomnia) interfere with her ability to work and enjoy daily activities. She denied falling asleep at inappropriate times or places.

History of Presenting Complaint. Mrs. McMuffin first experienced insomnia during her senior year in high school. She attributed this to the stress associated with trying to decide which university to attend. She has been intermittently bothered by sleep initiation and maintenance problems since. She indicated that she tolerated her sleep difficulties, which flared periodically during times of stress, until 1998. At this time, her sleep initiation problem worsened in association with her failure to be made a partner in her law firm. She stated that this failure was due to a conflict with one of the senior partners. Before the decision was made about the partnership, she began working longer hours, often not returning to her home until late at night, in hopes of influencing the decision. She attempted to cope with daytime fatigue by sleeping late on the weekends (1 P.M.) and by drinking large quantities of caffeine (16 to 18 cups a day) during the weekdays. In 2001, she decided to quit the firm and start her own private practice. At this time, she had gained 25 pounds (from 140 to 165 pounds), and her insomnia worsened to the point where it was a significant problem every night.

Prior Treatment for Sleep Disorders. In 2001, Mrs. McMuffin was evaluated by Dr. Nolieberger at her local sleep disorders center. She sought treatment because her husband complained she was snoring loudly, and she was experiencing severe daytime sleepiness in addition to fatigue and persistent insomnia. She underwent a nocturnal PSG study to evaluate the possibility of sleep disordered breathing. Mrs. McMuffin was found to have mild obstructive sleep apnea (OSA) with a sleep Respiratory Disturbance Index (RDI) of 8 events per hour (49 events per hour during REM sleep and 3 per hour during NREM sleep) without significant oxygen desaturation The events were primarily confined to REM sleep with the most substantial arousals being associated with the supine sleep position. On a follow-up study night, Mrs. McMuffin was tried on CPAP [continuous positive airway pressure] at an initial setting of 8 cm H_2O. Final treatment recommendations reportedly were (1) weight loss, (2) amitriptyline, 20mg, qhs, and (3) a trial of CPAP therapy. She was referred to her primary care physician and subsequently lost 25 pounds, with noticeable improvement in snoring and daytime sleepiness. She reportedly did not tolerate and discontinued CPAP, which she stated exacerbated her insomnia because of feelings of claustrophobia. According to her primary care physician, he believed that her sleep apnea had resolved. Her primary care physician referred her for behavioral sleep medicine treatment for persistent insomnia, after he had tried sleep hygiene education and amitriptyline (currently discontinued with no evidence of resurgence in sleep apnea symptoms) with little benefit.

Medical History. The patient denied any perinatal complications, reportedly achieving all developmental milestones within normal time frames. She described herself as having a relatively "healthy childhood" with the exception of frequent throat infections, which abated following a tonsillectomy/adenoidectomy (1952). Her two births were without complication and she is premenopausal. The patient's medical history is significant for frequent heartburn gastroesphageal reflux disease (GERD), which she developed in her early 30s. Her GERD symptoms are reliably worse after "rich" meals, and she reports nocturnal sequelae if she eats within a few hours of bedtime. The patient's GERD is treated with famotidine (Pepcid AC), prn. Mrs. McMuffin denies tobacco use and reports regular alcohol use (one martini per night). The patient reported that she used to smoke, but that she quit 10 years ago.

Personal and Family. Mrs. McMuffin lives with her husband of 30 years. She described herself as happily married. She has two children who are ages 20 (male) and 25 (female). Mrs. McMuffin herself is an only child. Both parents have been deceased for 10 years, having died from cardiovascular disease. Mrs. McMuffin's father was a prominent attorney, whom she described as a workaholic who frequently complained of insomnia but never sought treatment. Her mother worked as a part-time nurse. Mrs. McMuffin denied any family psychiatric history. The patient stated that she enjoyed a relatively happy childhood with no reported history of physical or sexual abuse. Mrs. McMuffin characterized herself as having been a hard-driving student as a teenager, who was active in sports. She graduated at the top of her high school and college classes before earning her JD degree from Harvard University.

Psychiatric History. Mrs. McMuffin denied previous psychiatric or psychological treatment, including hospitalizations. She also denied a history of suicidal ideation or attempts.

Current Medications. famotidine (Pepcid AC) 10mg prn.

Maladaptive Sleep-Related Behaviors. The patient endorsed a number of behaviors that may interfere with sleep and maintain her chronic insomnia. She reports that when she is unable to sleep, she usually lies in bed, aggravated by her inability to sleep. She also keeps an irregular sleep-wake schedule, going to bed two to three hours earlier when she has had trouble sleeping the previous night. On weekends, she reportedly sleeps late in an effort to catch up on lost sleep.

(continued)

Psychometric Indexes. In addition to clinical interview, the patient completed several self-report measures, including the Beck Depression and Anxiety Inventories, the Epworth Sleepiness Scale, and the Multidimensional Fatigue Inventory. The self-report measures were consistent with the findings of the clinical interview. On the Beck Depression Inventory, the patient reported symptoms at the mild level of severity (BDI = 10). On the Beck Anxiety Inventory, she reported symptoms in the minimal range (BAI = 4). The findings on both instruments are accounted for in part by the sleep disturbance item(s) on these measures. On the Multidimensional Fatigue Inventory, she reported a moderate degree of general fatigue (MFI = 14). On the Epworth Sleepiness Scale, she scored a 5, which is within normal limits.

Diagnostic Impressions

(307.42-0) Primary insomnia
History of mild obstructive sleep apnea

Treatment Plan—Follow-Up

Contact sleep disorders center to obtain full sleep report and discuss patient status.

Initiate a standard CBT regimen for primary insomnia. Monitor closely for worsening of OSA symptoms, particularly excessive daytime sleepiness (EDS) and snoring. CBT treatment to include stimulus control, sleep restriction therapy, sleep hygiene education, and cognitive therapy.

If insomnia symptoms are nonresponsive, more aggressive therapy for the GERD should be considered because this may not be adequately stabilized and partly responsible for the middle insomnia.

If the symptoms of OSA worsen (regardless of treatment outcome with the insomnia), consider a second PSG evaluation. If the OSA is mild and position related, (a) institute an exercise and weight loss program and/or (b) treat with positional therapy and/or consider a dental device. If the OSA is substantially worse and requires CPAP, undertake a CPAP desensitization regimen.

PHARMACOLOGIC TREATMENT OPTIONS

While most agree that monotherapy with pharmacologic agents is not ideal for the treatment of chronic insomnia, it is important to know about this form of intervention for at least two reasons. First, some patients may wish to be informed about their medical treatment options. Second, a sound knowledge about pharmacotherapy is required for a smooth interface with our sleep medicine colleagues.

There are a variety of empirically validated pharmacologic treatments for insomnia. The most commonly used therapies are benzodiazepine and the newer benzodiazepine receptor agonists such as zolpidem and zaleplon. In recent years, the use of sedating antidepressants and anticonvulsants has become increasingly popular in clinical practice despite a lack of mature literature on their use in primary insomnia. For a discussion of pharmacologic treatment approaches, see Buysse and Perlis (78). As for the clinical efficacy of the medical approach, it is clear that sedative hypnotics produce rapid results and about a 40% to 50% reduction in illness severity in the short term (two to four weeks; 91). Hypnotics, however, are generally not recommended for long-term use because of concerns about tolerance, possible daytime side effects, and rebound insomnia on discontinuation. While some of these concerns are mitigated by the newer benzodiazepine receptor agonists, no studies yet exist that demonstrate the long-term efficacy of these agents beyond 12 months or that treatment gains are maintained on withdrawal from medication. Of the studies that are as long as 12 months, though the data are suggestive, none of the studies are placebo controlled, and several do not use intent to treat-type statistical approaches.

Sedative Hypnotics

The most common hypnotic agents are benzodiazepines and imidazopyridines. Common examples of benzodiazepines that are marketed as hypnotics include estazolam (Prosom), quazepam (Doral), flurazepam (Dalmane), and temazepam (Restoril). The imidazopyridines that are marketed as hypnotics include zolpidem (Ambien) and zaleplon (Sonata). Both benzodiazepines and imidazopyridines purportedly bind selectively to GABA BZ1 and/or BZ2 receptor subtypes and have, to varying extents, myorelaxant, anticonvulsant, antianxiety, and amnestic properties. As hypnotics, these agents have low to moderate side effect profiles and good clinical efficacy relative to placebo.

The side effects, which vary largely as a function of elimination half-life, include daytime sedation; performance and cognitive impairment; and increases in daytime anxiety, nausea, and dizziness. Daytime sedation and cognitive impairments are thought to account for the increased risk of falls and automobile accidents that occur with the use of hypnotics.

The efficacy of these agents was addressed in a meta-analysis (91) showing that benzodiazepines and imidazopyridines produce significant changes in sleep latency (15- to 45-minute reductions), number of awakenings (one to three fewer), and total sleep time (15- to 60-minute increases). Of the various hypnotics evaluated in the meta-analysis, temazepam was found to have the largest effect on sleep latency and the second largest effect on total sleep time.

While benzodiazepines and imidazopyridines promote sleep, they often do not improve daytime performance. Thus, patients may take a sleeping pill in the hope that it will improve their sleep and their daytime function, but they may find that while their sleep is improved, their daytime function continues to be impaired (92–94). Impairment of function by hypnotics is well documented in short-term use, and there is no evidence that these impairments resolve with long-term use.

In the final analysis, the choice to prescribe sedative hypnotics must take into account:

1. There is little research concerning the long-term efficacy of these types of medications.

2. Sedative hypnotics do not appear to produce any long-term gains once the treatment regimen is discontinued.

In the case of benzodiazepines, the FDA guidelines explicitly recommend against long-term prescription. In addition, there is no research to suggest that benzodiazepines may be used effectively for periods longer than four to eight weeks, even with escalating the dosage. When patients discontinue using benzodiazepines, there appear to be no long-term benefits. Rather, a rebound insomnia occurs after withdrawal, a possible sign of dependence. Finally, like most medications, benzodiazepines alter sleep architecture, modestly suppressing REM sleep and substantially suppressing slow wave sleep. Given that the former is thought to be associated with mood and/or memory consolidation and the latter is thought to be associated with somatic restoration, suppression of these forms of sleep in favor of sleep continuity improvements may, in the long run, not be advisable.

In the case of imidazopyridines, the FDA guidelines also recommend against their long-term prescription. There is, however, some preliminary evidence suggesting that sleep-promoting effects of imidazopyridines may be maintained over time intervals up to 12 months (95–96). In addition, this class of hypnotics appears not to alter sleep architecture or result in rebound insomnia.

One final cautionary note is in order. Although there is little research on the long-term efficacy and/or safety of sedative hypnotics, epidemiologic data suggest that chronic use may be associated with increased mortality. In a study by Kripke et al. (97), nightly use of hypnotics was found to be associated with a 35% increased risk of mortality in men and a 22% increased risk of mortality in women. In a sample of more than 1 million people, these risks were approximately equivalent to those associated with smoking one to two packs of cigarettes per day. Thus, these data underscore the recommendation that chronic use of hypnotics should be avoided (97).

Antidepressants

Antidepressant medications are indicated for insomnia when sleep difficulties occur in association with mood or anxiety disorders. In practice, sedating antidepressants are often used to treat primary insomnia. The rationale for the off-label prescription by many practitioners is based on two beliefs: Chronic primary insomnia is not an independent clinical entity, but, rather, a symptom of a depression that is either not fully remitted or not yet an acute episode; and sedative antidepressants are more suitable for the long-term treatment of primary insomnia. This latter belief rests on the fact that sedative antidepressants have hypnotic value and the added advantages of long-term efficacy without habituation and low abuse profile (98).

Only two studies of sedating antidepressants have been undertaken in patients with primary insomnia (98–99). In one study, trimipramine increased total sleep time by about 65 minutes and increased sleep efficiency (TST/TIB) by about 10%; these effects were maintained for 30 days. Moreover, patients did not exhibit rebound insomnia when the medication was discontinued. In fact, the clinical gains appear to have persisted over a two-week withdrawal period.

The decision to use antidepressants to treat primary insomnia must take into account the risk of serious adverse consequences, including increased likelihood of cardiovascular effects (e.g., conduction changes, orthostatic hypotension) and anticholinergic side effects (e.g., blurred vision, constipation, dry mouth). In cases of overdose, death is far more likely with tricyclics than with benzodiazepines and imidazopyridines.

In summary, sedative antidepressants may represent a good alternative to long-term use of hypnotics in patients with primary insomnia. The lack of empirical validation and the potential for adverse events, however, suggest that other treatment options should be considered.

POSSIBLE RESEARCH AGENDA

Clinical Research

Over the past 10 to 15 years, substantial progress has been made with respect to establishing the efficacy, durability, and practicability of nonpharmacologic treatments for insomnia. We are fortunate that:

1. Several cognitive-behavioral treatments for insomnia have been developed (100–102).
2. A large number of clinical efficacy studies have been undertaken and summarized meta-analytically (14).

3. There is good evidence that the effects of CBT and medical treatment are comparable in the short term (61, 103).

4. CBT interventions appear to have significant long-term durability (15, 104).

Several important issues, however, remain.

First, how does effective treatment impact on clinical course, including time to recurrence, recurrence rates, and severity and/or duration of new episodes? While such studies have been undertaken in depression research, no long-term studies in insomnia have focused on these issues.

Second, does CBT impact on clinically relevant conditions beyond the disorder itself? As indicated early in this chapter, data now suggest that chronic untreated insomnia is associated with, and is a risk factor for, psychiatric (7–9, 43–45) and medical morbidity (11, 105). Of the two domains, less work has been undertaken concerning the medical correlates of insomnia. While several studies have shown that insomnia is associated with increased point prevalence of gastrointestinal, musculoskeletal, and central nervous system complaints (11), only one study has built on the associational data and provided relative risk assessments (11). Katz and colleagues found that patients with insomnia, when followed for two years, were 1.4 to 3.4 times more likely to develop problems with congestive heart failure, obstructive airway disease, and prostate, hip, and back problems. More research is needed. It would also be productive to extend our efforts beyond disease to system abnormalities (e.g., neuroendocrine and immune function abnormalities). If it is accepted that insomnia may be a risk factor for the subsequent development of medical and/or psychiatric disease, the question that needs to be directly addressed is: "Is insomnia a modifiable risk factor?" That is, when patients with insomnia are effectively treated, are these patients healthier than those not treated or not successfully treated?

Third, how is successful treatment related to personal and socioeconomic considerations? Does treatment result in better quality of life, enhanced work productivity, and/or less overall economic burden? Work by Zammit and colleagues (106) shows that insomnia is substantially associated with poorer quality of life and with increased absenteeism. Work by Johnson and Spinweber (107) indicates that insomnia is related to poorer work performance and fewer promotions. Data are needed to show that effective treatment diminishes such personal and socioeconomic costs.

In short, treatment intervention studies are needed that have, as outcome variables, not only improvement in sleep continuity, but also a broad spectrum of related clinical, personal, and social variables. Only in this way will we be able to demonstrate the broad-ranging, long-term value of behavioral sleep medicine interventions. Such demonstrations will provide the kind of information that will convince the larger medical and psychiatric communities of the value of CBT as a treatment for insomnia.

Experimental Research

The initial burst of physiologic and neurophysiologic research on insomnia that occurred during the 1970s and 1980s has all but come to a standstill—perhaps for several reasons. One possibility is that the discovery and validation of successful treatments may have diminished the press to better understand the biopsychosocial causes of insomnia. Alternatively, given effective treatment, we may have been too inclined to accept the theoretical models underlying CBT as having sufficient explanatory power. Another possibility is that early attempts to characterize insomnia with polysomnography presented us with a puzzle; that is, there were, and are, substantial discrepancies between self-report and polysomnographic measures of severity. To some, this may have suggested that the disorder was more psychological than biological in nature, which may have discouraged further exploration using physiologic measures. Finally, the dearth of funding for insomnia research, particularly in recent years, may have discouraged active investigation.

Whatever the reasons for the relative lack of biobehavioral research on insomnia, there is not a lack of interesting questions. Several directions are worth considering as targets for experimental research into the pathophysiology of insomnia. One direction would be to formally test the behavioral principles that are theorized to be operative in insomnia. For example, is it possible in humans to demonstrate that cues associated with the bed, bedroom, and/or bedtime do indeed produce arousal responses? Alternatively, conditioning experiments could be undertaken using animal models. Seligman's success with the conditioned helplessness paradigm suggests that an animal model of insomnia should be possible (108).

Another productive direction would be to expand on recent work on somatic (109) and cortical arousal (37, 110) by evaluating whether these domains are interrelated, how they produce sleep initiation and maintenance problems (DIMS), and/or how they contribute to sleep state misperception. Perhaps most important is that efforts are made to specify how somatic and/or cortical arousal are related to DIMS phenomena. It is not enough to say that arousal is incompatible with "relaxation" and thus incompatible with the ability to initiate and/or maintain sleep. We need to identify *how* the phenomena are incompatible.

In closing, we acknowledge that we have pointed out only a few possible avenues for research. Our intent is to stimulate investigators to renew their interests in both basic and clinical insomnia research. The questions are out there, and with the recent call for more insomnia research by the National Center on Sleep Disorders Research (111), perhaps the necessary funds are out there as well.

REFERENCES

1. Zorick, F. J. and J. K. Walsh. Evaluation and management of insomnia: An overview. In M. H. Kryger, T. Roth, and W. C. Dement, eds. *Principles and Practice of Sleep Medicine.* Philadelphia, PA: W.B. Saunders Company. 2000: 615–623.

2. Ohanyon, M. Epidemiological study on insomnia in the general population. *Sleep* 19: S7–S15, 1996.

3. Foley, D. J., A. Monjan, E. M. Simonsick, R. B. Wallace, and D. G. Blazer. Incidence and remission of insomnia among elderly adults: An epidemiologic study of 6,800 persons over three years. *Sleep* 22(Suppl. 2): S366–S372, 1999.

4. Ancoli-Israel, S. and T. Roth. Characteristics of insomnia in the United States: Results of the 1991 National Sleep Foundation Survey. I. *Sleep* 22(Suppl. 2): S347–S353, 1999.

5. Brabbins, C. J., M. E. Dewey, J. R. Copeland, and I. A. Davidson. Insomnia in the elderly: Prevalence, gender differences and relationships with morbidity and mortality. *International Journal of Geriatric Psychiatry* 8: 473–480, 1993.

6. Harvey, A. G. Insomnia: Symptom or diagnosis? *Clinical Psychology Review* 21: 1–22, 2001.

7. Dryman, A. and W. W. Eaton. Affective symptoms associated with the onset of major depression in the community: Findings from the U.S. National Institute of Mental Health Epidemiologic Catchment Area Program. *Acta Psychiatrica Scandinavica* 84: 1–5, 1991.

8. Breslau, N., T. Roth, L. Rosenthal, and P. Andreski. Sleep disturbance and psychiatric disorders: A longitudinal epidemiological study of young adults. *Biological Psychiatry* 39: 411–418, 1996.

9. Chang, P. P., D. E. Ford, L. A. Mead, L. Cooper-Patrick, and M. J. Klag. Insomnia in young men and subsequent depression. The Johns Hopkins Precursors Study. *American Journal of Epidemiology* 146: 105–114, 1997.

10. Wingard, D. and L. Berkman. Mortality risk associated with sleeping patterns among adults. *Sleep* 6: 102–107, 1983.

11. Kupperman, M., D. P. Lubeck, and P. D. Mazonson. Sleep problems and their correlates in a working population. *Journal of General Internal Medicine* 10: 25–32, 1995.

12. Katz, D. A. and C. A. McHorney. Clinical correlates of insomnia in patients with chronic illness. *Archives of Internal Medicine* 158: 1099–1107, 1998.

13. Morin, C. M., J. P. Culbert, and S. M. Schwartz. Nonpharmacological interventions for insomnia: A meta-analysis of treatment efficacy. *American Journal of Psychiatry* 151: 1172–1180, 1994.

14. Murtagh, D. R. and K. M. Greenwood. Identifying effective psychological treatments for insomnia: A meta-analysis. *Journal of Consulting and Clinical Psychology* 63: 79–89, 1995.

15. Edinger, J. D., W. K. Wohlgemuth, R. A. Radtke, G. R. Marsh, and R. E. Quillian. Cognitive behavioral therapy for treatment of chronic primary insomnia: A randomized controlled trial. *Journal of the American Medical Association* 285: 1856–1864, 2001.

16. Smith, M. T., M. L. Perlis, A. Park, M. S. Smith, J. Y. Pennington, D. E. Giles, et al. Behavioral treatment vs. pharmacotherapy for insomnia: A comparative meta-analysis. *American Journal of Psychiatry* 159: 1–5, 2002.

17. McClusky, H. Y., J. B. Milby, P. K. Switzer, V. Williams, and V. Wooten. Efficacy of behavioral versus triazolam treatment in persistent sleep-onset insomnia [see comments]. *American Journal of Psychiatry* 148: 121–126, 1991.

18. Morin, C. M., C. Colecchi, J. Stone, R. Sood, and D. Brink. Behavioral and pharmacological therapies for late-life insomnia: A randomized controlled trial *Journal of the American Medical Association* 281: 991–999, 1999.

19. McCrae, C. R. and K. L. Lichstein. Secondary insomnia: A heuristic model and behavioral approaches to assessment, treatment, and prevention. *Applied and Preventive Psychology* 10: 107–123, 2001.

20. Beasley, C. M., B. E. Dornseif, J. A. Pultz, J. C. Bosomworth, and M. E. Sayler. Fluoxetine versus trazodone: Efficacy and activating-sedating effects. *Journal of Clinical Psychiatry* 52: 294–299, 1991.

21. Beasley, C. M., Jr., M. E. Sayler, A. M. Weiss, and J. H. Potvin. Fluoxetine: Activating and sedating effects at multiple fixed doses. *Journal of Clinical Psychopharmacology* 12: 328–333, 1992.

22. Song, F., N. Freemantle, T. A. Sheldon, A. House, P. Watson, A. Long, et al. Selective serotonin reuptake inhibitors: Meta-analysis of efficacy and acceptability. *British Medical Journal* 306: 683–687, 1993.

23. de Wilde, J., R. Spiers, C. Mertens, F. Bartholome, G. Schotte, and S. Leyman. A double-blind, comparative, multicentre study comparing paroxetine with fluoxetine in depressed patients. *Acta Psychiatrica Scandinavica* 87: 141–145, 1993.

24. Bennie, E. H., J. M. Mullin, and J. J. Martindale. A double-blind multicenter trial comparing sertraline and fluoxetine in outpatients with major depression. *Journal of Clinical Psychiatry* 56: 229–237, 1995.

25. Morin, C. M., R. A. Kowatch, and J. B. Wade. Behavioral management of sleep disturbances secondary to chronic pain. *Journal of Behavior Therapy and Experimental Psychiatry* 20: 295–302, 1989.

26. Lichstein, K. L., N. M. Wilson, and C. T. Johnson. Psychological treatment of secondary insomnia. *Psychology and Aging* 15: 232–240, 2000.

27. Currie, S. R., K. G. Wilson, A. J. Pontefract, and L. deLaplante. Cognitive-behavioral treatment of insomnia secondary to chronic pain. *Journal of Clinical Psychology* 68: 407–416, 2000.

28. Savard, J., S. Simard, J. Blanchet, H. Ivers, and C. M. Morin. Prevalence, clinical characteristics, and risk factors for insomnia in the context of breast cancer. *Sleep* 24: 583–590, 2001.

29. Savard, J. and C. M. Morin. Insomnia in the context of cancer: A review of a neglected problem. *Journal of Clinical Oncology* 19: 895–908, 2001.

30. Dashevsky, B. A. and M. Kramer. Behavioral treatment of chronic insomnia in psychiatrically ill patients. *Journal of Clinical Psychiatry* 59: 693–699, 1998.

31. Smith, M. T., M. L. Perlis, M. S. Smith, D. E. Giles, and T. P. Carmody. Sleep quality and presleep arousal in chronic pain. *Journal of Behavioral Medicine* 23: 1–13, 2000.

32. World Health Organization. *The ICD-10 Classification of Mental and Behavioral Disorders: Clinical Descriptions and Diagnostic Guidelines.* Geneva, Switzerland: World Health Organization. 1992.

33. American Psychiatric Association. *Diagnostic and Statistical Manual of Mental Disorders* (4th ed.). Washington, DC: American Psychiatric Association. 1994.

34. American Sleep Disorders Association. *The International Classification of Sleep Disorders: Diagnostic and Coding Manual—Revised.* Rochester, MN: American Sleep Disorders Association. 1997.

35. Lichstein, K. L., H. H. Durrence, B. W. Riedel, D. J. Taylor, and A. J. Bush. *Epidemiology of Sleep: Age, Gender, and Ethnicity.* Mahwah, NJ: Erlbaum. Unpublished manuscript.

36. Perlis, M. L., M. T. Smith, H. J. Orff, P. J. Andrews, and D. E. Giles. Beta/Gamma EEG activity in patients with primary and secondary insomnia and good sleeper controls. *Sleep* 24: 110–117, 2001.

37. Merica, H., R. Blois, and J. M. Gaillard. Spectral characteristics of sleep EEG in chronic insomnia. *European Journal of Neuroscience* 10: 1826–1834, 1998.

38. Merica, H. and J. M. Gaillard. The EEG of the sleep onset period in insomnia: A discriminant analysis. *Physiology and Behavior* 52: 199–204, 1992.

39. Freedman, R. EEG power in sleep onset insomnia. *Electroencephalography and Clinical Neurophysiology* 63: 408–413, 1986.

40. Lamarche, C. H. and R. D. Ogilvie. Electrophysiological changes during the sleep onset period of psychophysiological insomniacs, psychiatric insomniacs, and normal sleepers. *Sleep* 20: 724–733, 1997.

41. Hall, M., D. J. Buysse, P. D. Nowell, E. A. Nofzinger, P. Houck, C. F. Reynolds III, et al. Symptoms of stress and depression as correlates of sleep in primary insomnia. *Psychosomatic Medicine* 62: 227–230, 2000.

42. Perlis, M. L., D. E. Giles, W. B. Mendelson, R. R. Bootzin, and J. K. Wyatt. Subjective-objective discrepancies in psychophysiologic insomnia: A neurocognitive perspective. *Journal of Sleep Research* 6: 179–188, 1997.

43. Ford, D. E. and D. B. Kamerow. Epidemiologic study of sleep disturbances and psychiatric disorders. An opportunity for prevention? *Journal of the American Medical Association* 262: 1479–1484, 1989.

44. Livingston, G., B. Blizard, and A. Mann. Does sleep disturbance predict depression in elderly people? A study in inner London. *British Journal of General Practice* 43: 445–448, 1993.

45. Perlis, M. L., D. E. Giles, D. J. Buysse, X. Tu, and D. J. Kupfer. Self-reported sleep disturbance as a prodromal symptom in recurrent depression. *Journal of Affective Disorders* 42: 209–212, 1997.

46. Warr, B. W. Organization of olivocochlear efferent systems in mammals. In R. Fay, A. Popper, and D. B. Webster, eds. *Mammalian Auditory Pathway: Neuroanatomy.* Springer Series in Auditory Research: Auditory Central Nervous System. New York, NY: Spring-Verlag. 1992: 410–448.

47. Association of Professional Sleep Societies. Guidelines for the Multiple Sleep Latency Test (MSLT): A standard measure of sleepiness. *Sleep* 9: 519–524, 1986.

48. Johns, M. W. A new method for measuring daytime sleepiness: The Epworth Sleepiness Scale. *Sleep* 14: 540–545, 1991.

49. Monk, T. H., C. F. Reynolds, and D. J. Kupfer. The Pittsburgh Sleep Diary (PghSD). *Journal of Sleep Research* 3: 111–120, 1994.

50. Carskadon, M., W. Dement, M. Mitler, C. Guilleminault, V. P. Zarcone, and R. Spiegel. Self-reports versus sleep laboratory findings in 122 drug-free subjects with complaints of chronic insomnia. *American Journal of Psychiatry* 133: 1382–1388, 1976.

51. Frankel, B. L., R. Coursey, R. Buchbinder, and F. Snyder. Recorded and reported sleep in primary chronic insomnia. *Archives of General Psychiatry* 33: 615–623, 1976.

52. Coates, T. J., J. Killen, J. George, E. Marchini, S. Hamilton, and C. Thoresen. Estimating sleep parameters: A multitrait-multimethod analysis. *Journal of Consulting and Clinical Psychology* 50: 345–352, 1982.

53. Kales, A., A. Caldwell, and T. Preston. Personality patterns in insomnia. *Archives of General Psychiatry* 33: 1128–1134, 1976.

54. Kales, A., E. Bixler, A. Vela-Bueno, R. Cadieux, C. Soldatos, and J. Kales. Biopsychobehavioral correlates of insomnia. III: Polygraphic findings of sleep difficulty and their relationship to psychopathology. *International Journal of Neuroscience* 23: 43–56, 1984.

55. Bonnet, M. H. and D. L. Arand. Physiological activation in patients with sleep state misperception. *Psychosomatic Medicine* 59: 533–540, 1997.

56. Perlis, M. L., D. E. Giles, W. B. Mendelson, R. R. Bootzin, and J. K. Wyatt. Psychophysiological insomnia: The behavioral model and a neurocognitive perspective. *Journal of Sleep Research* 6: 179–188, 1997.

57. Spielman, A., L. Caruso, and P. Glovinsky. A behavioral perspective on insomnia treatment. *Psychiatric Clinics of North America* 10: 541–553, 1987.

58. Stepanski, E. J. Behavioral therapy for insomnia. In M. H. Kryger, T. Roth, and W. C. Dement, eds. *Principles and Practice of Sleep Medicine.* Philadelphia, PA: W.B. Saunders Company. 2000: 647–656.

59. Bastien, C. H. and C. M. Morin. Familial incidence of insomnia. *Journal of Sleep Research* 9: 49–54, 2000.

60. Hall, M., D. J. Buysse, C. F. Reynolds III, D. J. Kupfer, and A. Baum. Stress-related intrusive thoughts disrupt sleep onset and contiguity. *Journal of Sleep Research* 25: 163, 1996. (Abstract).

61. Morin, C. M. *Insomnia: Psychological Assessment and Management.* New York, NY: Guilford Press. 1993.

62. Espie, C. A. *The Psychological Treatment of Insomnia.* New York, NY: John Wiley. 1991.

63. Harvey, A. G. A cognitive model of insomnia. *Behavioural Research and Therapy* 40(8): 869–893, 2002.

64. Morin, C. M., F. Blais, and J. Savard. Are changes in beliefs and attitudes about sleep related to sleep improvements in the treatment of insomnia? *Behavioural Research and Therapy* 40: 741–752, 2002.

65. Lichstein, K. and T. Rosenthal. Insomniacs' perceptions of cognitive versus somatic determinants of sleep disturbance. *Journal of Abnormal Psychology* 89: 105–107, 1980.

66. Nicassio, P. M., D. R. Mendlowitz, J. J. Fussell, and L. Petras. The phenomenology of the presleep state: The development of the pre-sleep arousal scale. *Behavioural Research and Therapy* 23: 263–271, 1985.

67. Van Egeren, L., S. N. Haynes, M. Franzen, and J. Hamilton. Presleep cognitions and attributions in sleep-onset insomnia. *Journal of Behavioral Medicine* 6(2): 217–232, 1983.

68. Kuisk, L. A., A. D. Bertelson, and J. K. Walsh. Presleep cognitive hyperarousal and affect as factors in objective and subjective insomnia. *Perceptual and Motor Skills* 69: 1219–1225, 1989.

69. Watts, F. N., K. Coyle, and M. P. East. The contribution of worry to insomnia. *British Journal of Clinical Psychology* 33: 211–220, 1994.

70. Perlis, M. L., H. Merica, M. T. Smith, and D. E. Giles. Beta EEG in insomnia. *Sleep Medicine Reviews* 5(5): 363–374, 2001.

71. Hall, M., D. J. Buysse, P. D. Nowell, E. A. Nofzinger, P. Houck, C. F. Reynolds III, et al. Symptoms of stress and depression as correlates of sleep in primary insomnia. *Psychosomatic Medicine* 62: 227–230, 2000.

72. Krystal, A. D., J. D. Edinger, W. K. Wohlgemuth, and C. Michaels. A within-subject study of the relationship of non-REM EEG spectral amplitude and the agreement between subjective and objective assessments of sleep time. *Sleep* 25(Abstract Suppl.): A33–A34, 2002.

73. Krystal, A. D., J. D. Edinger, W. K. Wohlgemuth, and G. R. Marsh. A pilot study of the sleep EEG power spectral effects of behavioral therapy in primary insomniacs. *Sleep* 24(Abstract Suppl.): A62, 2001.

74. Perlis, M. L., M. T. Smith, H. J. Orff, P. J. Andrews, and D. E. Giles. The mesograde amnesia of sleep may be attenuated in subjects with primary insomnia. *Physiology and Behavior,* 2001.

75. Chesson, A. L., Jr., W. M. Anderson, M. Littner, D. Davila, K. Hartse, S. Johnson, et al. Practice parameters for the nonpharmacologic treatment of chronic insomnia. An American Academy of Sleep Medicine report. Standards of Practice Committee of the American Academy of Sleep Medicine [In Process Citation]. *Sleep* 22: 1128–1133, 1999.

76. Shoham-Salomon, V. and R. Rosenthal. Paradoxical interventions: A meta-analysis. *Journal of Consulting and Clinical Psychology* 55: 22–28, 1987.

77. Harvey, A. G. and S. Payne. The management of unwanted presleep thoughts in insomnia: Distraction with imagery versus general distraction. *Behavioural Research and Therapy* 40: 267–277, 2002.

78. Buysse, D. J. and M. L. Perlis. The evaluation and treatment of insomnia. *Journal of Practical Psychiatry and Behavioral Health* March: 80–93, 1996.

79. Barlow, D. H., M. G. Craske, J. A. Cerny, and J. S. Klosko. Behavioral treatment of panic disorder. *Behavior Therapy* 20(2): 261–282, 1989.

80. Barlow, D. H. Cognitive-behavioral approaches to panic disorder and social phobia. *Bulletin of the Menninger Clinic* 56(2 Suppl A): A43–57, 1992.

81. Barlow, D. H. Cognitive-behavioral therapy for panic disorder: Current status. *Journal of Clinical Psychiatry* 58(Suppl 2): 32–36, 1997.

82. Lichstein, K. L., B. W. Riedel, N. M. Wilson, K. W. Lester, and R. N. Aguillard. Relaxation and sleep compression for late-life insomnia: A placebo-controlled trial. *Journal of Consulting and Clinical Psychology* 69: 227–239, 2001.

83. Haynes, S. N., S. Woodward, R. Moran, and D. Alexander. Relaxation treatment of insomnia. *Behavior Therapy* 5: 555–558, 1974.

84. Freedman, R. and J. D. Papsdorf. Biofeedback and progressive relaxation treatment of sleep-onset insomnia: A controlled, all-night investigation. *Biofeedback and Self Regulation* 1: 253–271, 1976.

85. Bootzin, R. R. Evaluation of stimulus control instructions, progressive relaxation, and sleep hygiene as treatments for insomnia. In W. P. Koella, E. Ruther, and H. Schulz, eds. *Sleep*. Stuttgart, Germany: Gustav Fischer Verlag. 1984: 142–144.

86. Borkovec, T. D. and D. C. Fowles. Controlled investigation of the effects of progressive and hypnotic relaxation on insomnia. *Journal of Abnormal Psychology* 82: 153–158, 1973.

87. Hauri, P. J. Can we mix behavioral therapy with hypnotics when treating insomniacs? *Sleep* 20: 1111–1118, 1997.

88. Milby, J. B., V. Williams, J. N. Hall, S. Khuder, T. McGill, and V. Wooten. Effectiveness of combined triazolam-behavioral therapy for primary insomnia. *American Journal of Psychiatry* 150: 1259–1260, 1993.

89. Morin, C. M., C. A. Colecchi, W. D. Ling, R. K. Sood, and H. Williams. Cognitive-behavioral therapy for benzodiazepine-dependent insomniacs. *Sleep Research* 23 (Abstract): 295, 1994.

90. Vallières, A., M. Le Blanc, B. Guay, and C. M. Morin. Sequential use of medication and behavioral therapies for chronic insomnia. *Sleep* 25(Abstract Suppl.): A69–A70, 2002.

91. Nowell, P. D., S. Mazumdar, D. J. Buysse, M. A. Dew, C. F. Reynolds III, and D. J. Kupfer. Benzodiazepines and zolpidem for chronic insomnia: A meta-analysis of treatment efficacy. *Journal of the American Medical Association* 278: 2170–2177, 1997.

92. Johnson, L. C. and D. A. Chernik. Sedative-hypnotics and human performance. *Psychopharmacology* 76: 101–113, 1982.

93. Wesensten, N. J., T. J. Balkin, and G. L. Belenky. Effects of daytime administration of zolpidem versus triazolam on memory. *European Journal of Clinical Pharmacology* 48: 115–122, 1995.

94. Berlin, I., D. Warot, T. Hergueta, P. Molinier, C. Bagot, and A. J. Puech. Comparison of the effects of zolpidem and triazolam on memory functions, psychomotor performances, and postural sway in healthy subjects. *Journal of Clinical Psychopharmacology* 13: 100–106, 1993.

95. Scharf, M. G., J. Mendels, M. Thorpy, and B. Weiss. Safety of long-term zolpidem treatment in patients with insomnia. *Current Therapeutic Research Clinical and Experimental* 55: 1100–1111, 1994.

96. Schlich, D., C. L'Heritier, J. Coquelin, and P. Attali. Long-term treatment of insomnia with zolpidem: A multicentre general practitioner study of 107 patients. *Journal of Internal Medicine Research* 19: 19–27, 1991.

97. Kripke, D. F., M. R. Klauber, D. L. Wingard, R. L. Fell, J. D. Assmus, and L. Garfinkel. Mortality hazard associated with prescription hypnotics. *Biological Psychiatry* 43: 687–693, 1998.

98. Hohagen, F., R. F. Montero, E. Weiss, S. Lis, E. Schonbrunn, H. Dressing, et al. Treatment of primary insomnia with trimipramine: An alternative to benzodiazepine hypnotics? *European Archives of Psychiatry and Clinical Neuroscience* 244: 65–72, 1994.

99. Hajak, G., A. Rodenbeck, L. Adler, G. Huether, B. Bandelow, G. Herrendorf, et al. Nocturnal melatonin secretion and sleep after doxepin administration in chronic primary insomnia. *Pharmacopsychiatry* 29: 187–192, 1996.

100. Bootzin, R. R. Stimulus control treatment for Insomnia. *Proceedings, 80th Annual Convention, APA:* 395–396, 1972.

101. Hauri P. *Current Concepts: The Sleep Disorders.* Kalamazoo, MI: The Upjohn Company. 1977.

102. Spielman, A. J., P. Saskin, and M. J. Thorpy. Treatment of chronic insomnia by restriction of time in bed. *Sleep* 10: 45–56, 1987.

103. Smith, M. T., M. L. Perlis, A. Park, M. S. Smith, J. Pennington, D. E. Giles, et al. Comparative meta-analysis of pharmacotherapy and behavior therapy for persistent insomnia. *American Journal of Psychiatry* 159: 5–11, 2002.

104. Morin, C. M., C. A. Colecchi, J. Stone, R. K. Sood, and D. Brink. Cognitive-behavior therapy and pharmacotherapy for insomnia: Update of a placebo-controlled clinical trial. *Sleep Research* 24: 303, 1995.

105. Bixler, E., A. Kales, C. R. Soldatos, E. C. Martin, and J. Kales. Physical and mental health correlates of insomnia. *Sleep Research* 6: 139, 1977.

106. Zammit, G. K., J. Weiner, N. Damato, G. P. Sillup, and C. A. McMillan. Quality of life in people with insomnia [In Process Citation]. *Sleep* 22(Suppl. 2): S379–S385, 1999.

107. Johnson, L. and C. Spinweber. Quality of sleep and performance in the navy: A longitudinal study of good and poor sleepers. In C. Guilleminault and E. Lugaresi, eds. *Sleep/Wake Disorders: Natural History, Epidemiology, and Long-Term Evaluation.* New York, NY: Raven Press. 1983: 13–28.

108. Seligman, M. E. Learned helplessness. *Annual Review Medicine* 23: 407–412, 1972.

109. Bonnet, M. H. and D. L. Arand. Hyperarousal and insomnia. *Sleep Medicine Reviews* 1: 97–108, 1997.

110. Smith, M. T., M. L. Perlis, V. U. Chengazi, J. Pennington, J. Socffing, J. M. Ryan, et al. Neuroimaging of NREM sleep in primary insomnia: A Tc-99-HMPAO single photon emission computed tomography study. *Sleep* 25: 325–335, 2002.

111. National Center on Sleep Disorders Research, National Heart Lung and Blood Institute. *Neurobiology of Sleep and Waking.* National Institutes of Health, Work Shop Report, Bethesda, MD. September 12, 2001.

Chapter 10 ————————————————————————

CURRENT STATUS OF COGNITIVE-BEHAVIOR THERAPY FOR INSOMNIA: EVIDENCE FOR TREATMENT EFFECTIVENESS AND FEASIBILITY

CHARLES M. MORIN, CÉLYNE BASTIEN, AND JOSÉE SAVARD

Significant advances have been made in the assessment and management of insomnia over the past decade (1–4). Insomnia is now recognized as a significant health problem, and there is increasing research evidence documenting the efficacy of cognitive-behavior therapy (CBT) for the management of this sleep disorder. Despite this progress, there is a persistent and troubling paradox that insomnia often remains untreated and CBT underutilized in clinical practice (5–7).

This chapter presents an updated summary of the evidence currently available in support of CBT for insomnia. Outcome findings from meta-analyses are summarized, and an overview of the most recent clinical trials is provided with a special emphasis on issues of clinical significance, long-term impact, generalizability of outcomes, and feasibility of implementing CBT in clinical settings. We conclude with suggestions about models of treatment implementation to overcome barriers that may impede a more widespread use of CBT for insomnia.

TREATMENT EFFICACY

Evidence from Meta-Analyses

The outcome evidence from more than 50 clinical trials (> 2,000 patients) evaluating nonpharmacological interventions for insomnia has been summarized in two meta-analyses (8, 9). The findings show that CBT produces reliable changes in several sleep parameters, including sleep onset latency (average effect size of 0.88), number of awakenings (0.53 to 0.63), duration of awakenings (0.65), total sleep time (0.42 to 0.49), and sleep quality ratings (0.94). According to Cohen's criteria, the magnitude of those treatment effects is considered large (i.e., $d > 0.8$) for sleep onset latency and sleep quality and moderate (i.e., $d > 0.5$) for other sleep parameters. For comparative purposes, the effect sizes of CBT are similar to those obtained for benzodiazepine-receptor agonists (3, 10). When transformed into a percentile rank, these data indicate that approximately 70% to 80% of insomnia patients benefit from CBT. While these data clearly show that CBT is efficacious for treating insomnia, they provide little information about the extent to which patients benefit from treatment.

Because patients are typically selected on the basis of a sleep latency and/or time awake after sleep onset exceeding 30 minutes per night, it is useful to examine the absolute changes on those sleep parameters as indicators of success. The findings from meta-analyses indicate that the overall effect of treatment is to reduce subjective sleep onset latency from an average of 60 to 65 minutes at baseline to about 35 minutes at posttreatment. Similar results are obtained for the duration of nocturnal awakenings, which is reduced from an average of 70 minutes at baseline to about 38 minutes following treatment. The number of awakenings is decreased from an average of two per night at baseline to about one at posttreatment. Total sleep time is increased by 30 minutes, from 6 hours to 6.5 hours after treatment, and ratings of sleep quality are significantly enhanced with treatment. Thus, for the average insomnia patient, treatment effects may be expected to reduce sleep onset latency and wake after sleep onset by an average of about 50% and to bring the absolute values of those sleep parameters below or near the 30-minute cutoff criterion initially used to define sleep onset or maintenance insomnia. Treatment effects are similar for sleep-onset and sleep-maintenance problems, although few studies have yet examined the effect of treatment specifically for early morning awakening problems. Overall, findings from meta-analyses represent fairly conservative estimates of treatment effects because they are based on averages computed across all nonpharmacological interventions, of which efficacy varies considerably.

Empirically Validated Therapies

A task force of the American Psychological Association has developed several criteria to determine the level of empirical evidence available to support the efficacy of psychological treatments (11). Some of those criteria include evidence that treatment is superior to control and that treatment effect is documented by at least two independent investigators. According to these criteria, treatment efficacy for a given intervention can be graded as either well established or as probably efficacious. In a review of nonpharmacological interventions for insomnia (2), stimulus control therapy, progressive-muscle relaxation, and paradoxical intention were judged to meet criteria for well-established treatments, while sleep restriction, EMG biofeedback, and multicomponent CBT met criteria for probably efficacious therapies. Since then, additional evidence has been published to upgrade CBT from probably efficacious to a well-established treatment (12–14). Although sleep restriction is often considered one of the most effective single therapies for insomnia, along with stimulus control, there is still a lack of evidence for upgrading its status. Aside from the Friedman et al. study (16), there is no other randomized controlled study that has shown sleep restriction alone to be more effective than placebo control or another active treatment. Such stamps of approval as "empirically supported" or "probably efficacious" are useful in identifying treatments with adequate validation, but they provide no information for guiding clinicians in selecting the most appropriate interventions based on the specific profiles of individual patients. In addition, they do not inform clinicians about the relative efficacy of different therapies for insomnia.

Comparative Efficacy of Treatment Modalities

Table 10.1 provides a list of treatment outcome studies evaluating the efficacy of at least one nonpharmacological intervention for insomnia. Only group studies published since 1990 are listed. For each study, the main methodological features (design, patients, diagnosis, treatment) and outcome findings are summarized. Of those investigations, several comparative studies have found that stimulus control therapy was slightly more effective (50% to 60% improvement rates) than other single therapies such as relaxation (40%) or paradoxical intention (30%; see 2, 8–9, 15–18). Relaxation-based interventions have been extensively evaluated and probably remain the most widely used treatment for insomnia. Clinical studies have shown that relaxation methods focusing on cognitive arousal may yield better outcomes than those targeting somatic arousal (19). The evidence also shows that sleep hygiene education produces little impact on sleep, particularly when it is the only intervention (20). Formal cognitive therapy has not been evaluated as a single treatment modality, but excellent outcomes have been reported in clinical studies that have incorporated cognitive restructuring of dysfunctional sleep cognitions (12–14, 21–23). There is also evidence that reductions of dysfunctional sleep cognitions are correlated with sleep improvements at posttreatment, and fewer dysfunctional cognitions at posttreatment are associated with better maintenance of sleep changes over time (24, 25). In their clinical series of 89 patients with mixed primary and secondary insomnias, Verbeek and her colleagues (26) found more nonresponders among those who did not receive the cognitive therapy component. As shown in Table 10.1, numerous studies have evaluated the effect of

Table 10.1 Studies of Nonpharmacological Treatments of Insomnia

Author(s) (Year)	Design (Control)	Patients N, % of Female, Mean Age	Diagnosis/ Characteristics*	Treatment Conditions	Format of Treatment	Treatment (Weeks/ Hours) Follow-Up (Months)	Outcomes
Backhaus et al. (2001)*	NRCT (no)	20 65.0 43.0	Primary insomnia	CBT and a self-help manual (stimulus control, relaxation, cognitive restructuring)	Group	6/9 24	Increased TST and SE, reduced SOL and negative sleep-related cognitions. Reductions of depression and anxiety symptoms. Treatment effects remained stable up to 36-month FU.
Campbell et al. (1993)	RCT (control)	16 56 70.4	Phase-advanced disorder	Bright light exposure (4,000 lux; active); dim light (50 lux; control)	Individual	12 days/2 No	Decreased WASO by one hour and increased SE.
Chambers & Alexander (1992)*	CRS	103 67.0 39.9	Mixed primary and secondary insomnia	CBT (stimulus control, sleep restriction, sleep hygiene, cognitive restructuring)	Individual	1/2.5 6	Treatment reduced reported SOL and WASO by 30 and 50 minutes, respectively. 58% of patients rated their sleep as significantly improved.
Currie et al. (2000)*	RCT (wait-list)	60 55.0 45.0	Insomnia secondary to chronic pain	CBT (stimulus control, sleep restriction, education, cognitive therapy, relaxation) Waiting list control	Group	7/14 3	Treated patients improved more than controls on SOL, SE, WASO, and sleep quality. They also showed less motor activity on nocturnal actigraphy recordings. Benefits well maintained at FU.
Dashevsky & Kramer (1998)*	CRS (no)	48 75.0 47.3	Insomnia secondary to psychiatric disorders	Multicomponent behavioral treatment (sleep hygiene, relaxation, stimulus control, sleep restriction)	Individual	6/5 12	Significant improvements in subjective sleep parameters; changes sustained after 6 and 12 months. 69% achieved moderate/important clinical changes at 12-month FU. 53% of medicated participants reduced or stopped their hypnotics.

(continued)

Table 10.1 *Continued*

Author(s) (Year)	Design (Control)	Patients N, % of Female, Mean Age	Diagnosis/ Characteristics*	Treatment Conditions	Format of Treatment	Treatment (Weeks/ Hours) Follow-Up (Months)	Outcomes
Edinger et al. (2001)	RCT (placebo)	75 46.7 55.8	Primary insomnia	CBT (sleep restriction, stimulus control, cognitive therapy/education) Progressive muscle relaxation Placebo therapy	Individual	6/6 6	CBT produced larger subjective reductions of WASO (54%) than relaxation training (16%) or placebo (12%). PSG changes were smaller but CBT was also more effective. Sleep changes maintained at 6 months FU.
Engle-Friedman et al. (1992)	RCT (wait-list)	53 66.0 59.6	N/A	Sleep hygiene Sleep hygiene/relaxation Sleep hygiene/stimulus control Waiting list	Individual	4/4 24	Improvements on measures of SOL and number of awakenings in all treatments but not in the control condition. Stimulus control more effective at post- and 2-year FU. No changes on PSG measures.
Espie, Inglis, Tessier et al. (2001)*	RCT (control)	139 68.3 51.4	Primary insomnia	CBT (stimulus control, sleep restriction, relaxation, cognitive therapy) Wait-list control	Group	6/5	Significant reductions of SOL (61 to 28 min) and WASO in CBT but not in control. Significant increase of TST at FU, and 84% of patients initially using hypnotics remained drug-free.
Friedman et al. (1991)*	RCT (no)	22 63.6 69.2	Primary insomnia	Sleep restriction Relaxation	Individual	4/4 3	Improvement rates for sleep restriction were twice that of relaxation (33% vs. 16% for WASO). SE was increased from 67% to 83% with sleep restriction; total sleep time was increased by 51 minutes at FU relative to baseline.

Study	Design	N / Age	Diagnosis	Treatment conditions	Format	Sessions/FU	Outcome
Guillemi-nault et al. (1995)	RCT (no)	30 56.3 44.0	Primary insomnia	Stimulus control/sleep hygiene Stimulus control/sleep hygiene/exercise Stimulus control/sleep hygiene/bright light	Individual	4/NA 9–12	All three conditions improved on measures of SOL and TST, but only the bright light condition showed statistically significant changes over time. Outcome corroborated with actigraphy.
Gustafson (1992)*	CRS (no)	22 54.5 42.0	N/A	Relaxation	Self-administered	NA 12	86% rated the treatment as successful; 27% felt they still needed additional treatment. 32% reported a reduction in the use of sleep medications.
Hauri (1997)	RCT (wait-list)	26 73.1 47.7	Primary insomnia	Sleep hygiene/relaxation Sleep hygiene/relaxation/medication Waiting list	Individual	6/6 10	The two active treatments were more effective than control at post; however, at FU, subjects treated with the behavioral approach alone had a higher SE (83%) than the combined intervention (79%). Actigraphy used to document outcome.
Jacobs et al. (1996)*	CRS	102 61.0 39.3	Primary insomnia	CBT (sleep restriction, modified stimulus control, relaxation, education, cognitive restructuring, medication withdrawal)	Group	10/14 6	58% of patients reported significant sleep improvement, 33% moderate and 9% slight improvement. 91% of sleep medication users eliminated or reduced medication use. 90% of patients maintained or enhanced their sleep at FU.
Jacobs, Benson, et al. (1993)	NRCT (good sleepers)	26 58.3 37.8	Primary insomnia	Multicomponent (sleep restriction, modified stimulus control, relaxation) Good sleepers	Individual	10/2.5 6	Significant improvements on measures of SOL and TST based on sleep diary and PSG. No significant difference between treated patients and good sleepers at posttreatment. Significant reductions of anxiety and depressive symptoms.

(continued)

Table 10.1 Continued

Author(s) (Year)	Design (Control)	Patients N, % of Female, Mean Age	Diagnosis/ Characteristics*	Treatment Conditions	Format of Treatment	Treatment (Weeks/ Hours) Follow-Up (Months)	Outcomes
Jacobs, Rosenberg, et al. (1993)	RCT (no)	20 80.0 36.7	Primary insomnia	Sleep education/stimulus control / Sleep education/stimulus control/relaxation	Individual	10/3 1	Combined stimulus control and relaxation reduced SOL by 77% compared to the 63% for stimulus control alone.
Lack & Wright (1993)	NRCT (no)	9 44 53.4	Advanced circadian phase (EMA)	Bright light exposure (2,500 lux)	Individual	2 days/4 no	Final wake-up time shifted one hour later, SOL remained unchanged, TST increased. Temperature and melatonin rhythms phase markers were delayed.
Lichstein & Johnson (1993)*	NRCT (good sleepers)	57 100.0 66.2	Primary and hypnotic-dependent insomnia	Relaxation	Individual	2/3 1.5	Relaxation improved SE equally for unmedicated (64% to 72%) and medicated (62% to 70%) insomniacs. Medication reduced by 47%.
Lichstein et al. (1999)*	RCT (wait-list)	40 57.5 52	Primary and hypnotic-dependent insomnia	Medication withdrawal + relaxation / Medication withdrawal alone / Wait-list control	NA	2/2 2	Sleep medication was reduced by nearly 80%. Participants who received relaxation obtained additional benefits in sleep efficiency, sleep quality, and reduced withdrawal symptoms.
Lichstein et al. (2000)*	RCT (wait-list)	44 50 68.6	Secondary insomnia	Multicomponent behavioral treatment (sleep hygiene, stimulus control, relaxation) / Wait-list control	Individual	4/4 3	Treated participants showed significantly greater improvement on WASO, SE, and sleep quality than control participants.

Study	Design	Sample	Diagnosis	Treatment	Format	FU	Results
Lichstein et al. (2001)	RCT (placebo)	74 72.6 68.03	Primary insomnia	Relaxation Sleep restriction Placebo desensitization	Individual	6/5 12	All three conditions improved subjective but not PSG-defined sleep parameters. Sleep restriction was the most effective treatment.
McClusky et al. (1991)	RCT (no)	30 56.7 32.0	Primary insomnia	Stimulus control/relaxation training Triazolam	Group	3/NA 1	Triazolam produced a faster reduction of SOL, whereas the behavioral condition yielded better outcome at FU.
Mimeault & Morin, 1999	RCT (wait-list)	54 59.2 50.8	Primary insomnia	Self-help CBT manual Self-help CBT manual plus weekly phone consultation Waiting-list control	Self-help or Individual	NA/6 3	The two treatments showed significant changes on SE and TWT, whereas the control did not. The addition of a phone consultation provided a slight advantage during treatment but not at follow-up.
Morin et al. (1993)	RCT (waiting list)	24 70.8 67.1	Primary insomnia	CBT (stimulus control, sleep restriction, cognitive therapy, education) Waiting list	Group	8/12 12	CBT was effective in reducing WASO and in increasing SE (69% à 83%). Results were corroborated by PSG data. Therapeutic gains were maintained at 3- and 12-month FU.
Morin et al. (1994)*	CRS (none)	100 64.0 45.1	Primary, secondary, and hypnotic-dependent insomnia	CBT (stimulus control, sleep restriction, cognitive therapy, education, medication withdrawal)	Individual	14/NA 24	Reported SE improved from 68% to 80% for the total sample. Significant reductions in usage of sleep aids (46% to 28% medicated nights). Sleep clinic patients.
Morin, Colecchi, et al. (1999)	RCT (placebo)	78 64.0 65.0	Primary insomnia	CBT (stimulus control, sleep hygiene, cognitive therapy) Pharmacotherapy Both (CBT + Pharmacotherapy) Placebo	Group (CBT); Individual (Pharm.)	8/12 24	The 3 active treatments were more effective than placebo at posttreatment. The combined approach improved sleep more than either of its two single components. CBT participants sustained their clinical gains at FU, whereas those treated with pharmacotherapy alone did not.

(continued)

Table 10.1 *Continued*

Author(s) (Year)	Design (Control)	Patients N, % of Female, Mean Age	Diagnosis/ Characteristics*	Treatment Conditions	Format of Treatment	Treatment (Weeks/ Hours) Follow-Up (Months)	Outcomes
Perlis et al. (2000)	CRS (no)	116 57 39.2	Primary insomnia	CBT (sleep restriction, stimulus control, sleep hygiene, cognitive therapy, relaxation)	Individual	4–9/NA	61% of patients completed therapy and reported significant global improvements. Subjects who completed a minimum adequate trial reduced their SOL (65%) and WASO (47%) and increased their TST (13%).
Riedel et al. (1995)	RCT (waiting list)	75 65.6 67.4	Primary insomnia	Education/sleep restriction (video) Education/sleep restriction (video/therapist guidance) Waiting list	Self-help or Group	Video: 2/ 30min Therapist: 2/4 2	Sleep restriction and education administered by video with or without therapist guidance. The video yielded reductions in only WASO (92 to 63 minutes), but the addition of therapist guidance enhanced outcome on measures of SOL and WASO (68 to 37 minutes).
Riedel et al. (1998)*	NRCT (wait-list)	41 54 56.6	Primary insomnia and hypnotic-dependent insomnia	Medication withdrawal + stimulus control Medication withdrawal alone Stimulus control Wait-list control	Individual	2/2 2	Stimulus control participants, unlike controls, showed an improvement at FU for TST, SE, and sleep quality. Nonmedicated participants presented a more positive response to stimulus control therapy than medicated participants.

Sanavio et al. (1990)	RCT (waiting list)	40 65.0 39.6	Primary insomnia	EMG biofeedback Cognitive therapy Stimulus control/ relaxation Waiting list	Individual	2/6 36	All three treatments more effective than control in reducing SOL (37% vs. 1%) and WASO (50% vs. 1%). Benefits were maintained at 1- and 3-year FU.
Verbeek et al. (1999)*	NRCT (no)	86 65.1 49.6	Primary and secondary insomnia	CBT (sleep hygiene, relaxation, cognitive therapy, behavioral techniques)	Individual	6/5–6 1	Subjective improvement of sleep: reduction of time in bed, SOL, and WASO and increase in SE. 19% of the participants became good sleepers.

*Use of sleep medication on entering treatment was permissible.

CBT = Cognitive-behavior therapy; CRS = Clinical replication series; FU = Longest available follow-up; NA = Information not available; NRCT = Nonrandomized clinical trial; PSG = Polysomnography; RCT = Randomized clinical trial; SE = Sleep efficiency; SOL = Sleep onset latency; TST = Total sleep time; TWT = Total wake time; WASO = Wake after sleep onset.

multicomponent interventions, with or without cognitive therapy. Although such interventions are not always more effective than stimulus control alone, it seems that multicomponent therapy is becoming a fairly standard approach for insomnia. This approach typically includes a behavioral (stimulus control, sleep restriction, and, sometimes, relaxation), a cognitive (cognitive restructuring therapy), and an educational component (sleep hygiene). The appeal for this multimodal approach may come from the fact that it addresses different facets of insomnia and may actually lead to changes in domains that are not always targeted for assessment in insomnia research (e.g., psychological distress, daytime functioning, treatment satisfaction/acceptability).

Combined Behavioral and Pharmacological Approaches

Combined behavioral and pharmacological therapies should theoretically optimize treatment outcome by capitalizing on the more immediate and potent effects of the medication and the more sustained effects of behavior therapy. The limited evidence available, however, is not entirely clear as to whether a combined approach has an additive or subtractive effect on long-term outcome. Only a few studies have directly evaluated the combined or differential effects of behavioral (relaxation, stimulus control, CBT) and pharmacological (benzodiazepines) therapies for insomnia (14, 27–30). Collectively, those studies indicate that drug therapy produces quicker and slightly better results in the acute phase (first week) of treatment, whereas behavioral and drug therapies are equally effective in the short-term interval (four to eight weeks). Combined behavioral plus medication seems to have a slight advantage over single treatment modalities during the initial course of treatment, but it is unclear whether a combined approach produces a better long-term outcome than behavioral therapy alone. For instance, sleep improvements are well sustained after behavioral therapy, and those obtained with hypnotic drugs are quickly lost after discontinuation of the medication. The long-term effects of combined biobehavioral interventions are more equivocal. Some of those patients treated with a combined approach retain their initial sleep improvements over time whereas others return to their baseline values. Thus, despite the intuitive appeal in combining drug and nondrug interventions, it is not entirely clear when, how, and for whom it is indicated to combine behavioral and drug treatments for insomnia. In light of the mediating role of psychological factors in chronic insomnia, behavioral and attitudinal changes appear essential to sustain improvements in sleep patterns. When combining behavioral and drug therapies, patients' attributions of the initial benefits may be critical in determining long-term outcomes. Attribution of therapeutic benefits to the drug alone, without integration of self-management skills, may place a patient at greater risk for insomnia recurrence after the drug is discontinued. Additional research is needed to evaluate the effects of combined treatments for insomnia and to examine potential mechanisms of changes mediating short- and long-term outcomes.

Efficacy versus Specificity of Treatment

Although there is ample evidence supporting the *efficacy* of CBT for insomnia, there is still little information about the *specificity* of this treatment modality and the active mechanisms responsible for sleep improvements.

With a few notable exceptions that have used attention-placebo conditions (13, 15), most clinical trials of cognitive-behavioral approaches have used waiting-list control groups, precluding the unequivocal attribution of treatment effects to any specific ingredient of CBT. The lack of a pill-placebo control equivalent in psychological outcome research makes it difficult to determine what percentage of the variance in outcomes is due to specific therapeutic ingredients (i.e., restriction of time in bed, cognitive restructuring), the measurement process (i.e., self-monitoring), or to nonspecific factors (e.g., therapist attention, patients' expectations). There is a need for using more sophisticated, yet practical, comparative conditions to control for nonspecific factors and to identify the psychological and biological mechanisms responsible for sleep changes.

Initial Treatment Response versus Sustained Efficacy

A fairly robust finding across studies is that CBT produces stable changes in sleep patterns over time (8–9). Most studies with follow-up data indicate that changes in sleep latency and wake after sleep onset observed at posttreatment are well maintained up to 12, 24, and even 36 months later (14, 21, 31). On the other hand, interventions that incorporate a procedure restricting time spent in bed may yield only modest increases in sleep time after the initial treatment period. These gains are typically enhanced at follow-ups, with total sleep time often exceeding 6.5 hours. Follow-up data must be interpreted cautiously, however, because few studies report long-term follow-ups, and, among those that do, attrition rates increase substantially over time. In addition, it is important to keep in mind that a substantial proportion of those patients with chronic insomnia who benefit from short-term therapy may remain vulnerable to recurrent episodes of insomnia in the long term. As such, there is a need to develop and evaluate the effects of long-term, maintenance therapies to minimize the frequency and severity of those episodes.

TREATMENT EFFECTIVENESS
AND GENERALIZABILITY

Until recently, treatment studies focused predominantly on highly selected individuals with primary insomnia, who were specifically solicited from the community to participate in a research study. An important issue often raised was whether the findings obtained from those efficacy studies would generalize to patients seen in primary care practice (effectiveness studies), the main entry point for most patients seeking treatment for insomnia. A few studies have recently addressed this important issue of generalizability. Espie and his colleagues (12) recruited 139 patients with primary insomnia from primary care practices in Scotland; the results showed an average reduction of sleep onset latency from 61 to 28 minutes following CBT with similar reductions on time awake after sleep onset. In addition, 84% of patients initially using hypnotics remained drug-free at a one-year follow-up. A very innovative feature was the implementation of treatment by nurse practitioners in general medical practices. Another study conducted in Germany (21) showed that group CBT was effective in treating 20 patients, who were referred by their primary care physicians specifically for insomnia to a sleep clinic. Significant reductions of sleep onset latency (67 min to 30 min) and increases of total sleep time (298 min to 351 min) and sleep efficiency (59% to 77%) were reported from baseline to posttreatment, and those gains were well maintained at several follow-ups conducted up to 36 months after treatment. The proportion of patients using hypnotic medications was decreased from 60% to 35% after therapy and to 22% at long-term follow-up. Similar findings were reported in another study of 30 clinical patients with primary insomnia seeking treatment from a sleep clinic (32).

Additional large clinical case series have also shown that the treatment response of unsolicited clinical patients is comparable to that of insomnia participants solicited for clinical trials (22, 26, 33–35). Because of their more naturalistic focus, those studies are not as tightly controlled as randomized clinical trials; however, they typically include a more heterogeneous group of patients with various subtypes of insomnias and with significant medical and psychiatric comorbidity. The findings from these case series indicate that baseline and endpoint scores on insomnia symptom measures are usually more severe among patients with comorbid psychiatric and medical disorders, but the absolute changes on those outcome measures during treatment are compa-rable to patients with primary insomnia.

Treatment of Medicated Patients

While some investigators exclude medicated patients to enroll a more homoge-neous sample, others have directly compared treatment response of medicated and unmedicated insomniacs. Studies by Lichstein and his colleagues (36–37) have shown that medicated insomniacs can benefit from behavioral interventions such as stimulus control and relaxation training, even though their overall treatment re-sponse may be smaller than unmedicated patients. These findings are similar to those obtained with medicated patients seen in sleep disorders clinics (22, 26). While reductions of hypnotic medications are also reported in studies with med-icated insomniacs, patients meeting criteria for hypnotic-dependent insomnia often require a systematic and supervised withdrawal plan to achieve clinically meaningful and durable reductions of hypnotic medications (18, 37–39).

Secondary Insomnia

The treatment of secondary insomnia has received very little attention in the re-search literature (40), presumably because of the assumption that if the pri-mary disorder is treated adequately, the secondary insomnia will automatically be alleviated. Clinical evidence shows that this assumption is not always valid. Early clinical studies were mostly exploratory case studies conducted with pa-tients who suffered from insomnia secondary to cancer (41) or chronic pain (42). In the only group study conducted before 2000 (43), 30 cancer patients (mixed cancer sites) were randomly assigned to a three-session relaxation treat-ment or to routine care. Among the sleep variables assessed, only sleep latency improved significantly in the treatment group (reductions from 124 min to 20 min) compared to the control group. Although those exploratory studies yielded promising findings, methodological limitations (e.g., small sample, use of sub-jective and global measures, no clear definition of secondary insomnia) pre-cluded unequivocal conclusions about the efficacy of psychological treatments for secondary insomnia.

It is only recently that more rigorous research has been conducted in this field. The first study, conducted in 60 patients suffering from insomnia secondary to chronic pain, showed that a multimodal treatment combining sleep restriction and stimulus control therapy, relaxation training, cognitive therapy, and sleep hy-giene education was effective to improve several subjective sleep parameters and nocturnal motor activity measured by actigraphy (44). Therapeutic gains were well maintained at a three-month follow-up. The second study, conducted in 44 elderly persons with insomnia secondary to a medical or psychiatric condition, provided additional evidence supporting the efficacy of a treatment combining relaxation and stimulus control procedures (45). Treated participants experienced greater improvements in subjective time spent awake at night, sleep efficiency, and sleep quality compared to control participants.

There is also additional evidence that insomnia secondary to cancer can be effectively treated with psychological interventions. In a preliminary study using a multiple baseline experimental design, eight participants received CBT for insomnia secondary to breast cancer (46). Time series analyses of daily sleep diary data revealed significant improvements of sleep efficiency and total wake time in all patients. These results were corroborated by polysomnographic data. In addition, treatment was associated with significant improvements of mood, fatigue, and quality of life. A randomized trial comparing the same treatment protocol to a waiting list control condition is underway to replicate these findings in a larger sample. Preliminary results of this study are promising (47).

Two clinical case series have examined treatment effectiveness for insomnia secondary to psychiatric disorders. In an early study (48), multimodal intervention (individual and group psychotherapy, occupational therapy) produced some improvements in self-rated sleep quality among 20 psychiatric inpatients. More recently, Dashevsky and Kramer (49) have documented further the efficacy of behavioral treatment (stimulus control, sleep restriction, relaxation) for insomnia in psychiatric patients. Forty-eight patients, mostly with depressive and somatoform disorders, showed some improvements on sleep parameters and reductions of hypnotic medications. Finally, Blais, Mimeault and Morin (50) used a single-case/crossover design to evaluate treatment efficacy in 10 patients with insomnia associated with a generalized anxiety disorder (GAD). Half of the patients first received CBT for insomnia, followed by CBT for GAD, while the other half received the same interventions but in the reverse order. The results showed that treatment targeting anxiety during the initial phase of treatment was more effective to improve both anxiety and insomnia symptoms.

In summary, there is evidence that psychological interventions are efficacious to treat insomnia secondary to medical conditions such as chronic pain and cancer and, to a lesser extent, secondary to some psychiatric disorders. Additional research is needed to study separately the efficacy of interventions for insomnia secondary to psychiatric and medical conditions because the appropriate course of action may differ for those conditions. Sequential intervention studies, targeting the primary and secondary conditions in different sequences, represent promising lines for future research. Future studies also need to use more stringent criteria to define secondary insomnia (40). Although this is a challenging task, it is crucial to distinguish patients in whom the accompanying condition had a causal role on the development of insomnia from patients in whom it constitutes only a comorbid condition because both situations may react differently to treatment.

Circadian Rhythm Disorders

Some circadian rhythms disorders (i.e., delayed and advanced sleep phase syndromes) may overlap with insomnia in their clinical presentation. Although bright light exposure (BLE) is not a behavioral intervention, it is reviewed here because it is the only nonpharmacological intervention that has received some empirical support for those conditions. BLE in the morning advances the timing of the circadian phase, while exposure in the evening delays the circadian phase. In one study with 16 elderly patients suffering from sleep maintenance insomnia (51), BLE was used to delay the circadian phase of core body temperature. Eight patients were exposed to a bright white light of 4,000 lux, and eight control patients were exposed to dim red light of approximately 50 lux. Both groups were exposed to bright light for a period of two hours in the evening during 12 consecutive days. The results showed that BLE reduced the amount of time awake after sleep onset by about one hour, and sleep efficiency was increased from 78% at baseline to 90%. The core body temperature curve was also moved later during the night. Similar results were reported in another study conducted with 13 elderly patients with sleep maintenance insomnia (52). BLE (4,000 lux) scheduled in the evening was superior to BLE in the afternoon for improving sleep efficiency and delaying core body temperature. There was no follow-up of long-term effects of BLE in these studies. In another study (53), BLE was used with nine middle-age subjects with early morning awakenings. BLE (2,500 lux), administered over two consecutive days from 8 P.M. to midnight, produced a shift to about one hour later in the final wake-up time, which resulted in an increase in total sleep time. These preliminary findings suggest that BLE can be useful for patients with sleep maintenance insomnia of a circadian rhythm origin. However, more studies are needed to document further the efficacy, utility, and long-term impact of this intervention for insomnia.

CLINICAL SIGNIFICANCE OF TREATMENT OUTCOME

Evidence of treatment efficacy is typically documented by examining average changes on parameters such as sleep onset latency, time awake after sleep onset, and total sleep time. An important issue that needs to be addressed is the extent to which those sleep changes are clinically meaningful. Because there is currently no consensus as to what represents a clinically meaningful outcome, investigators use different markers of clinical significance. Those include the proportion of patients who reach a 50% or greater improvement rate on the main target symptoms, an absolute value of those symptoms falling below the 30-minute cutoff criterion used to define insomnia, the proportion of patients reaching a sleep efficiency of 80%, or who discontinue/reduce hypnotic medications. Using those criteria, Morin, Stone, and colleagues (22) reported that half of their 100 clinical patients achieved a 50% or better improvement rate, and between 37% and 40% reached a dual criterion of clinical improvement, that is, 50% reduction of their target symptom, while the absolute value of that symptom also fell below the 30-minute cutoff criterion. There were 38 patients whose sleep efficiency increased to more than 80% at posttreatment. Espie et al. (31) reported that two-thirds of the 109 patients treated with CBT in general practice, and who completed follow up, achieved normative values (i.e., < 30 min) on measures of sleep onset latency and time awake after sleep onset, 50% reduced their scores on those variables by more than 50%, and 84% of those using hypnotic medications initially were drug-free at a one-year follow-up. These findings obtained from clinical patients are comparable to those reported earlier by Lacks and Powlishta (54), who found that 39% of their 216 treated subjects achieved reliable change, whereas 23% became good sleepers. At the one-year follow-up, 49% showed reliable change, 32% became good sleepers, and 76% were medication free (compared to 35% at baseline).

Methods and Targets of Outcome Assessment

Treatment efficacy has been documented primarily with prospective daily sleep diaries and focused almost exclusively on sleep parameters. Several studies have complemented those findings with data from polysomnography (13–14, 55) and wrist actigraphy (12, 32). Although the magnitude of improvements is usually smaller on those objective measures, they tend to parallel clinical changes reported on daily sleep diaries. For example, in a study of sleep onset insomnia (55), baseline sleep latencies were 77 minutes (diary) and 84 minutes (polysomnography); at posttreatment, these values had decreased to 19 minutes and 21 minutes, respectively, on both measurement methods. In another study of late-life insomnia (14), average baseline values for wake after sleep onset were 62 minutes for daily diaries and 73 minutes for polysomnographic measures. Posttreatment means were 29 minutes for the diary and 35 minutes for polysomnography, yielding improvement rates of 54% and 51%, respectively, for the two assessment methods.

Edinger and colleagues (13) reported average sleep efficiency increases of 8% and 12% for PSG and diary measures, respectively, following CBT. Collectively, these findings indicate that CBT not only alters sleep perception on daily diaries, but also produces objective changes on EEG sleep continuity measures.

While promising, those results fail to address the extent to which treatment improves other important domains such as daytime functioning, alertness, mood and psychological well-being, and quality of life. Insomnia is more than a sleep problem, and patients often seek treatment because of the perceived consequences of sleep disturbances rather than because of the sleep problem per se. Hence, it is essential to document outcome beyond the mere reductions of insomnia symptoms. Investigators often incorporate a battery of self-report measures to assess changes on psychological variables (anxiety, depression), but because patients with significant anxiety and/or depressive disorders are usually excluded, it is no surprise that there is little change on those variables. Perhaps it would be important in the future to develop and obtain a consensus on a standardized assessment battery that would be used in randomized clinical trials of insomnia. Such a battery could incorporate multiple measures of sleep, daytime functioning (attention, memory, concentration), fatigue, psychological symptoms, functional impairments, satisfaction with treatment, and quality of life (56).

Cost-Effectiveness

Insomnia entails significant costs, both for the individual and for society. In the United States only, $1.7 billion and $11.96 billion are attributed to the direct costs of insomnia for sleep-promoting substances and health care services, respectively. Indirect costs, which include expenses not directly related to insomnia treatment, are even higher. According to Chilcott and Shapiro (57), combining direct and associated expenses leads to a yearly estimation of $30 billion to $35 billion of total cost of insomnia in the United States.

The direct costs of CBT for insomnia may seem higher initially because it is a more time-consuming intervention than prescribing a sleep medication. However, preliminary findings (58) suggest that insomniacs treated with CBT use health care services less frequently after treatment than those treated with pharmacotherapy. Participants in that study completed a brief health survey inquiring about the number of illnesses, the use of health services, and the quantity of medication prescribed for sleep difficulties and other medical conditions. The results showed that fewer insomniacs treated with CBT had used health care services at three-month follow-up compared to those receiving medications. These findings suggest that CBT, while more expensive in the short run, may become a more cost-effective solution in the long term. It is plausible that patients learn to use newly learned self-management skills to treat their insomnia and, perhaps, other health-related conditions. These results need replication on a larger scale.

Feasibility—Treatment Implementation Models

Despite the extensive evidence supporting their efficacy, nonpharmacological interventions for insomnia are underused in clinical practice. Several barriers (e.g., time, cost, access) seem to compromise a larger utilization by practitioners (59). Several studies have examined cost-reducing strategies such as brief consultations (60), group therapy, and self-help interventions (61–64). Group therapy has been used in several studies (see Table 10.1), and it represents an appealing and cost-effective alternative to individual therapy (8–9). Self-help treatment is the most inexpensive approach because it involves no therapist time, no transportation, and minimal costs for written materials. Mimeault and Morin (62) reported that a cognitive-behavioral bibliotherapy was efficacious for the treatment of chronic insomnia, although the addition of professional guidance produced slightly superior results to self-help therapy alone. Another cost-reducing strategy for implementing therapy is via telephone consultations. A "Sleep Service Line" offering clinical advice about sleep hygiene and behavioral practices for insomnia improved sleep in more than 25% of callers in the Netherlands (65). Only one study has compared the relative effectiveness of phone (20 minutes per session), group (90 minutes per session), and individual (45 minutes per session) therapy for chronic primary insomnia (66). The findings showed that CBT was equally effective when implemented on an individual or a group format or in the context of telephone consultations. Clinical improvements were maintained at the three-month follow-up in all three conditions. Collectively, these findings provide evidence about the feasibility of implementing insomnia treatment at minimal cost. The next challenging step will be to find effective methods to disseminate those minimal interventions to clinicians and their patients. Additional research is also needed to determine who is likely to benefit from self-help interventions and the appropriate treatment dosage required for different insomnia severity and subtypes (67).

CONCLUSIONS AND FUTURE DIRECTIONS

Significant advances have been made in the cognitive-behavioral management of insomnia in the past decade. Evidence from clinical trials indicates that approximately 70% to 80% of individuals with primary insomnia are likely to benefit from cognitive-behavior therapy. The majority of patients with primary insomnia achieve meaningful reduction of insomnia symptoms, although not all treatment responders become good sleepers. In addition, there is still limited evidence that improvements in sleep lead to meaningful changes in other important areas of functioning such as daytime performance, mood, and quality of life. Thus, additional clinical research is essential to design strategies to optimize treatment response and to broaden the scope of outcome. In addition, despite the evidence supporting the efficacy of multimodal CBT, there is still little information about the specificity of its therapeutic ingredients and about the mechanisms of changes associated with sleep improvements.

There is some evidence that treatment is effective for not only highly selected and motivated patients participating in clinical trials but also those who spontaneously present to primary care practices and sleep specialty clinics. There is, nonetheless, a need for additional randomized clinical trials conducted specifically in primary care practices.

The evidence also shows that patients with some coexisting medical and psychiatric conditions are likely to benefit from treatment as well, although treatment expectations/prognosis may need to be adjusted according to the nature and severity of those comorbid conditions. Finally, despite the increasing evidence that CBT is an effective method for treating various subtypes of insomnia, there are still important barriers compromising their routine use by clinical practitioners. An important challenge for the future will be to design and validate cost-effective treatment protocols that will be more readily accessible and more widely used by clinicians and patients.

REFERENCES

1. Edinger, J. D. and W. K. Wohlgemuth. The significance and management of persistent primary insomnia: The past, present and future of behavioral insomnia therapies. *Sleep Medicine Reviews* 3: 101–118, 1999.

2. Morin, C. M., P. J. Hauri, C. A. Espie, A. J. Spielman, D. J. Buysse, and R. R. Bootzin. Nonpharmacologic treatment of chronic insomnia. *Sleep* 22: 1134–1156, 1999.

3. Smith, M. T., M. L. Perlis, A. Park, M. S. Smith, J. Pennington, D. E. Giles, et al. Comparative meta-analysis of pharmacotherapy and behavior therapy for persistent insomnia. *American Journal of Psychiatry* 159: 5–11, 2002.

4. Sateia, M. J., K. Doghramji, P. J. Hauri, and C. M. Morin. Evaluation of chronic insomnia. An American Academy of Sleep Medicine review. *Sleep* 23: 243–308, 2000.

5. Morin, C. M. *Insomnia: Psychological Assessment and Management.* New York, NY: Guilford Press. 1993.

6. Mellinger, G. D., M. B. Balter, and E. H. Uhlenhuth. Insomnia and its treatment: Prevalence and correlates. *Archives of General Psychiatry* 42: 114–232, 1985.

7. Simon, G. and M. VonKorff. Prevalence, burden, and treatment of insomnia in primary care. *American Journal of Psychiatry* 154: 1417–1423, 1997.

8. Morin, C. M., J. P. Culbert, and S. M. Schwartz. Nonpharmacological interventions for insomnia: A meta-analysis of treatment efficacy. *American Journal of Psychiatry* 151: 1172–1180, 1994.

9. D. R. R. Murtagh and K. M. Greenwood. Identifying effective psychological treatments for insomnia: A meta-analysis. *Journal of Consulting and Clinical Psychology* 60: 79–89, 1995.

10. Nowell, P. D., S. Mazumdar, D. J. Buysse, M. A. Dew, C. F. Reynolds III, and D. J. Kupfer. Benzodiazepines and zolpidem for chronic insomnia: A meta-analysis of treatment efficacy. *Journal of the American Medical Association* 278: 2170–2177, 1997.

11. Chambless, D. L. and S. D. Hollon. Defining empirically supported therapies. *Journal of Consulting and Clinical Psychology* 66: 7–18, 1998.

12. Espie, C. A., S. J. Inglis, S. Tessier, and L. Harvey. The clinical effectiveness of cognitive behavior therapy for chronic insomnia: Implementation and evaluation of a sleep clinic in general medical practice. *Behaviour Research and Therapy* 39: 45–60, 2001.

13. Edinger, J. D., W. K. Wohlgemuth, R. A. Radtke, G. R. Marsh, and E. Quillian. Cognitive behavioral therapy for treatment of chronic primary insomnia: A randomized controlled trial. *Journal of the American Medical Association* 285: 1856–1864, 2001.

14. Morin, C. M., C. Colecchi, J. Stone, R. Sood, and D. Brink. Behavioral and pharmacological therapies for late-life insomnia: A randomized clinical trial. *Journal of the American Medical Association* 281: 991–999, 1999.

15. Lichstein, K. L., B. W. Riedel, N. M. Wilson, K. W. Lester, and R. N. Aguillard. Relaxation and sleep compression for late-life insomnia: A placebo-controlled trial. *Journal of Consulting and Clinical Psychology* 69: 227–239, 2001.

16. Friedman, L., D. Bliwise, J. A. Yesavage, and S. R. Salom. A preliminary study comparing sleep restriction and relaxation treatments for insomnia in older adults. *Journal of Gerontology* 46: 1–8, 1991.

17. Jacobs, G. D., P. A. Rosenberg, R. Friedman, J. Matheson, G. M. Peavy, A. D. Domar, et al. Multifactorial behavioral treatment of chronic sleep-onset insomnia using stimulus control and the relaxation response: A preliminary study. *Behavior Modification* 17: 498–509, 1993.

18. Lichstein, K. L. and R. Johnson. Relaxation for insomnia and hypnotic medication use in older women. *Psychology and Aging* 8: 103–111, 1993.

19. Harvey, A. G. and S. Payne. The management of unwanted presleep thoughts in insomnia: Distraction with imagery versus general distraction. *Behaviour Research and Therapy* 40:267–277, 2002.

20. Engle-Friedman, M., R. R. Bootzin, L. Hazlewood, and C. Tsao. An evaluation of behavioral treatments for insomnia in the older adult. *Journal of Clinical Psychology* 48: 77–90, 1992.

21. Backhaus, J., F. Hohagen, U. Voderholzer, and D. Riemann. Long-term effectiveness of a short-term cognitive-behavioral group treatment for primary insomnia. *European Archives of Psychiatry and Clinical Neuroscience* 25: 35–41, 2001.

22. Morin, C. M., J. Stone, K. McDonald, and S. Jones. Psychological management of insomnia: A clinical replication series with 100 patients. *Behavior Therapy* 25: 291–309, 1994.

23. Sanavio, E., G. Vidotto, O. Bettinardi, T. Rolletto, and M. Zorzi. Behavior therapy for DIMS: Comparison of three treatment procedures with follow-up. *Behavioural Psychotherapy* 18: 151–167, 1990.

24. Edinger, J. D., W. K. Wohlgemuth, R. A. Radtke, G. R. Marsh, and E. Quillian. Does cognitive-behavioral insomnia therapy alter dysfunctional beliefs about sleep? *Sleep* 24: 591–599, 2001.

25. Morin, C. M., F. C. Blais, and J. Savard. Are changes in beliefs and attitudes about sleep related to sleep improvements in the treatment of insomnia? *Behaviour Research and Therapy* 47: 741–752, 2002.

26. Verbeek, I., K. Schreuder, and G. Declerck. Evaluation of short-term nonpharmacological treatment of insomnia in a clinical setting. *Journal of Psychosomatic Research* 47: 369–383, 1999.

27. Hauri, P. J. Insomnia: Can we mix behavioral therapy with hypnotics when treating insomniacs? *Sleep* 20: 1111–1118, 1997.

28. McClusky, H. Y., J. B. Milby, P. K. Switzer, V. Williams, and V. Wooten. Efficacy of behavioral versus triazolam treatment in persistent sleep-onset insomnia. *American Journal of Psychiatry* 148: 121–126, 1991.

29. Rosen, R. C., D. S. Lewin, R. L. Goldberg, and R. L. Woolfolk. Psychophysiological insomnia: Combined effects of pharmacotherapy and relaxation-based treatments. *Sleep Medicine Reviews* 1: 279–288, 2000.

30. Milby, J. B., V. Williams, J. N. Hall, S. Khuder, T. McGill, and V. Wooten. Effectiveness of combined triazolam-behavioral therapy for primary insomnia. *American Journal of Psychiatry* 150: 1259–1260, 1993.

31. Espie, C. A., S. J. Inglis, and L. Harvey. Predicting clinically significant response to cognitive behavior therapy for chronic insomnia in general medical practice: Analyzes of outcome data at 12 months posttreatment. *Journal of Consulting and Clinical Psychology* 69: 58–66, 2001.

32. Guilleminault, C., A. Clerk, J. Black, M. Labanowski, R. Pelayo, and D. Claman. Nondrug treatment trials in psychophysiological insomnia. *Archives of Internal Medicine* 155: 838–844, 1995.

33. Chambers, M. J. and S. D. Alexander. Assessment and prediction of outcome for a brief behavioral insomnia treatment program. *Journal of Behavior Therapy and Experimental Psychiatry* 23: 289–297, 1992.

34. Jacobs, G. D., H. Benson, and R. Friedman. Perceived benefits in behavioral-medicine insomnia program: A clinical report. *American Journal of Medicine* 100: 212–216, 1996.

35. Perlis, M., M. Aloia, A. Millikan, J. Boehmler, M. Smith, D. Greenblatt, et al. Behavioral treatment of insomnia: A clinical case series study. *Journal of Behavioral Medicine* 23: 149–161, 2000.

36. Lichstein, K. L., B. A. Peterson, B. W. Riedel, M. K. Means, M. T. Epperson, and R. N. Aguillard. Relaxation to assist sleep medication withdrawal. *Behavior Modification* 23: 379–402, 1999.

37. Riedel, B., K. L. Lichstein, B. A. Peterson, M. T. Epperson, M. K. Means, and R. N. Aguillard. A comparison of the efficacy of stimulus control for medicated and nonmedicated insomniacs. *Behavior Modification* 22: 3–28, 1998.

38. Morin, C. M., C. Bastien, B. Guay, M. Radouco-Thomas, J. Leblanc, and A. Vallières. *Insomnia and chronic use of benzodiazepines: A randomized clinical trial of supervised tapering, cognitive-behavioral therapy, and a combined approach to facilitate benzodiazepine discontinuation.* Manuscript submitted for publication. 2003.

39. Baillargeon, L., P. Landreville, R. Verreault, J.-P. Beauchemin, and C. M. Morin. *Discontinuation of benzodiazepines among older insomniacs adults treated through cognitive-behavioral therapy combined with gradual tapering: A randomized trial.* Canadian Medical Association Journal in press.

40. McCrae, C. S. and K. L. Lichstein. Secondary insomnia: Diagnostic challenges and intervention opportunities. *Sleep Medicine Reviews* 5: 47–61, 2001.

41. Stam, H. J. and B. D. Bultz. The treatment of severe insomnia in a cancer patient. *Journal of Behavior Therapy and Experimental Psychiatry* 17: 33–37, 1986.

42. Morin, C. M., R. A. Kowatch, and J. B. Wade. Behavioral management of sleep disturbances secondary to chronic pain. *Journal of Behavior Therapy and Experimental Psychiatry* 20: 295–302, 1989.

43. Cannici, J., R. Malcom, and L. A. Peek. Treatment of insomnia in cancer patients using muscle relaxation training. *Journal of Behavior Therapy and Experimental Psychiatry* 14: 251–256, 1983.

44. Currie, S. R., K. G. Wilson, A. J. Pontefract, and L. deLaplante. Cognitive-behavioral treatment of insomnia secondary to chronic pain. *Journal of Consulting and Clinical Psychology* 68: 407–416, 2000.

45. Lichstein, K. L., N. M. Wilson, and C. T. Johnson. Psychological treatment of secondary insomnia. *Psychology and Aging* 15: 232–240, 2000.

46. Quesnel, C., J. Savard, S. Simard, H. Ivers, and C. M. Morin. *Efficacy of cognitive-behavioral therapy for insomnia in women treated for nonmetastatic breast cancer.* Journal of Consulting and Clinical Psychology 71: 189–200, 2003.

47. Savard, J., S. Simard, C. Quesnel, H. Ivers, and C. M. Morin. Treatment of insomnia secondary to breast cancer. *Psycho-Oncology* 12: S93, 2003.

48. Tan, T. L., J. D. Kales, A. Kales, et al. Inpatient multidimensional management of treatment-resistant insomnia. *Psychosomatics* 28: 266–272, 1987.

49. Dashevsky, B. and M. Kramer. Behavioral treatment of chronic insomnia in psychiatrically ill patients. *Journal of Clinical Psychiatry* 59: 693–399, 1998.

50. Blais, F. C., V. Mimeault, and C. M. Morin. *Treatment of comorbid insomnia and generalized anxiety disorders.* Sleep 23 (Suppl 2): A312, 2000.

51. Campbell, S. S., D. Dawson, and M. W. Anderson. Alleviation of sleep maintenance insomnia with timed bright light exposure. *Journal of the American Geriatrics Society* 41: 829–836, 1993.

52. Murphy, P. and S. Campbell. Enhanced performance in elderly subjects following bright light treatment of sleep maintenance insomnia. *Journal of Sleep Research* 5: 165–172, 1996.

53. Lack, L. and H. Wright. The effect of evening bright light in delaying the circadian rhythms and lengthening the sleep of early morning awakening insomniacs. *Sleep* 16: 436–443, 1993.

54. Lacks, P. and K. Powlishta. Improvement following behavioral treatment for insomnia: Clinical significance, long-term maintenance, and predictors of outcome. *Behavior Therapy* 20: 117–134, 1989.

55. Jacobs, G. D., H. Benson, and R. Friedman. Home-based central nervous system assessment of a multifactorial behavioral treatment of chronic sleep-onset insomnia. *Behavior Therapy* 24: 159–174, 1993.

56. Morin, C. M. Measuring outcomes in randomized clinical trials of insomnia treatments. Sleep Medicine Reviews, in press.

57. Chilcott, L. A. and C. M. Shapiro. The socioeconomic impact of insomnia: An overview. *PharmacoEconomics* 10: 1–14, 1996.

58. Bastien, C. H., F. C. Blais, and C. M. Morin. *Use of health services as a cost-efficacy indicator of cognitive-behavioral treatment for insomnia.* Paper presented at the meeting of the Association for the Advancement of Behavior Therapy (AABT), Washington, DC. 1998, November.

59. National Institutes of Health. NIH releases statement on behavioral and relaxation approaches for chronic pain and insomnia. *American Family Physician* 53: 1877–1880, 1996.

60. Hauri, P. J. Consulting about insomnia: A method and some preliminary data. *Sleep* 16: 344–350, 1993.

61. Morawetz, D. Behavioral self-help treatment for insomnia: A controlled evaluation. *Behavior Therapy* 20: 365–379, 1989.

62. Mimeault, V. and C. M. Morin. Self-help treatment for insomnia: Bibliotherapy with and without professional guidance. *Journal of Consulting and Clinical Psychology* 67: 511–519, 1999.

63. Riedel, B. W., K. L. Lichstein, and W. O. Dwyer. Sleep compression and sleep education for older insomniacs: Self-help versus therapist guidance. *Psychology and Aging* 10: 54–63, 1995.

64. Gustafson, R. Treating insomnia with a self-administered muscle relaxation training program: A follow-up. *Psychological Reports* 70: 124–126, 1992.

65. Verbeek, I., G. Declerck, A. Knuistingh Neven, and A. Coenen. Sleep service by telephone: Positive effects on insomnia. *Sleep and Hypnosis* in press.

66. Bastien, C. H., C. M. Morin, M. C. Ouellet, F. Blais, and S. Bouchard. *Cognitive-behavioral treatment for insomnia: A comparison of three treatment modalities.* Manuscript under editorial review 2003.

67. Edinger, J. D., W. K. Wohlgemuth, R. A. Radtke, and G. R. Marsh. Dose response effects of behavioral insomnia therapy. *Sleep* 23: 310, 2000.

68. Morin, C. M., R. Kowatch, T. Barry, and E. Walton. Cognitive-behavior therapy for late life insomnia. Journal of Consulting and Clinical Psychology 61: 137–146, 1993.

Chapter 11

SECONDARY INSOMNIA: DIAGNOSTIC ISSUES, COGNITIVE-BEHAVIORAL TREATMENT, AND FUTURE DIRECTIONS

KENNETH L. LICHSTEIN, CHRISTINA S. McCRAE, AND NANCY M. WILSON

There are numerous varieties of insomnia. The *International Classification of Sleep Disorders* (ICSD; 1) identifies at least seven types of insomnia. Examples are psychophysiological insomnia (due to worry or arousing associations with the bedroom), inadequate sleep hygiene (due to disruptive habits such as excessive napping or irregular sleep schedule), and environmental sleep disorder (due to environmental noise or discomfort). The ICSD also lists about a dozen psychiatric and medical disorders that may cause insomnia. The *Diagnostic and Statistical Manual of Mental Disorders,* fourth edition (*DSM-IV*; 2) is less copious. It lists one insomnia diagnosis, primary insomnia (comparable to psychophysiological insomnia from the ICSD), one general category for insomnia associated with mental disorders, and one general category for insomnia associated with medical disorders. The *International Classification of Diseases* (3) treats insomnia with frugality. It refers only to nonorganic insomnia but acknowledges that this may occur as a symptom of a mental or physical disorder.

This somewhat complex and confusing state of affairs may be distilled into a more compact nomenclature. When poor sleep is thought to arise from conditioned aversion to the bedroom or from subclinical emotional/cognitive turmoil, the disturbance may be termed *primary insomnia* (PI). However, when poor sleep is associated with an intrusive agent such as a psychiatric disorder, medical condition, or medication, the terms *secondary insomnia* (SI) or *comorbidity* applies. A large body of literature attests to the successful behavioral management of PI in middle-aged (4) and older (5) groups, but much less is known about the clinical management of SI. It is likely that one factor that has dampened interest in SI clinical trials is the commonly held belief that direct psychological treatment of SI is futile (6–8). Presumably, the primary condition would replenish the insomnia at the same pace as the behavioral intervention improved sleep. Not surprisingly, when sleep specialists confer the diagnosis of SI, they are less likely to treat the insomnia directly and more likely to focus treatment on the primary condition (9).

The diagnosis of SI is conferred if the offending agent, termed the *primary condition,* is believed to own a causal relationship with the insomnia, such that the primary condition instigated and sustains poor sleep. A corollary of this definition presumes the insomnia will resolve when the primary condition is successfully treated. However, if the suspicious agent shares more of an egalitarian relationship with the insomnia such that the insomnia and the other condition vacillate between (1) reciprocal exacerbation and (2) parallel coexistence absent of bearing influence one on the other, the term *comorbid* insomnia would be more appropriate.

SI is of critical clinical concern, because the majority of all insomnias are thought to be secondary to a psychiatric disorder, medical condition, or medication (10). Sleep is a vulnerable, fragile phenomenon. There is no limit to the number of primary conditions that could induce insomnia through some idiosyncratic interaction with an individual's physiological sensitivities, polypharmacy profile, personality, occupational demands, and interpersonal relationships.

EPIDEMIOLOGY

Diagnosis

Discerning the presence of an external agent that holds the potential to disrupt sleep is easy. Discriminating between SI and comorbid insomnia is difficult. The critical issue distills down to the philosophy of science question of causal inference. Whether co-occurrences are reviewed in the clinic or the laboratory, three conditions must be met to assert A (primary condition) causes B (insomnia; 11):

1. A must precede B.
2. Variations in A and B must covary.
3. Plausible alternative explanations for conditions 1 and 2 have been ruled out.

Establishing the presence of a causal relationship between the primary condition and the insomnia is the weak link in SI theory and practice.

Common Diagnostic Procedures

The *DSM-IV* (2) provides the most detailed guidance on the diagnosis of SI. To qualify as insomnia secondary to a mental disorder, the insomnia must be "temporally and causally (p. 592)" related to the mental disorder. As to medical SI, the *DSM* instructs there should be an association between the "onset, exacerbation, or remission of the general medical condition and that of the sleep disturbance (p. 598)." Further, the presence of atypical characteristics of the insomnia and a rationale for the mechanism of action of the primary condition on sleep strengthen the diagnosis. However, the *DSM* does not specify how the evaluator ascertains the presence of these salient characteristics.

Differentiating between SI and comorbidity is usually difficult. Aside from modestly reliable REM and delta sleep indicators associated with some forms of depression (12), there are no physical indicators of SI. Information on the history of the primary condition and the history of the insomnia are obtained by interview, and these are the data that discern a temporal relationship, covariation, and rule out competing explanations. The only study to evaluate agreement in diagnosing SI between two independent clinicians found weak reliability, kappa = 0.42 (13).

Clinical interview questions that can be expected to maximize diagnostic validity are presented in Table 11.1. Notice that the questions avoid steering the response toward confirmation of SI. The longer the SI has been present, the more difficult it would be for the patient to produce historically accurate information. We make no claims as to the actual level of validity attained by this approach. A response contrary to the prescribed response for *any one* of the five questions would rule out SI in the strict definition of the label.

Table 11.1   Interview Questions to Establish SI Using Depression as the Primary Condition

Question	Response that Would Be Positive for SI
1. Which started first, depression or insomnia?	1. Depression
2. How long after the depression started did insomnia begin?	2. Shortly thereafter
3. Have you noticed changes in your insomnia during periods when your depression gets worse?	3. Insomnia gets worse
4. Have you noticed changes in your insomnia during periods when your depression gets better?	4. Insomnia gets better
5. Have you noticed influences unrelated to your depression that make your insomnia better or worse?	5. No

Diagnostic Reconceptualization

A recently introduced heuristic diagnostic model of SI (10) specified three modified SI states: *absolute, partial,* and *specious* (see Table 11.2). Absolute SI refers to the common use of the term *SI.* That is, a primary condition instigates and sustains the poor sleep, but this subtype must satisfy several criteria:

1. The evaluator must be convinced that the informant is providing a reliable historical account.
2. The primary condition must have preceded the onset of the insomnia.
3. The time offset between the initiation of the primary condition and the insomnia must be brief (otherwise causal influence could be ascribed to other intervening variables).
4. Variations in the severity of the primary condition over time must be accompanied by like changes in sleep.
5. Insomnia changes do not occur in the absence of changes in the primary condition.

Logic mandates that the absence of any one of these criteria would preclude the diagnosis of absolute SI. Even when absolute SI exists, it would be difficult to collect enough information to reliably establish the presence of these five criteria.

Partial SI requires a subset of these same criteria. Foremost, the evaluator must still be convinced that the informant is providing a reliable historical account;

Table 11.2   Hypothesized Trichotomy of Secondary Insomnia

Type	Definition	Plausible Alternative Diagnoses
Absolute SI	A primary disorder or substance caused the initiation and controls the course of the insomnia.	Partial SI Specious SI
Partial SI	A primary disorder or substance may have initiated the insomnia or exacerbated a preexisting insomnia, but some proportion of the insomnia is functionally independent from the *primary disorder.*	Specious SI
Specious SI	There is the false appearance that a primary disorder or substance controls the insomnia. This is comorbidity mistaken for SI.	

otherwise, he or she would be at a loss to determine which part of the information to use. Two varieties of partial SI can be discerned. First, partial SI can be established when poor sleep shortly followed the onset of the primary condition (criteria 2 and 3), but criteria 4 and 5 did not hold. Apparently, having been instigated by an external agent, the insomnia subsequently assumed part or full functional independence. Second, the insomnia could have preexisted the onset of the primary condition, but subsequently the course of the insomnia did partially or fully track variations in the severity of the primary condition. In this SI subtype, the primary condition mainly serves to exacerbate the insomnia. McCrae and Lichstein (14) labeled these two subtypes *origin partial SI* and *severity partial SI,* respectively.

Finally, *specious SI* refers to cases where the conditions of either absolute or partial SI appear to be satisfied, but nevertheless, there is no SI, only comorbidity. This occurs when the evaluator is unable to discriminate the level of reliability of the patient's historical account, and such ambiguity commonly prevails. Even when the diagnosis of absolute or partial SI is confidently conferred, the evaluator still lacks unequivocal knowledge as to the causal relationship between the primary condition and poor sleep, and specious SI cannot be ruled out.

It is important to appreciate the complexity of the diagnosis of SI because it directly invites behavioral intervention. If clinicians accept the premise that absolute, partial, and specious SI are difficult to discriminate, they never really know what they are treating. Absolute SI would be a poor candidate for direct behavioral intervention because the primary condition would replenish the treated insomnia. However, partial SI, particularly of the origin subtype, would be expected to show at least a moderate treatment response and specious SI should respond as well as PI. Indeed, the magnitude of the treatment response to behavioral intervention may provide diagnostic insight in clarifying what type of SI is present.

Diagnostic Reciprocity

The role of the *primary condition* and the insomnia may transform over time. For delimited periods, it may be clear that the primary condition is moving the insomnia, but at other times, the reverse may be equally clear. Within the same individual, there may also be times when the relationship appears more egalitarian: Both are affecting the other or neither is affecting the other.

There are several hypothetical mechanisms by which insomnia may instigate or aggravate psychiatric or medical conditions. PI is commonly associated with elevated, but subclinical, anxiety, depression, and fatigue (15). Such conditions render the individual more vulnerable to psychiatric or medical challenge. There is also evidence that insomnia can compromise immunocompetence (16–18), again leading to heightened vulnerability. Further, we (19) have recently hypothesized that insomnia may function as a health risk factor in a diathesis-stress model. Individuals predisposed to a psychiatric or medical disorder are less able to defend against health challenge while contending with insomnia.

There are numerous clinical reports of variations in SI effecting change in the primary condition (20–23). In a clear example of reciprocity, pain during the day disturbed nighttime sleep in women with fibromyalgia, but poor sleep also intensified daytime pain (24). Basic research also supports the assertion that poor sleep compromises daytime pain tolerance (25).

Alcohol relapse is more likely with precedent insomnia (26), as is the onset of depression (27). Morawetz (28) presented dramatic data consistent with the primary role of insomnia. He behaviorally treated 84 individuals referred for insomnia, and two-thirds of these individuals had comorbid depression. Of the 84 patients, 87% exhibited substantial sleep improvement. Among the group of insomnia responders, 70% of those with depression also showed significant depression improvement, though the depression was untreated. Among insomnia nonresponders who were also depressed, none showed depression improvement.

COMMON CAUSES OF SECONDARY INSOMNIA

Sleep is highly reactive to irritants, including a broad range of psychiatric disorders (8), medical conditions (29–30), and medications (31). Conversely, it is worth noting that having a condition notorious for disrupting sleep does not necessarily condemn an individual to insomnia. No primary condition (except acute, severe intrusions such as surgery) produces universal insomnia.

There are four paths by which the primary condition can alter sleep. These mechanisms and examples are summarized in Table 11.3. Other documented examples include:

1. *Direct effects*—neurological diseases may produce muscle tremors and stiffness that disrupt sleep (32).
2. *Physical side effects*—pain associated with a wide range of disorders is a high risk factor for insomnia (33).
3. *Psychological side effects*—stress associated with cancer is one factor contributing to the high rate of insomnia in this group (34).
4. *Medications*—a broad range of nonprescription (e.g., caffeine, nicotine, and alcohol; 6, 35) and prescription (e.g., energizing antidepressants,

Table 11.3   Mechanisms that Produce Secondary Insomnia

Type	Description	Example
1. Direct effects	The primary disorder directly works on sleep.	Depression disrupts the psychophysiology of sleep.
2. Physical side effects	The primary condition produces physical side effects that disturb sleep.	Cancer may produce pain that disrupts sleep.
3. Psychological side effects	The primary condition produces stress that disturbs sleep.	Any medical or psychiatric condition that causes worry, disrupts relationships, increases financial burden, and so on, may also induce insomnia.
4. Medications	Prescription and over-the-counter medications taken for the primary condition may disturb sleep.	A long list of medications for physical (e.g., cancer chemotherapy) and psychiatric (e.g., SSRI antidepressants) disorders may disturb sleep.

antihypertensives, bronchodilators, diuretics, beta-blockers, and corticosteroids; 36–38) medications can induce insomnia.

It is not unusual for multiple causal mechanisms to simultaneously operate in a given case (39).

PREVALENCE

Estimating the prevalence of SI (either absolute or partial) is difficult because epidemiological studies rarely collect enough information to distinguish SI from comorbidity. Given our earlier discussion of the difficulty in making this distinction in the clinic, ambiguous diagnostic discrimination at the epidemiological level should be expected. This important constraint notwithstanding, some level of insight into SI prevalence can be achieved. Epidemiological research typically finds comorbidity rates of 40% to 60% between insomnia and serious psychiatric disorders (40–43). Ohayon's (44) epidemiological study conducted the most extensive interviews to date to establish SI. He found a 65% rate of SI—51.8% psychiatric SI, 8.9% medical SI, and 3.6% substance SI. Ohayon found a 9 to 1 ratio of medical SI in older adults compared to middle-aged individuals but found psychiatric SI was slightly more common in younger groups. Among older adults, medical SI probably accounts for the majority of insomnia complaints (45). Lichstein (10) reviewed diagnostic data from six sleep disorders centers. Nearly 75% of their insomnia patients were diagnosed as SI, including psychiatric, medical, and substance versions.

Several factors increase the likelihood that SI is more common and more severe in older adults. First, lighter sleep makes this group more sensitive to medical and psychiatric irritants. Second, higher rates of medical illness in older adults produce greater exposure to potential sources of SI. Third, normal physiologic changes associated with aging retard drug absorption, distribution, metabolism, and elimination and elevate target site sensitivity (38, 46). Fourth, bereavement is a risk factor for insomnia and is more likely to occur in this age group (45, 47, 48).

BEHAVIORAL TREATMENT OF SECONDARY INSOMNIA

Rationale for Treating Secondary Insomnia

Three lines of reasoning support the conclusion that SI is amenable to direct psychological intervention. First, as discussed earlier, therapists are usually not sure if they are treating absolute, partial, or specious SI. Partial and specious SI represent misdiagnosing comorbidity for SI, and there is little reason to hesitate treating insomnia with comorbid conditions. Second, we have previously cited research showing that treating SI will sometimes benefit the *primary condition.* Under such circumstances, it would be inadvisable to withhold insomnia treatment. Third, there is a recently emerging line of basic research showing that the polysomnography profile (49), subjective sleep disturbance (50), and presleep cognitive arousal (51) associated with SI do not significantly differ from PI. Therefore, the nature of the sleep disturbance in SI appears similar to that of PI, and these findings are consistent with the assumption that SI would be responsive to the same interventions used for PI.

Summary of Treatment Research

Our recent reviews provide an adequate summary of behavioral treatment for SI (10, 14, 29). Herein, we present an abbreviated review of this topic, emphasizing the studies with the strongest methodologies.

Several case studies dating to the early 1970s reported success applying a variety of behavioral interventions with different types of SI (21, 52–56). Morin et al. (22) presented a carefully done multiple baseline design demonstrating the effectiveness of stimulus control and sleep restriction for insomnia secondary to chronic pain in three individuals. Six-month follow-up revealed good maintenance of gains.

Dashevsky and Kramer (57) reported on the treatment of a group of individuals with *DSM-IV* psychiatric diagnoses who were unresponsive to hypnotic treatment of their insomnia. They were then offered behavioral treatment. About a third dropped out, but the 48 completers received a package of six sessions comprising sleep hygiene instruction, progressive relaxation, stimulus control, and sleep restriction. Significant improvement occurred at posttreatment and one-year follow-up on about a dozen self-report sleep and quality-of-life measures. About half the patients eliminated or reduced hypnotic use during behavioral treatment.

It is perhaps worthwhile to again note the Morawetz (28) data summarized previously (Diagnostic Reciprocity section)—the unique situation of indirectly treating *secondary depression* by intervening with PI.

There are only three randomized studies in this area. The first one evaluated a mixed age sample of cancer patients (58). Thirty patients were randomly assigned to usual medical care for their cancer or usual care plus three sessions of progressive relaxation (PR). Latency to sleep was dramatically improved in the PR group, going from 124 minutes at pretreatment to 29 minutes post. This variable was unchanged in the comparison group. Three-month follow-up found that both groups changed little from posttreatment. Other measures of sleep and pain favored the PR group but were not statistically significant.

Nearly two decades later, Currie, Wilson, Pontefract, and deLaplante (59) evaluated cognitive-behavioral therapy (CBT) in 60 patients suffering chronic pain from a variety of sources. Participants were randomized to CBT, consisting of sleep restriction, stimulus control, cognitive restructuring, and relaxation or to a wait-list control (WLC). Compared to WLC, CBT participants demonstrated significant improvement from baseline to three-month follow-up on self-reported sleep onset latency (54.7 min to 27.8 min), wake time after sleep onset (88.9 min to 51.6 min), sleep efficiency (72% to 84%), and sleep quality (Pittsburgh Sleep Quality Index score of 13.6 to 7.9).

Last, our group (20) reported a randomized study of SI in older adults. Forty-four volunteers who satisfied the SI interview screening presented in Table 11.1 were randomized to four sessions of combined hybrid passive relaxation, stimulus control, and sleep hygiene instructions or to a WLC. Our sample was evenly divided between insomnia secondary to psychiatric and to medical disorders. There was significantly greater improvement at posttreatment and three-month follow-up for the treated group on three self-report sleep measures: wake time during the night, sleep efficiency percent, and rated quality of sleep (from 1 = very poor to

5 = excellent). From baseline to follow up for the treated group, wake time went from 87.3 minutes to 56.4 minutes, sleep efficiency percent went from 66.7% to 77.7%, and rated quality of sleep went from 2.7 to 3.2. Participants with medical and psychiatric SI did not differentially respond.

Prevention

Based on a search of PsychLit and MedLine, there is no prior literature on prevention of SI. We (14) recently initiated a discussion of this matter. The following summarizes and extends our previous comments.

Figure 11.1 presents a hypothetical model for the ontogeny of SI. The common prevalence of insomnia is about 10%, and this is referred to as the premorbid phase with respect to onset of a threatening psychiatric or medical condition. For example, with pain, incident insomnia abruptly jumps with severe pain onset, and most of these new cases are probably absolute SI. The acute phase is distinguished by intense symptoms or intense treatment. The acute phase may last days or years. When the primary condition assumes chronic status (marked by stable, decreased symptomatology) or is alleviated altogether, some proportion of the SI group will revert to normal sleep (shown by the striped segment in Figure 11.1). Individuals

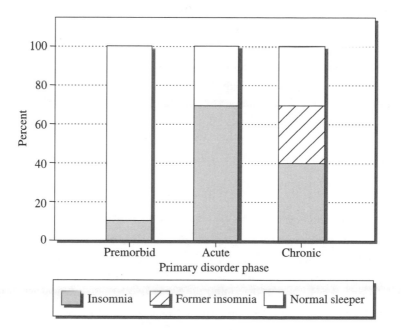

Figure 11.1   Hypothetical Course of Secondary Insomnia over the Life of the Primary Condition

with enduring SI extending into the chronic phase are now more likely character-ized by partial or specious SI.

We can derive a number of insights from this model:

1. It would be useful to identify premorbid characteristics that differentially predict who will preserve normal sleep, who will exhibit insomnia only during acute challenge, and who will acquire chronic insomnia.

2. Behavioral intervention for insomnia is likely to have greater success dur-ing the chronic phase than during the acute phase.

3. The treatment response of the primary condition may be inhibited by per-sistent insomnia during the chronic phase.

Four principles, summarized in Table 11.4, should guide SI prevention efforts. The remainder of this section explores these four concepts.

Minimize Impact of Primary Condition Treatment on Sleep

When an individual is diagnosed with a primary condition known to produce SI, it is important to try to minimize the impact of such treatment on sleep. The at-tending physician is in the best position to assess threats to sleep, and patients should be encouraged to assertively express their concerns to their physician about sleep impact. Under the best of circumstances, the physician will incorpo-rate sleep considerations into his or her treatment plan.

Medication prescribed for the primary condition is often the chief culprit in dis-rupting sleep and may be amenable to sleep-friendly revision. In some cases, it may be possible to substitute a sedating, nonalerting, or less alerting, medication. For example, mirtazapine (Remeron), an antidepressant that may improve insomnia (60), could be used in place of fluoxetine (Prozac). When there is no appropriate

---

Table 11.4 Four Principles for Guiding SI Prevention

1. Treatment of psychiatric and medical conditions should be orchestrated to mini-mize impact on sleep.
2. Identify individuals who might be at risk for SI and prepare them for approaching initiation or exacerbation of insomnia.
3. Identify disorders notorious for instigating SI and prepare individuals for approaching initiation of insomnia.
4. Early intervention with emergent SI.

substitute, other steps may be available to minimize the impact of medication on sleep. For example, it may be possible to alter time of administration. Taking alerting medication in the morning sometimes spares nighttime sleep.

Identifying Individuals at Risk for Secondary Insomnia

Individuals with a history of insomnia, even intermittent mild insomnia, who are newly diagnosed with a disorder that poses at least a minor irritant to sleep, are probably at risk for partial SI of the severity subtype. This assumption, like most others in the prevention section, is untested. There is little research profiling who is at risk for either PI or SI.

In some cases, individuals with a history of insomnia happen to encounter a disorder that raises the threat of worsening sleep. In other cases, insomnia is a known risk factor for the disorder, and it is expected that a substantial number of individuals diagnosed with this disorder (e.g., depression) will present with insomnia (40).

Although preventive behavioral interventions for insomnia have not been studied, models for such approaches exist in other domains. Anxiety and depression have been shown to be responsive to prevention efforts (61). University students at risk for depression had fewer episodes of generalized anxiety disorder and showed a trend toward fewer major depressive episodes following CBT than did controls. Similarly, individuals who have exhibited subclinical levels of panic disorder were randomized to CBT or WLC (62). Subsequently, treated individuals suffered significantly fewer panic attacks.

Relapse prevention (RP; 63) is a model worth testing with individuals at risk for SI. Originally developed for individuals with a history of alcohol abuse, RP has been successfully used with a wide range of disorders including sexual aggression, obsessive-compulsive disorder, and depression (summarized in 63). RP uses an array of CBT techniques to nurture self-efficacy in individuals confronting return of unwanted behaviors in high-risk situations. Individuals are prepared with coping responses and taught to distinguish lapses (temporary return) from relapses (full-blown return) of unwanted behaviors.

As adapted to SI, individuals with a history of insomnia might encounter intensification of sleep disturbance during spells of exacerbation of the primary disorder. Rather than invigorate former attitudes of worry and exacerbation cycling, individuals would summon up insomnia coping skills (e.g., stimulus control, relaxation) to self-manage instances of poor sleep and embrace an optimistic, self-confident attitude (self-efficacy). Such coping skills would be trained before the appearance of SI.

High-Risk Primary Disorders

Conditions such as depression, anxiety, cancer, and chronic pain have earned a notorious label for SI. Details about the causal path and discriminating between absolute and partial SI aside, we know that a substantial portion of individuals with these and other disorders will develop insomnia. Studies of patients experiencing pain from varied sources report 50% to 70% of these individuals suffer insomnia (64–66). Sleep difficulties occur in 40% to 60% of outpatients and up to 90% of inpatients with major depression (2). Insomnia prevalence of 20% to 50% occurs among cancer patients (67).

Factors that might elevate SI risk among individuals with no history of insomnia are unknown, although a history of psychiatric disturbance would plausibly be relevant. There is little empirical basis to guide the clinician in identifying individuals who will actually develop insomnia from among those exposed to high-risk comorbid conditions.

The clinician may consider asking the patient to periodically maintain a sleep diary to monitor sleep. The sleep diary serves a dual purpose:

1. It helps to raise the individual's awareness of his or her sleep pattern.
2. If the patient begins to develop a problem sleeping, the clinician can identify and treat it before it develops into a chronic problem.

As a cautionary note, for some patients, self-monitoring may foster performance anxiety that obstructs sleep.

The RP model could be adapted to the present circumstance as well, although this section is distinguished by individuals who have been asymptomatic for insomnia before the onset of the primary condition. Perhaps a more relevant model is stress inoculation (68). Individuals may be trained to better cope with anticipated stressors to avert expected noxious consequences. Stress inoculation comprises three steps:

1. Education
2. Training CBT coping skills
3. Practice

Steps 1 and 2, more so than step 3, could readily be accommodated within an SI framework. Education and training would commence as soon as the threatening primary condition was diagnosed. Practice would naturally occur if insomnia gradually emerged.

Early Intervention with Emergent Secondary Insomnia

When primary prevention fails, secondary prevention or early SI intervention may prove helpful in circumventing the reciprocal escalation of symptoms between the insomnia and the primary condition. This requires some degree of vigilance on the part of the provider and/or the patient. SI tends to be a persistent rather than a short-lived disorder (69). Ignoring emergent SI is not likely to be rewarded by its natural demise. When SI is detected, our advice is to aggressively treat it as you would PI.

SUMMARY AND FUTURE DIRECTIONS

Though difficult to estimate the prevalence of SI, it probably accounts for 50% to 70% of all insomnia cases. A critical problem in diagnosing SI is distinguishing between comorbidity and true SI wherein a primary condition owns a causal relationship with the insomnia. We hypothesized that SI is more accurately conceived of as a trichotomy: absolute, partial (with origin and severity subtypes), and specious. These components usually defy diagnostic differentiation, absolute is probably the least common form, and aggressive behavioral management of SI, the same as that for PI, is usually justified.

Unidimensional conceptions of SI will fail to appreciate the role of comorbidity, will lead to overdiagnosis of SI, and will result in lost opportunities for effective insomnia intervention. When considering the SI diagnosis, the clinician/researcher is obliged to scrutinize relationships and processes between the *primary* condition and the sleep disturbance. There may evolve an upward spiraling, reciprocal relationship between the insomnia and the primary disorder, whereby each aggravates the other, and each subsequently suffers as the other worsens (23, 66). A downward spiraling, beneficial version of this reciprocity has also been reported (20–22). At other times, the insomnia may precede and instigate the *primary* disorder (23, 40).

Accelerating interest by psychologists in SI barely extends back a decade. This is an area with recent exciting results in both the basic research and clinical trial domains. There are prime opportunities just on the horizon for important behavioral sleep medicine (BSM) research. Three areas appear to be particularly compelling. First, more systematic research on the effect of treating either the insomnia or the primary condition and the effect on the other is warranted. Morawetz' (28) research is a stunning example of successful insomnia treatment garnering significant improvement in the primary condition. Is it possible that focusing on insomnia treatment could routinely obtain substantial improvement in the primary condition? Pain, depression, and anxiety are perhaps particularly ripe for such studies. The reverse, focusing on the primary condition, is also of concern. It is interesting that there has never been a single published report of a controlled investigation obtaining insomnia relief following treatment of the primary condition. Second, and related to the first, if reciprocity often exists between the insomnia and the primary condition, might it not be clinically useful to treat both simultaneously? It may be that greater gains can be obtained by treating both disorders than either one separately. There has never been a single published report of a controlled investigation testing this plausible thesis. Third, primary and secondary prevention of SI is an important topic and is wide open for investigation. The relapse prevention and stress inoculation models could be easily adapted to SI. Experimental designs used in other areas (62) would fit well in SI research. Individuals on the threshold of a threatening primary disorder could be randomized to treatment or WLC/placebo conditions, and prospective evaluations would determine the preventive utility of the intervention.

REFERENCES

1. American Sleep Disorders Association. *International Classification of Sleep Disorders: Diagnostic and Coding Manual.* Rochester, MN: American Sleep Disorders Association. 1990.

2. American Psychiatric Association. *Diagnostic and Statistical Manual of Mental Disorders* (4th Edition). Washington, DC: American Psychiatric Association. 1994.

3. World Health Organization. *International Statistical Classification of Diseases and Related Health Problems,* tenth revision. Geneva, Switzerland: World Health Organization. 1992.

4. Lichstein, K. L. and C. M. Morin, eds. *Treatment of Late-Life Insomnia.* Thousand Oaks, CA: Sage. 2000.

5. Lichstein, K. L. and B. W. Riedel. Behavioral assessment and treatment of insomnia: A review with an emphasis on clinical application. *Behavior Therapy* 25: 659–688, 1994.

6. Mendelson, W. B. and B. Jain. An assessment of short-acting hypnotics. *Drug Safety* 13: 257–270, 1995.

7. National Institutes of Health. The treatment of sleep disorders of older people, March 26–28, 1990. *Sleep* 14: 169–177, 1991.

8. Walsh, J. K. and J. L. Sugerman. Disorder of initiating and maintaining sleep in adult psychiatric disorders. In M. H. Kryger, T. Roth, and W. C. Dement, eds. *Principles and Practice of Sleep Medicine.* Philadelphia, PA: W.B. Saunders Company. 1989: 448–455.

9. Buysse, D. J., C. F. Reynolds III, D. J. Kupfer, M. J. Thorpy, F. Bixler, A. Kales, et al. Effects of diagnosis on treatment recommendations in chronic insomnia: A report from the APA/NIMH *DSM-IV* field trial. *Sleep* 20: 542–552, 1997.

10. Lichstein, K. L. Secondary insomnia. In K. L. Lichstein and C. M. Morin, eds. *Treatment of Late-Life Insomnia.* Thousand Oaks, CA: Sage. 2000: 297–319.

11. Shadish, W. R., T. D. Cook, and D. T. Campbell. *Experimental and Quasi-Experimental Designs for Generalized Causal Inference.* Boston, MA: Houghton Mifflin. 2002.

12. Perlis, M. L., D. E. Giles, D. J. Buysse, M. E. Thase, X. Tu, and D. J. Kupfer. Which depressive symptoms are related to which sleep electroencephalographic variables? *Biological Psychiatry* 42: 904–913, 1997.

13. Buysse, D. J., C. F. Reynolds III, P. J. Hauri, T. Roth, E. J. Stepanski, M. J. Thorpy, et al. Diagnostic concordance for *DSM-IV* sleep disorders: A report from the APA/NIMH *DSM-IV* field trial. *American Journal of Psychiatry* 151: 1351–1360, 1994.

14. McCrae, C. S. and K. L. Lichstein. Secondary insomnia: A heuristic model and behavioral approaches to assessment, treatment and prevention. *Applied and Preventive Psychology* 10: 107–123, 2001.

15. Riedel, B. W. and K. L. Lichstein. Insomnia and daytime functioning. *Sleep Medicine Reviews* 4: 277–298, 2000.

16. Cover, H. and M. Irwin. Immunity and depression: Insomnia, retardation and reduction of natural killer cell activity. *Journal of Behavioral Medicine* 17: 217–223, 1994.

17. Hall, M., A. Baum, D. J. Buysse, H. G. Prigerson, D. J. Kupfer, and C. F. Reynolds III. Sleep as a mediator of the stress-immune relationship. *Psychosomatic Medicine* 60: 48–51, 1998.

18. Irwin, M., M. Fortner, C. Clark, J. McClintick, C. Costlow, J. White, et al. Reduction of natural killer cell activity in primary insomnia and in major depression. *Sleep Research* 24: 256, 1995.

19. Taylor, D. J., K. L. Lichstein, and H. H. Durrence. Insomnia as a Health Risk Factor. *Behavioral Sleep Medicine* in press.

20. Lichstein, K. L., N. M. Wilson, and C. T. Johnson. Psychological treatment of secondary insomnia. *Psychology and Aging* 15: 232–240, 2000.

21. Morin, C. M., R. A. Kowatch, and G. O'Shanick. Sleep restriction for the inpatient treatment of insomnia. *Sleep* 13: 183–186, 1990.

22. Morin, C. M., R. A. Kowatch, and J. B. Wade. Behavioral management of sleep disturbances secondary to chronic pain. *Journal of Behavior Therapy and Experimental Psychiatry* 20: 295–302, 1989.

23. Paiva, T., A. Batista, P. Martins, and A. Martins. The relationship between headaches and sleep disturbances. *Headache* 35: 590–596, 1995.

24. Affleck, G., S. Urrows, H. Tennen, P. Higgins, and M. Abeles. Sequential daily relations of sleep, pain intensity, and attention to pain among women with fibromyalgia. *Pain* 68: 363–368, 1996.

25. Onen, S. H., A. Alloui, A. Gross, A. Eschallier, and C. Dubray. The effects of total sleep deprivation, selective sleep interruption and sleep recovery on pain tolerance thresholds in healthy subjects. *Journal of Sleep Research* 10: 35–42, 2001.

26. Brower, K. J., M. S. Aldrich, E. A. R. Robinson, R. A. Zucker, and J. F. Greden. Insomnia, self-medication, and relapse to alcoholism. *American Journal of Psychiatry* 158: 399–404, 2001.

27. Perlis, M. L., D. E. Giles, D. J. Buysse, X. Tu, and D. J. Kupfer. Self-reported sleep disturbance as a prodromal symptom in recurrent depression. *Journal of Affective Disorders* 42: 209–212, 1997.

28. Morawetz, D. Depression and insomnia: Which comes first? *Australian Journal of Counseling Psychology* 3(1): 19–24, 2001.

29. McCrae, C. S. and K. L. Lichstein. Secondary insomnia: Diagnostic challenges and intervention opportunities. *Sleep Medicine Reviews* 5: 47–61, 2001.

30. Wooten, V. Medical causes of insomnia. In M. H. Kryger, T. Roth, and W. C. Dement, eds. *Principles and Practice of Sleep Medicine.* Philadelphia, PA: W.B. Saunders Company. 1989: 456–475.

31. Schweitzer, P. K. Drugs that disturb sleep and wakefulness. In M. H. Kryger, T. Roth, and W. C. Dement, eds. *Principles and Practice of Sleep Medicine* (3rd Edition). Philadelphia, PA: W.B. Saunders Company. 2000: 441–461.

32. Aldrich, M. S. Insomnia in neurological diseases. *Journal of Psychosomatic Research* 37(Suppl. 1): 3–11, 1993.

33. Moldofsky, H. Sleep and pain. *Sleep Medicine Reviews* 5: 387–398, 2001.

34. Hu, D. S. and P. M. Silberfarb. Management of sleep problems in cancer patients. *Oncology* 5(9): 23–27, 1991.

35. Moran, M. G. and A. Stoudemire. Sleep disorders in the medically ill patient. *Journal of Clinical Psychiatry* 53(Suppl.): 29–36, 1992.

36. Becker, P. M. and A. O. Jamieson. Common sleep disorders in the elderly: Diagnosis and treatment. *Geriatrics* 47(3): 41–42, 45–48, 51–52, 1991.

37. Mitler, M. M., S. Poceta, S. J. Menn, and M. K. Erman. Insomnia in the chronically ill. In P. J. Hauri, ed. *Case Studies in Insomnia.* New York, NY: Plenum Press. 1991: 223–236.

38. Monane, M. Insomnia in the elderly. *Journal of Clinical Psychiatry* 53(Suppl.): 23–28, 1992.

39. Smith, M. C., H. Ellgring, and W. H. Oertel. Sleep disturbances in Parkinson's disease patients and spouses. *Journal of the American Geriatrics Society* 45: 194–199, 1997.

40. Ford, D. E. and D. B. Kamerow. Epidemiologic study of sleep disturbances and psychiatric disorders: An opportunity for prevention? *Journal of the American Medical Association* 262: 1479–1484, 1989.

41. Klink, M., S. F. Quan, W. T. Kaltenborn, and M. D. Lebowitz. Risk factors associated with complaints of insomnia in a general adult population: Influence of previous complaints of insomnia. *Archives of Internal Medicine* 152: 1634–1637, 1992.

42. Mellinger, G. D., M. B. Balter, and E. H. Uhlenhuth. Insomnia and its treatment. *Archives of General Psychiatry* 42: 225–232, 1985.

43. Ohayon, M. M., M. Caulet, and P. Lemoine. Comorbidity of mental and insomnia disorders in the general population. *Comprehensive Psychiatry* 39: 185–197, 1998.

44. Ohayon, M. M. Prevalence of *DSM-IV* diagnostic criteria of insomnia: Distinguishing insomnia related to mental disorders from sleep disorders. *Journal of Psychiatric Research* 31: 333–346, 1997.

45. Hoch, C. C., D. J. Buysse, T. H. Monk, and C. F. Reynolds III. Sleep disorders and aging. In J. E. Birren, R. B. Sloane, and G. D. Cohen, eds. *Handbook of Mental Health and Aging* (2nd Edition). San Diego, CA: Academic Press. 1992: 557–581.

46. Gottlieb, G. L. Sleep disorders and their management: Special considerations in the elderly. *American Journal of Medicine* 88(Suppl. 3A): 29S–33S, 1990.

47. Hall, M., D. J. Buysse, M. A. Dew, H. G. Prigerson, D. J. Kupfer, and C. F. Reynolds III. Intrusive thoughts and avoidance behaviors are associated with sleep disturbances in bereavement-related depression. *Depression and Anxiety* 6: 106–112, 1997.

48. Monjan, A. and D. Foley. *Incidence of Chronic Insomnia Associated with Medical and Psychosocial Factors: An Epidemiological Study among Older Persons.* Paper presented at the meeting of the Association of Professional Sleep Societies, Washington, DC. 1996, June.

49. Schneider-Helmert, D., I. Whitehouse, A. Kumar, and C. Lijzenga. Insomnia and alpha sleep in chronic nonorganic pain as compared to primary insomnia. *Neuropsychobiology* 43: 54–58, 2001.

50. Lichstein, K. L., H. H. Durrence, B. W. Riedel, and U. J. Bayen. Primary versus secondary insomnia in older adults: Subjective sleep and daytime functioning. *Psychology and Aging* 16: 264–271, 2001.

51. Smith, M. T., M. L. Perlis, M. S. Smith, D. E. Giles, and T. P. Carmody. Sleep quality and presleep arousal in chronic pain. *Journal of Behavioral Medicine* 23: 1–13, 2000.

52. French, A. P. and J. P. Tupin. Therapeutic application of a simple relaxation method. *American Journal of Psychotherapy* 28: 282–287, 1974.

53. Kolko, D. J. Behavioral treatment of excessive daytime sleepiness in an elderly woman with multiple medical problems. *Journal of Behavior Therapy and Experimental Psychiatry* 15: 341–345, 1984.

54. Stam, H. J. and B. D. Bultz. The treatment of severe insomnia in a cancer patient. *Journal of Behavior Therapy and Experimental Psychiatry* 17: 33–37, 1986.

55. Tan, T. L., J. D. Kales, A. Kales, E. D. Martin, L. D. Mann, and C. R. Soldatos. Inpatient multidimensional management of treatment-resistant insomnia. *Psychosomatics* 28: 266–272, 1987.

56. Varni, J. W. Behavioral treatment of disease-related chronic insomnia in a hemophiliac. *Journal of Behavior Therapy and Experimental Psychiatry* 11: 143–145, 1980.

57. Dashevsky, B. A. and M. Kramer. Behavioral treatment of chronic insomnia in psychiatrically ill patients. *Journal of Clinical Psychiatry* 59: 693–699, 1998.

58. Cannici, J., R. Malcolm, and L. A. Peek. Treatment of insomnia in cancer patients using muscle relaxation training. *Journal of Behavior Therapy and Experimental Psychiatry* 14: 251–256, 1983.

59. Currie, S. R., K. G. Wilson, A. J. Pontefract, and L. deLaplante. Cognitive-behavioral treatment of insomnia secondary to chronic pain. *Journal of Consulting and Clinical Psychology* 68: 407–416, 2000.

60. Thase, M. E. Antidepressant treatment of the depressed patient with insomnia. *Journal of Clinical Psychiatry* 60: 28–31, 1999.

61. Seligman, M. E. P., P. Schulman, R. J. DeRubeis, and S. D. Hollon. The prevention of depression and anxiety. *Prevention and Treatment* 2: article 8, 1999.

62. Gardenswartz, C. A. and M. G. Craske. Prevention of panic disorder. *Behavior Therapy* 32: 725–737, 2001.

63. Marlatt, G. A. and W. H. George. Relapse prevention and the maintenance of optimal health. In S. A. Shumaker, E. B. Schron, J. K. Ockene, and W. L. McBee, eds. *The Handbook of Health Behavior Change* (2nd Edition). New York, NY: Springer. 1998: 33–58.

64. Atkinson, J. H., S. Ancoli-Israel, M. A. Slater, S. R. Garfin, and J. C. Gillin. Subjective sleep disturbance in chronic back pain. *Clinical Journal of Pain* 4: 225–232, 1988.

65. Morin, C. M., D. Gibson, and J. Wade. Self-reported sleep and mood disturbance in chronic pain patients. *Clinical Journal of Pain* 14: 311–314, 1998.

66. Pilowsky, I., I. Crettenden, and M. Townley. Sleep disturbance in pain clinic patients. *Pain* 23: 27–33, 1985.

67. Savard, J. and C. M. Morin. Insomnia in the context of cancer: A review of a neglected problem. *Journal of Clinical Oncology* 19: 895–908, 2001.

68. Meichenbaum, D. *Cognitive-Behavior Modification: An Integrative Approach*. New York, NY: Plenum. 1977.

69. Katz, D. A. and C. A. McHorney. Clinical correlates of insomnia in patients with chronic illness. *Archives of Internal Medicine* 158: 1099–1107, 1998.

Chapter 12

CIRCADIAN RHYTHM FACTORS IN INSOMNIA AND THEIR TREATMENT

LEON C. LACK AND RICHARD R. BOOTZIN

Earlier chapters have discussed insomnia in terms of being primary or secondary. In other words, its etiology either cannot be explained or can be explained by other contributing factors. Although the distinction between primary and secondary may have some merit for purposes of categorization, it is dependent on the current degree of understanding of the causes of insomnia. As new correlates or causes of insomnia continue to be discovered, some have questioned whether the entity of "primary" insomnia will survive, thereby making the primary/secondary distinction uninformative. In any case, to conceptualize in simple cause and effect terms is not helpful in understanding a complex system such as a human interacting with a complex physical/social environment. This environment impinges on the individual, but it, in turn, changes because of the responses of the individual. The following discussion shows that a circadian rhythm phase or timing abnormality can lead to insomnia but also that insomnia can lead to a circadian abnormality. Thus, a feedback loop can be established, which perpetuates and exacerbates both aspects of the problem.

FACTORS THAT AFFECT SLEEP PROPENSITY

To appreciate the role of circadian rhythm factors in insomnia, it is necessary to understand how our circadian rhythms normally influence sleep propensity. By *sleep propensity,* we mean the ease or speed of falling asleep. Subjective sleepiness and its inverse, subjective alertness, are imperfectly related to the behavioral measure of sleep propensity and are thus somewhat different measures. Because insomnia is a difficulty in initiating and maintaining sleep when attempting to sleep, the determinants of sleep propensity are more relevant to this discussion.

First, it is useful to put the circadian rhythm factor into the context of all the ways in which sleep propensity can be influenced. These influences include external stimuli such as noise, light, and pain. There are internal processes such as emotional responses, motivation to resist sleep, drugs that are stimulants or sedatives, and learned or conditioned responses to external stimuli that raise or lower arousal level. The latter example may be implicated in *psychophysiological* insomnia in the form of bedroom stimuli and intentions to fall asleep. For the good sleeper, these stimuli associated with bedtime are probably conditioned stimuli eliciting an increase in sleep propensity. However, as mentioned in earlier chapters, for the insomniac, the stimuli are presumed to be conditioned stimuli that elicit sympathetic nervous system activation and result in decreased sleep propensity. It is this putative contribution to psychophysiological insomnia that is addressed by the behavioral therapies of stimulus control and bedtime restriction.

Homeostatic Sleep Propensity

A group of factors, called *endogenous biological factors,* include those biological effects inherent to the neurological mechanisms that generate sleep as well as those that vary sleep propensity in a rhythmical way. Probably the most commonly understood of these influences is increasing sleep propensity with accumulated time awake. The commonly held notion is that we need sleep simply to compensate for our time awake, and the longer we stay awake, the greater becomes our sleep propensity and the longer we need to sleep to recover. This is seen to operate similar to the increase of hunger and food-seeking behavior with increasing abstinence from food. The maintenance of a stable body weight illustrates a homeostatic process, which roughly balances nutriment intake with energy expenditure over the long term. Similarly, the maintenance of a relatively fixed ratio of sleep to wakefulness (a ratio of about 1 to 2) or about 8 hours sleep to 16 hours wakefulness every 24 hours of time represents a homeostatic sleep-wake process. It does this by building up sleep pressure or propensity during wakefulness and reducing it during sleep.

The homeostatic process, *Process S,* is a major determiner of sleep propensity (1). Until the last couple of decades, this was the only endogenous biological influence that had common acceptance. Two more influences have been relatively recently elucidated: sleep inertia and the circadian influence. *Sleep inertia* or *Process W* (for wakening) is the label given to a postsleep effect. Immediately after awakening from sleep, there is a depression of alertness, which has both subjective and objective consequences. It is more intense and lasts longer when prior sleep has been longer and is stronger if awoken from deeper sleep stages. However, this effect dissipates within two to four hours and, thus, is relatively short lived (2).

Endogenous Circadian Determination of Sleep Propensity

Over the past two decades, a large range of research studies has shown the influence of circadian rhythms on sleep propensity to be robust and predictable. *Circadian rhythms* refer to oscillations of some measure (physiological, hormonal, behavioral) with one complete oscillation or period of about (circa) 24 hours or one day (dian). Circadian rhythms are ubiquitous. Virtually every biological or psychological measure taken on an individual repeatedly over time shows a circadian rhythm. This is true for biochemical measures such as sodium and potassium levels; physiological measures such as core body temperature and metabolic rate; hormonal measures such as melatonin, cortisol, and testosterone; and cognitive-behavioral measures such as short-term memory capacity, reaction times, and sleep propensity. For example, core body temperature normally reaches its peak in the early evening (6 to 8 P.M.) and trough in the early morning (4 to 6 A.M.), cortisol hormone normally reaches its peak in the last few hours of nocturnal sleep, short-term memory capacity is greatest in the morning (4 to 10 A.M.), and least sleep propensity or longest sleep latency is normally in the early evening (6 to 8 P.M.) and greatest sleep propensity in the early morning (4 to 6 A.M.).

It is felt that the complex of biochemical, physiological, and hormonal rhythms (the endogenous circadian system) influences the cognitive-behavioral rhythms including sleep propensity. The circadian system does not categorically enforce the state of wake or sleep; instead, it varies sleep propensity or the likelihood and ease of falling asleep. The question is: What is the relative strength of the circadian effect? For example, even though the sleep propensity from circadian processes would normally be high and strongly predispose toward sleep in the early morning, it is possible to remain awake with counteracting psychological motivation and drugs. This impetus may arise, for example, in a truck driver with the need to reach a shipping destination by dawn. However, despite motivation and help from stimulant drugs, even in potentially dangerous circumstances, wakefulness is not always maintained in opposition to the circadian effect, as witnessed by some notable early morning disasters such as those at the Chernobyl and Three Mile Island nuclear reactors. Those on a night shift of work regularly report great difficulty remaining awake during the hours of 3 to 6 A.M. If that were not enough of a problem, the night worker then usually experiences difficulty in obtaining satisfactory sleep during the day. Part of that difficulty arises from the circadian rhythm predisposition for alertness during the day.

People who cross several time zones on intercontinental flights often experience difficulty sleeping at the nighttime of their destination and difficulty staying awake during their destination daytime. This experience, called *jet lag,* may continue for up to several days or weeks following the flight. The explanation is that our circadian rhythms are still timed according to our normal home time zone and may take several days to weeks to resynchronize with the destination day- or nighttimes.

Experimental Support for the Circadian Effect on Sleep Propensity

The strength of the circadian rhythm effect on sleep propensity has been experimentally investigated in several interesting and sometimes Herculean ways. In the normally entrained individual, sleep occurs consistently in one phase of the circadian cycle. If core body temperature (usually measured with a rectal thermistor) is used as a marker for the circadian system, the sleep phase normally coincides with the period of decreasing and lowest core temperatures. However, to test the strength of the circadian effect on sleep propensity independent of prior time awake, the homeostatic Process S needs to be dissociated from its normal phase relationship to the circadian rhythm system.

The earliest studies in which this dissociation occurred were the so-called "free-running" studies in time-free environments in which individuals lived alone for weeks at a time in isolation of time cues from the environment. They were allowed to eat, sleep, and be active (to the extent possible in an underground bunker or confined experimental studio apartment) at whatever time they preferred. Thus, their circadian systems were "free-running" and determined by endogenous rhythms rather than any external environmental time cues. An interesting finding of these studies was that most of the participants maintained coherence between their circadian rhythms and sleep-wake cycles, but the period length extended to a mean of about 24.5 hours. That is, their choices of bedtimes and wake-up times delayed by about 30 minutes in every 24 hours. Why the average endogenous period length of humans appears to be somewhat longer than 24 hours is an interesting but unresolved question. Of more practical import is the fact that most of us manage to remain synchronized with the daily rhythm when exposed to the normal 24-hour world. However, most young adults who participated in this type of time-free study showed a tendency to phase delay with respect to the 24-hour world when they were freed from its influences. This is an important fact to remember when we later consider delayed sleep phase syndrome (DSPS), a sleep-wake problem common in adolescents and young adults.

However, despite the coherence between the sleep-wake cycle and other circadian rhythms in most participants, after the first few weeks or several days of the free-running experiment, many participants showed an uncoupling or dissociation between the sleep-wake cycle and the circadian system. While most rhythms such as core body temperature, cortisol, and melatonin remained circadian (close to 24 hours in period), the sleep-wake cycle (and a few other rhythms such as growth hormone) adopted a relatively consistent but different period length. Most individuals who dissociated the sleep-wake cycle adopted a longer period length (e.g., 28 to 36 hours) while a few adopted shorter than 24-hour sleep-wake cycles (3). This dissociation, while it was not an experimental manipulation but was spontaneous and endogenous, nevertheless allowed the possibility of exploring the influence of the circadian system on the sleep-wake cycle. More specifically, it allowed the examination of the timing of participants' choices of bedtimes and the timing of spontaneous awakenings from sleep. Because the two rhythms then had different period lengths, choices of bedtimes and sleep periods could occur at various circadian phases. If the circadian system had no effect on sleep propensity, choices of bedtime and arousals from sleep should, over the long term, occur equally in all phases.

The examination of these studies showed that bedtimes and awakenings from sleep were not equally distributed across all circadian phases (4). Bedtimes, and thus sleep onsets, were significantly more likely when the circadian temperature rhythm was in the phase of descending and low core temperature, which in a normal environment would correspond to the hours from about 12 midnight to 7 A.M. There was also a secondary peak of sleep onsets about nine hours after the core temperature minimum (CTmin). This second peak of sleep onsets normally corresponds to the early afternoon period when there is a recognizable increase of sleep propensity in many individuals (siesta or afternoon nap period).

Of most relevance to the question of sleep disorders was the discovery of two circadian phases during which the participants rarely chose to go to bed, presumably because they did not feel sleepy. This was largely independent of how long they had been awake up to that point and thus independent of the value of the homeostatic Process S. These two phases were called *wake-maintenance* zones because wakefulness was maintained during them (4–5). The more intense of these zones occurred around the time of maximum core temperature, which was about eight hours before the CTmin. This corresponds to the period from about 6 to 10 P.M. in a normally entrained individual (an individual who sleeps well in the normal nocturnal period of about 11 P.M. to 7 A.M.). A second, less intense, wake-maintenance zone was apparent about four to seven hours after the CTmin when core temperature is rising and corresponds to 8 to 11 A.M. in a normally entrained individual. It was also the period during which most wake-ups from sleep occurred largely independent of the time of sleep onset and thus length of prior sleep. Therefore, the most sleep-preferred circadian phase was shown to be the low core temperature period. However, this 8- to 10-hour sleep-conducive period is surrounded by periods during which participants chose not to go to bed or had an increased tendency to awake from sleep.

While the free-running studies established that participants avoided bed during these wake-maintenance zones, the studies did not determine whether sleep would be inhibited if subjects were instructed to attempt sleep during these zones. Because the sleep disorder of insomnia is associated with difficulty initiating sleep when the individual is clearly attempting to do so, the ability to initiate sleep across all circadian phases needed to be tested directly. This was done in a number of different studies by alternating fixed times of enforced wakefulness with fixed times of sleep opportunity. Although the different studies used different cycling periods (0.33, 0.50, 1.5, and 28 hours), in all cases, the ratio of wake to sleep durations was two to one, which maintained the normal ratio of wake time (16 hours) to sleep time (8 hours). Furthermore, all period lengths were outside the range of circadian rhythm entrainment. Therefore, the temperature rhythm followed a circadian period length while sleep propensity could be tested at all phases of the circadian rhythm. In this sense, these were "forced desynchrony" experiments in contrast to the spontaneous desynchrony occurring in the free-running studies.

Weitzman et al. ran a three-hour "day" experiment in which subjects were allowed one hour to sleep every three hours (6). This was continued over a period of five days. They found that the most sleep was generally obtained in the one-hour sleep opportunities around the CTmin and least sleep around the body temperature maximum. However, with only eight data points across the 24-hour period, it was not possible to investigate the presence of the secondary sleep period and second wake-maintenance zone predicted from the free-running studies.

Carskadon and Dement doubled the number of data points to 16 across the 24-hour period by running the 90-minute "day" experiment (60-min enforced wakefulness, 30-min allowed sleep) across several consecutive days (7). Strogatz's analysis of the Carskadon and Dement sleep data with respect to the measured core temperature showed a low sleep propensity corresponding with the predicted wake-maintenance zone six to nine hours before the CTmin and high sleep propensity around the time of the CTmin (4). However, evidence for the other zones was not apparent from this analysis, possibly because there were still too few data points across the 24-hour period. Furthermore, the masking effects of body activity (8–9) and evoked decreases of body temperature (10) from sleeps of up to 30 minutes long may have lowered the reliability of temperature rhythm phase determination.

Lavie (11) used seven-minute sleep trials every 20 minutes (20-minute "days") measured 72 times across a 24-hour period. The amount of sleep obtained in each trial plotted over this period resulted in a "sleep propensity function." It generally showed high sleep propensity over the hours from 12 midnight to about 7 A.M. and a less prominent peak of sleep propensity in the mid-afternoon. There was also a period of low sleep propensity in the early evening (named the *forbidden sleep zone*) when little or no sleep was obtained in the sleep trials despite prior sleep deprivation. This zone coincided with the evening wake-maintenance zone evident in the free-running studies. There was also a secondary nadir of sleep propensity in the late morning coinciding in clock time with the wake-up zone found in the earlier free-running studies. Therefore, Lavie's studies, with more frequent sampling of sleep propensity across the circadian period, confirmed the presence of the two sleep inhibition periods surrounding the nocturnal sleep-conducive period. However, because Lavie was not able to record core body temperature in his studies, it was not possible to confirm the direct relationship of these sleep inhibition zones to the circadian temperature rhythm.

Lack and Lushington (12) provided this confirmation in a 30-minute "day" study (10-minute sleep opportunity alternating with 20 minutes enforced wakefulness). Fourteen participants were sleep deprived for 24 hours and then sampled for sleep propensity (sleep latency) 48 times across another circadian period of enforced bed rest and continuous core temperature measurement. They confirmed the presence of the two sleep inhibition zones, one centered eight hours before the CTmin (at about 8 P.M.) and the second centered six hours after the CTmin (at about 10 A.M.). Furthermore, the timing of these zones was significantly correlated with the timing of the core temperature minimum. Therefore, these very short "day" studies have confirmed a reduced ability, even of sleep-deprived individuals, to initiate sleep in these wake-maintenance or sleep-forbidden and wake-up zones that surround the sleep-conducive period and are timed by the circadian system.

Other Herculean studies have tended to confirm at least parts of this model. Instead of rapid cycling of sleep and wake periods, some studies have enforced slow cycling or long enforced periods of wakefulness (e.g., 19 hours), alternating with proportionately long sleep opportunities (keeping the ratio of 2 to 1; 13). In these slow-cycling "forced-desynchrony" studies, the circadian system simply maintains a relatively consistent period length of about 24.4 hours despite an enforced 28-hour sleep-wake cycle. Over a period of about 34 continuous days of measurement (thus the Herculean label), sleep onsets occurred at all circadian phases after wakeful periods of about the same length (19 hours), thus controlling the length of prior wakefulness and intensity of the homeostatic Process S.

They confirmed that the endogenous circadian effect (independent of prior wakefulness) produced a peak sleep latency or minimum sleep propensity about eight hours before the CTmin. When the amount of wakefulness was examined in ongoing sleep, it showed a rapid increase a few hours following the CTmin. This was particularly dramatic in older individuals, who showed a secondary peak of wakefulness about six hours following the CTmin (14). Therefore, both the rapid cycling and slow cycling-forced desynchrony experiments have confirmed the difficulty in initiating sleep 6 to 10 hours before the core body temperature minimum and difficulty maintaining sleep, particularly for older people, four to eight hours following the CTmin.

CIRCADIAN RHYTHM INVOLVEMENT IN INSOMNIA

Publications as early as 1971 have suggested a possible involvement of circadian rhythm abnormalities in sleep disorders (15). Similar suggestions also came from a number of other authors (5, 16–24). Circadian rhythm factors may be involved in insomnia in several ways. The previous section has implied a difficulty with circadian rhythm phase or the timing of rhythms with respect to desired sleep times. The amplitude of the rhythms (the difference between maximum and minimum extent of the rhythm) may also be implicated in sleeping difficulties. The third way more recently suggested is with respect to the overall mean level of the rhythm; for example, it may be elevated over the entire period (day and night) in chronic insomniacs. Because most research has been on phase considerations in etiology and treatment, these are discussed in most detail and the other rhythm aspects of amplitude and overall mean are discussed briefly later.

Phase-Delayed Circadian Rhythms and Sleep Onset Insomnia

A phase delay of the circadian system with respect to the desired sleep period could possibly lead to sleep onset insomnia. For example, if the circadian system were delayed two to three hours, the evening wake-maintenance would also be delayed, extending until 1 A.M. and should delay sleep onsets attempted before that time. If a conventional arising time was still required (e.g., 6 to 7 A.M. as during a normal working weekday), delayed sleep onset would result in reduced and insufficient total sleep. An earlier similar suggestion from Weitzman and colleagues was that delayed sleep phase syndrome, often leading to sleep onset insomnia, resulted from a delayed circadian rhythm (25–26). Moreover, from a comprehensive analysis of the free-running studies as mentioned previously, Strogatz and colleagues suggested that a circadian phase delay could lead to sleep onset insomnia (4, 23).

How can an individual's circadian system lose its normal entrainment and become phase delayed? It may arise from an intentional realignment of the sleep-wake cycle and the endogenous circadian system such as occurs in transmeridian jet travel or in night shift work. For example, an eastward plane trip across three time zones would result in a three-hour phase delay of the traveler's circadian rhythms with respect to the destination clock (solar) time. The traveler's circadian timing would remain initially linked with home time. The circadian system has considerable inertia and is not easily retimed or phase changed. Therefore, the normal bedtime, for example, 11 P.M., in the destination would be 8 P.M. in the home time zone and would coincide with the evening wake-maintenance zone of the traveler's circadian rhythm. Sleep onset would be inhibited and result in a long sleep onset latency—perhaps the one to two hours that it takes to pass beyond the wake-maintenance zone. Thus, sleep onset may not occur until 1 A.M. in the destination. Then, if a 6 A.M. wake-up time is required in the destination, the traveler obtains only five hours sleep that night. It is very difficult to arise at that time, not only after insufficient sleep but because it is 3 A.M. with respect to the traveler's home-based circadian rhythm, the period of lowest circadian alertness and behavioral competence. If, instead, the traveler succumbs to this combination of biological sleep imperatives and sleeps past the intended wake-up time, there is little chance of resynchronizing to the destination environment.

Another increasingly common way of losing the normal entrainment of circadian rhythms results from a period of shift work, especially late or night shift. These work shifts may require work until late at night (12 midnight to 2 A.M.) or as late as 7 A.M. in the morning. Shift workers then usually attempt to sleep soon after their shift work with sleep periods extending until very late morning or early afternoon. If there is some circadian rhythm adjustment to this shift work-enforced sleep-wake schedule, it will phase delay the worker's rhythm. Attempts to reestablish a conventional sleep period (11 P.M. to 7 A.M.) after the period of shift work will confront the shift worker with the same type of phase delay as the previous example of the jet-lagged traveler (19). Sleep onsets at the conventional bedtime will be inhibited, and arousals at conventional times will be very difficult. If adjustment back to normal circadian entrainment does not occur rapidly, the several nights of sleep onset difficulty may develop into sleep onset insomnia.

Even without transmeridian plane flights or shift work, many individuals become phase delayed in their normal environments. Remember that most individuals have endogenous circadian period lengths longer than 24 hours. The average endogenous period length is estimated at about 24.3 hours with many individuals at 24.5 hours or greater. In other words, without the cues or entraining forces to keep synchronized to the 24-hour solar clock and social world, circadian rhythms would become increasingly phase delayed by 20 to 30 minutes per day in most individuals. After a couple of days (e.g., a weekend), a phase delay of an hour can occur. After a week of 30-minute nightly delays, the final phase delay could be about three hours and produce as much difficulty for sleep onsets at conventional bedtimes as the two previous examples. The cues or entraining forces (called *Zeitgebers* or *time givers*) that operate to keep the large majority of us appropriately synchronized to the 24-hour world is discussed next.

Light as a Zeitgeber

At one time, it was felt that what keeps us normally entrained and puts the brakes on this unrelenting tendency to phase delay is the combination of social cues (family, work, etc., requirements) and its effect on the timing of our behavior. However, now it is appreciated that the most potent entraining cue of our circadian rhythms is the light/dark cycle (for a recent review, see 27). Light stimulation of the retinas of the eyes activates phototransducers, which then stimulate the suprachiasmatic nucleus (SCN) of the hypothalamus (thought to be the circadian clock) to effect retiming or phase changes of the circadian system. These retinal phototransducers have yet to be identified, but it appears that they are most sensitive to the shorter wavelengths of the visible spectrum (blue at 450 nm to blue/green at 500 nm wavelengths; 28–31). Besides wavelength, the other characteristics of light that determine the strength of the phase change effect are the intensity, duration, and timing of the light with respect to the individual's present circadian phase.

In the initial studies with humans, light was not found to be an entraining stimulus—probably because the intensity of the light tested was too low. Low-intensity light (less than 100 lux illuminance, which is about normal for indoor room lighting) could entrain many species of rodents and birds but appeared ineffective with humans (20). However, it was then found that higher intensity light (> 2,000 lux) had a significant phase-changing effect (20, 32–35). Although the early studies did not find significant phase shifts in humans with low-light intensity, more carefully controlled recent studies have found that even moderate to lower intensity light (1,200 lux to 100 lux) can produce phase delays (36–37) and even phase advances with moderate to high indoor lighting of about 400 lux (38). Therefore, although bright light (> 2,000 lux) is more effective in circadian phase shifting, lower intensities can still be significantly effective.

The dose response curve showed an exponential decelerating function relating intensity to degree of phase change. That is, equal linear increments of intensity produced diminishing increments of phase change. For example, a doubling of phase change would have to be effected by much more than a doubling of intensity (36). This may be a similar response of the visual system to its normal intensity coding function for vision, which determines the relation between physical and subjectively experienced light intensity.

The timing of visual light stimulation is another dimension that determines circadian phase change effect. For a normally entrained individual, bright light stimulation during the middle of the day (as would be experienced from outdoor sunlight) has very little effect on changing the timing of a normally entrained circadian system. However, if bright light stimulation occurs during the normal nighttime, it can have the effect of retiming the circadian system (resetting the biological clock). More precisely, it appears that the effectiveness of the time of light stimulation is in relation to an individual's presently timed circadian system rather than nighttime per se. The critical reference point is the minimum phase of the endogenous core body temperature rhythm (CTmin). Bright light visual stimulation before the time of the CTmin will phase delay the circadian rhythm. For example, if the endogenous CTmin is at 4 A.M. and if bright light stimulation occurs from 12 midnight to 4 A.M., the subsequently measured endogenous CTmin will show a later temperature minimum, perhaps delayed by as much as three to four hours. Alternatively, if bright light visual stimulation occurs following the 4 A.M. time of CTmin (e.g., 5 A.M. to 7 A.M.), a phase advance will be produced in which the subsequently measured CTmin may then occur one to two hours earlier at 2 to 3 A.M.

Several studies have tested various time relationships between the light stimulation and initial CTmin time to explore how this relationship determines the magnitude and direction of the phase change effect (20, 32–36, 39–41). In general, the closer in time between the light stimulation and the time of the CTmin, the greater is the magnitude of phase change. This relationship is illustrated in Figure 12.1 by what has been termed the *phase response curve* (PRC) to the timing of light stimulation. Thus, the greatest phase delays occur for light timed immediately before the CTmin and the greatest advances for light immediately after the CTmin. The figure shows three PRCs for the effects of three different levels of light intensity.

The duration of the light stimulation is also of importance. Just as many species have shown phase-change effects to low-intensity light, they have shown effects to very brief durations (pulses) of light. Whereas in humans the intensity of light has to be greater to be noticeably effective, the duration of light "pulse" needs to be comparably longer. Generally, the longer the duration, the greater the magnitude of effect. In this sense, variation of duration has a similar effect to the variation of intensity of light. For long durations of light stimulation (e.g., four to five hours), the "timing" of the pulse is taken as its time-weighted average. For constant intensity, this would be the midpoint in time of the stimulation. For example, it is found that a phase advance was obtained even for light stimulation beginning 1.5 hours before the temperature minimum as long as the duration of the pulse was five hours, in which case the midpoint of the pulse followed the CTmin (42).

Spontaneous Phase Delay

We return to the individual who is not a jet-lagged traveler nor a night shift worker, but who may, nevertheless, become phase delayed. An individual with an endogenous period length of 24.5 hours must effectively phase advance by

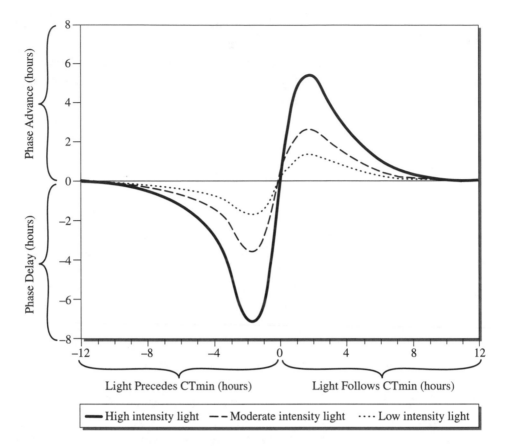

Figure 12.1   Phase Response Curves to Light. The curves indicate the amount of phase delay or advance (earlier) in hours produced by a pulse of light timed before or after the time when the core body temperature reaches its minimum. The curves show greater delaying and advancing effects for more intense light.

0.5 hours each day to stay synchronized with respect to the 24-hour world. Bright light stimulation is the most effective phase change tool and can naturally provide the brakes on this individual's tendency to sleep later each day. Awakening at a regular time each morning and getting visual exposure to moderately intense light will have a phase-advancing effect and can provide this brake to the delaying tendency. Awakening usually occurs soon after the body temperature minimum, during which time light stimulation has a strong phase-advancing effect.

However, sleeping later in the morning (common on weekends) effectively blocks retinal stimulation until later when the phase-advancing effect of light is diminished. This desire to sleep late may be understandable to catch up on lost sleep after a late night and exhausting week. However, this late sleep releases the phase-delay brake and can allow at least a half hour of circadian phase delay to occur after two sleep-ins over a weekend (43).

Later bedtimes and, especially, later waking times on weekends, are particularly common in high school and university students (43–46). Those who show the greatest weekend delay pattern also have the most difficulty on weekdays with scholastic demands and mood (44, 47–48).

A circadian phase delay in combination with recovery sleep over the weekend (from long sleep-ins) and the fact that by 11 P.M. on Sunday night, the individual may have been awake for only 12 instead of 16 hours may make sleep onset at 11 P.M. very difficult and most likely delayed (43). The return to early rising on Monday morning following a shorter than normal sleep and at an earlier circadian phase with its impairment to alertness may contribute to the depressed mood of the "Monday morning blues" (45, 49–50). Even with the attempt to maintain consistent wake times during weekdays, a delayed circadian rhythm may be difficult to fully phase advance back to preferred entrainment, especially if bright light is avoided in the mornings, for example, with the use of dark glasses. This phase delay will continue to be an obstruction for early enough sleep onsets to allow sufficient sleep by the necessary weekday wake-up time.

In addition to a period length longer than 24 hours, the tendency to phase delay may also arise from a reduced sensitivity of the phase advance portion of the phase response curve. This is implied in Figure 12.1 by a smaller amplitude of the PRC in the advance direction than delay direction for each of the three intensities. Both the longer period length and reduced advance response have been suggested as explanations of the finding that circadian phase adjustments requiring phase delays, such as westward time zone changes and "coming off" daylight savings time, are made more quickly than equal phase advance adjustments (51–53).

The critical role played by visual stimulation as the entraining cue ("brakes" to spontaneous phase delay) is dramatized in the example of individuals who are totally blind by the absence of eyes with functioning retinas (54). Despite regular lifestyles with daytime jobs and normal physical and social circadian cues other than retinal activation, they progressively phase delay. As a result, they show poor sleep for a period of one to two weeks, followed by a period of normal sleep and daytime functioning when their circadian rhythms periodically resynchronize with the 24-hour world (55). This is not the case with functionally blind individuals possessing intact retino-hypothalamic tracts who maintain synchrony and do not report recurrent insomnia (56).

Any cause of sleeping difficulty, even if it is relatively short lived, can lead to the development of perpetuating factors and chronic psychophysiological insomnia. The model presumes that experiencing difficulty falling asleep elicits a number of negative emotions such as frustration, anger, and anxiety. All of these increase arousal, both cortical and autonomic, and delay sleep onset further. There are always a number of cues consistently associated with this arousal, including the bedroom, turning out the lights, lying down, the bedclothes, the pillow, the bed, a sleeping partner, the time of night, and even the intention and desire to fall asleep. Gradually, these cues, through an association or conditioning process, can become triggers or conditioned stimuli, which can elicit the arousal response.

The development of psychophysiological sleep onset insomnia is most likely, then, to exacerbate the circadian phase delay component. Indeed, with increasingly late sleep onset times, there is an increased tendency to sleep late to obtain sufficient sleep. However, this later arising time avoids morning light exposure and thus leads to further phase delay, which, in turn, increases the sleep onset difficulty. In fact, the initial cause of sleep onset difficulty may not be a circadian phase delay. Whatever the initial cause, sleep onset insomnia may lead to a phase delay, which then becomes one of the perpetuating factors.

In summary, an individual's circadian rhythm can become chronically delayed for several reasons. Once delayed, it can inhibit sleep onset at the time the individual needs to initiate sleep to avoid sleep loss. This difficulty with sleep onset, although it may arise initially from a circadian phase delay, can lead to perpetuating psychological factors and the development of psychophysiological insomnia. Even in cases in which the initial causes of sleep onset difficulty may not be a circadian phase delay, a phase delay is likely to develop and become one of the perpetuating factors.

This hypothesized delay is illustrated in Figure 12.2. Sufferers of sleep onset insomnia, indicated with open circles, have a delayed circadian rhythm with respect to their intended sleep period as indicated by their lights-out time (LOT). As a result, their LOT occurs in their evening wake-maintenance zone (WMZ, as indicated by vertical hatching) inhibiting and delaying their sleep onset. This can be the initial cause or a perpetuating contributor to the sleep onset insomnia.

Empirical Support for the Circadian Phase Delay in Sleep Onset Insomnia

Monroe's classic finding of elevated core body temperature in poor sleepers across the sleep period suggested the possibility that the total circadian rhythm may be abnormal (57). However, without measures across at least 24 hours, it was not clear whether the poor sleepers' rhythms were reduced in amplitude or elevated across the total 24-hour period. Early evidence from groups undifferentiated as to the type of insomnia supported the notion in general of circadian rhythm abnormalities associated with the insomnia (58–59). However, these studies included a mixture of characteristics: sleep onset insomnia, sleep maintenance insomnia, and early morning awakening insomnia. Furthermore, physiological data were collected on ambulatory subjects, which possibly masked differences in endogenous circadian rhythms such as core temperature. When

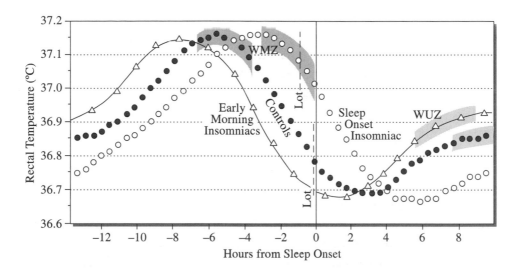

Figure 12.2   Circadian Core Temperature Rhythms of Sleep Onset Insomniacs and Early Morning Awakening Insomniacs in Comparison with Good Sleeping Controls. The curves have been adjusted to a common time of sleep onset. With respect to the time of sleep onset, sleep onset insomniacs have phase delayed circadian rhythms with a wake maintenance zone (WMZ) present at bedtime. Early morning awakening insomniacs are phase advanced with a wake up zone (WUZ) beginning only about five hours after sleep onset.

specific types of insomnia were selected, predicted circadian abnormalities were confirmed.

Morris et al. selected those with sleep onset insomnia to compare with age-matched good sleepers in the carefully controlled conditions of the constant routine methodology (60). This procedure controlled for activity and sleep-wake state to reveal the endogenous circadian temperature rhythm. The overall mean core temperature and circadian rhythm amplitude did not differ between the groups. However, the time of the core temperature minimum for the good sleepers was 3:15 A.M. but was four hours later at 7:18 A.M. for those with sleep onset insomnia. The good sleepers' normal bedtime was at 11:06 P.M., estimated to be two hours following their wake-maintenance zones, and they took only 11 minutes to fall asleep on the average. Those with sleep onset insomnia went to bed at 12:02 A.M., estimated to be still within their wake-maintenance zone, and they took 42 minutes to fall asleep on the average. This phase delay associated with longer sleep latency has been confirmed more recently (61). Therefore, sleep onset insomnia is associated with phase-delayed circadian rhythms, which would be expected to be a significant contribution to the insomnia.

Delayed sleep phase syndrome (DSPS) is estimated to account for about 10% of the insomnias presenting to sleep disorder clinics (Diagnostic Classification Steering Committee, 1990). However, it could have a higher prevalence in the general population, especially among younger age groups. The *International Classification of Sleep Disorders* (ICSD) nosology and generally accepted conceptualization of DSPS requires a consistent but rather extremely late sleep onset time between 2 and 6 A.M. (62–63). It has long been recognized that DSPS would result in sleep onset insomnia if sleep were attempted at a conventional time (e.g., 10 P.M. to 1 A.M.; 19, 63–65). There is also considerable evidence that DSPS arises from a delayed circadian rhythm (61, 65–71).

Does this evidence linking extreme phase delay to the extreme sleep onset latencies in DSPS support the Morris et al. finding that a circadian phase delay contributes to the more common type of sleep onset insomnia? This depends on whether sleep onset insomnia and DSPS are considered to be the same type of problem, with DSPS being a more extreme but less common version. This has not been recognized by the ICSD nosology (Diagnostic Classification Steering Committee, 1990) nor some early studies (26), which suggested that DSPS patients had normal sleep with little sleep onset difficulty when sleep was attempted at the usually delayed period (e.g., 4 A.M. to 12:00 P.M.). However, even at the usual delayed sleep time, DSPS sufferers are shown to have sleep onset latencies, which, although less than when sleep is attempted earlier in the night, are still significantly and clinically lengthened (32 minutes versus 10 minutes for controls; 65). Therefore, it appears that DSPS may not only be a phase delay problem, but there may be some degree of psychophysiological or learned insomnia contributing to their sleep onset difficulties. This would not be surprising given that the DSPS sufferer would make at least occasional attempts at earlier bedtimes and experience frustratingly long sleep latencies.

Chronic sleep onset insomnia is usually considered a form of psychophysiological or learned insomnia and is treated best with stimulus control therapy. However, as shown in the Morris et al. study, without nearly as much phase delay of sleep onset time as in DSPS, sleep onset insomnia also is associated with a phase delay of the endogenous circadian rhythm. Thus, it appears that sleep onset insomnia is a less extreme version of DSPS and should, therefore, be treated for its circadian abnormality as well as learned component.

Morning Bright Light Therapy for Sleep Onset Insomnia

It follows from the earlier discussion of the phase-advancing effects of morning bright light that this would be the indicated circadian treatment for phase-delayed sleep onset insomnia. Only a few studies have used this potential treatment. An early study compared eight controls with nine patients suffering mid-winter sleep onset insomnia in the subarctic region (72). It was found that the patients had a predicted phase delay of their melatonin and cortisol rhythms compared to the good sleepers. Five mornings of half-hour bright light therapy resulted in evidence of phase advances of these two rhythms as well as a decreased sleep onset latency for the insomnia group.

Another study randomly allocated 16 individuals with sleep onset insomnia to a week of one-hour exposures of morning bright white light or control condition of dim red light (73). While the control group showed no changes in the timing of the melatonin rhythm or sleep measures, the bright light group showed a significant phase advance of melatonin rhythm and sleep onset time (75 minutes) as well as a reduction of sleep latency from 75 to 40 minutes and an increase in total sleep time of 30 minutes. The bright light group also reported easier morning arousals and reduced daytime sleepiness.

A more recent larger study compared morning bright light, stimulus control therapy, and the combination of both with control conditions of dim morning light and no treatment (74). All active treatments showed significant and comparable reductions of sleep onset latency (from about 70 minutes at pretreatment to 35 minutes at posttreatment), which were maintained during the follow-up period. Although the combination treatment was not superior to either morning bright light or stimulus control therapy alone, it supported the earlier result that morning bright light therapy alone is efficacious for sleep onset insomnia.

Because the more extreme sleep onset insomnia of DSPS is also associated with circadian phase delays, treatments of morning bright light and other chronobiotics or substances with phase-shifting capacity have been recommended (75–78). There are only a few clinical trials of morning bright light therapy for DSPS. Rosenthal et al. (69) treated 20 DSPS patients with two hours (between 6 and 9 A.M.) of morning bright light (2,500 lux) over a two-week period. The treatment resulted in a significant phase advance of the body temperature rhythm, increased alertness in the morning, and improved subjective sleep. However, without objective measures of sleep, it is difficult to assess the total benefits of morning bright light for the treatment of DSPS. More recently, Cole et al. (79) used light masks applied while DSPS patients were in their last few hours of sleep before awakening. They found phase advances of temperature rhythms after 28 days of therapy and advances of sleep onset of more than an hour in the more extremely delayed patients. While the masks produced white light of 2,500 lux illuminance on closed eyelids, it is difficult to know the effective illuminance or wavelength of the light at the retinas after the light has passed through the eyelids. While it seems likely that morning bright light could be used effectively to treat DSPS, carefully controlled clinical trials with objective sleep measures have yet to be conducted.

Evening Melatonin Treatment for Sleep Onset Insomnia

In addition to bright light stimulation, a chronobiotic that has received considerable attention for its circadian phase shifting capacity is melatonin. In fact, a phase response curve for melatonin administration has been established (80–81). Administration of melatonin at certain circadian phases can phase advance and at other phases can delay the endogenous melatonin and other circadian rhythms. However, in contrast to bright light, melatonin taken in the early evening produces a phase advance and in the morning produces a phase delay. Its effects are opposite to that of bright light and about 12 hours different in phase (82). Therefore, melatonin administration in the early evening (8 to 11 P.M.) has been recommended for the treatment of DSPS (77, 80).

As well as successful treatment of an animal model of DSPS (83), evening melatonin administration has been used successfully to treat DSPS in humans (66, 84–85). It was found generally that 5 mg of melatonin administered nightly at about 10 P.M. (which was about five hours before their pretreatment sleep onset times) resulted in significant phase advances of the melatonin rhythm as well as sleep onset and wake times in the order of one to two hours. Melatonin has been likened to a dose of extreme darkness in its phase-shifting effects (82). Recently, it has been shown that, in fact, a period of complete darkness preceding the normal sleep period can have phase-advancing effects (86–87).

Because research has not directly compared the relative effects of melatonin administration with complete darkness, it is not clear if the effect of melatonin is to simulate darkness or if it is additive to darkness. It has been shown that melatonin administration cannot counteract the phase-delaying effects of evening bright light administration (88–89). Therefore, if a phase advance is desired, it would be advisable to administer evening melatonin in a dark or dimly lit environment. In addition, it would be suggested that phase advance may be maximized with the combined use of evening melatonin administration in a dark environment and the administration of bright light in the morning. This proposal should be experimentally and clinically evaluated.

Phase-Advanced Circadian Rhythms and Early Morning Awakening Insomnia

The other way in which a circadian phase abnormality may lead to chronic insomnia is the case of a phase advance or body clock timed too early. The "free-running" studies found a late morning wake-maintenance zone and a "wake-up" zone, which covered the period from about four to seven hours following the time of the core body temperature minimum (4). The timing of this zone was also consistent with the rapid sleep-wake alternating studies and the slow alternating "forced desynchrony" studies (11–12, 90). Most important for this discussion is the finding that this second alert zone was associated with an increased probability of awakening from sleep.

It is conceivable that this zone could result in an awakening before sufficient sleep is obtained. This could be the case if an individual's circadian rhythm were phase advanced with respect to the desired sleep period. For example, the desired sleep period may be from 10 P.M. to 6 A.M. In a normally entrained individual with core temperature minimum timed at 4 A.M., there would be no tendency for premature awakening because the "wake-up" zone would not start until about 8 A.M. If, however, the individual's CTmin were timed at 12 midnight, the "wake-up" zone would occur at about 4 A.M. and tend to wake up the individual after only six hours of sleep. This individual is likely to feel very sleepy before 10 P.M. and could fall asleep much earlier than 10 P.M. but chooses to remain out of bed until a more conventional bedtime. The result is a reduction of total sleep time to perhaps only six hours per night.

The hypothesized phase advance of early morning insomnia is indicated with open triangles in Figure 12.2. Relative to their intended sleep period, as indicated by lights-out time (LOT), their circadian temperature rhythm is phase advanced. If their bedtime occurs only two to three hours before their CTmin, they experience a rapid sleep onset. However, after only five to six hours of sleep, they enter their wake-up zone (WUZ, as indicated by horizontal hatching) and have difficulty maintaining sleep.

The insufficient sleep can be distressing and lead to the same types of arousal on awakening too early in the morning as experienced in sleep onset insomnia when trying to fall asleep initially. This arousal response can become a perpetuating factor in the development of psychophysiological sleep maintenance or early morning awakening insomnia. Thus, a circadian rhythm phase advance can lead to sleep maintenance or early morning awakening insomnia, sometimes alarmingly referred to as *terminal insomnia*. Strogatz and colleagues suggested this possibility early in this research area (4, 23).

The circadian rhythm may become phase advanced for the same types of reasons that can lead to a phase delay (jet travel, shift work, and natural phase shift arising from less than 24-hour period length). In the case of jet travel, a westward flight results in a phase advance of the traveler's circadian rhythm with respect to the destination clock time. A common experience is early evening sleepiness and a premature early awakening. If the individual has difficulty resynchronizing with the destination environment (perhaps because of too little evening light exposure during the winter months), the early morning awakening difficulty may persist for long enough to develop psychophysiological insomnia.

An early morning work shift schedule (e.g., one that starts at 4 A.M. requiring a 3 A.M. awakening) can result in some adjustment after several days on that schedule. This adjustment is a circadian phase advance relative to the worker's original rhythm phase. At the end of the shift work when the individual tries to readjust to a normal entrainment of the sleep period (e.g., 10 P.M. to 6 A.M.), the resultant phase advance may cause early morning awakening earlier than desired. This would result in the same internal phase advance experienced by the westward traveler and the same possibility of developing early morning awakening insomnia.

A phase advance of an individual's endogenous circadian phase relative to the external world may also arise spontaneously without transmeridian plane flights or shift work schedules. Remember that individuals with a long endogenous circadian period (> 24.5 hours) have their tendency to phase delay realized if the phase advance entraining cues such as morning bright light are absent ("brakes released"). Although there appear to be far fewer people with endogenous circadian period lengths less than 24 hours, they should, nevertheless, have a tendency to phase advance in the absence of phase-delaying entraining cues. The strongest phase-delaying cue would be evening bright light. Therefore, individuals with shorter than 24-hour period lengths have a tendency to become phase advanced if they are exposed only to dim light (< 80 lux) from the late afternoon to bedtime. This is indeed possible in a dimly lit domestic environment in which considerable time is spent watching television, particularly in the winter months when late afternoon sunlight is less available.

In summary, an individual's circadian rhythm can become chronically advanced for several different reasons. Once advanced, it can contribute to sleep disruption in the latter part of the sleep period and to early premature awakening, thus resulting in sleep loss. This difficulty with maintaining sleep, although it may arise initially from a circadian phase advance, can lead to perpetuating psychological factors and the development of psychophysiological insomnia. Even in cases in which the initial causes of early morning awakening difficulty may not be a circadian phase advance, a phase advance is likely to develop and become one of the perpetuating factors. If continued sleep seems impossible, making productive use of the early morning hours (such as walking the dog or gardening) may be laudable, but the potential early sunlight exposure can unwittingly incur an increased phase advance.

What is the evidence for a circadian phase advance in early morning awakening insomnia? These sufferers are typically very sleepy in the evening and have difficulty remaining awake in sedentary activities until a conventional bedtime (e.g., 10 P.M.), at which time they have a short sleep latency. They tend to experience increasing awake time in the latter part of the sleep period until they eventually cannot return to sleep despite insufficient total sleep time. They also tend to be relatively alert and active in the morning, even after an early final awakening (e.g., 4 A.M.).

Just such a group of individuals experiencing early morning awakening insomnia ($n = 10$) was compared with an age- and gender-matched group of good sleepers (91). The groups did not differ in lights-out time (about 11 P.M.) or sleep latency (both groups, about 15 minutes). However, the insomnia group had a mean final awakening at 4:49 A.M. after only 5.5 hours sleep while the good sleepers had an average of 7.75 hours sleep until 7:24 A.M. Their endogenous circadian rhythms of core temperature, melatonin, objective sleep propensity, and subjective sleepiness were evaluated in a 26-hour ultradian bed rest routine. Compared with the control group, the insomnia group had circadian rhythms phase advanced by two to four hours with a mean temperature minimum as early as 12:20 A.M. It would be predicted that they would be entering their endogenous wake-up zone by about 4:20 A.M. At this time, their core body temperature was increasing rapidly, melatonin was decreasing, and objective and subjective sleepiness was decreasing. This phase of their endogenous circadian rhythm corresponded closely with their habitual wake-up time of 4:49 A.M.

Treatment of Early Morning Awakening Insomnia with Evening Bright Light Therapy

If early morning awakening (EMA) insomnia is caused by, or at least exacerbated by, a phase-advanced circadian rhythm, the use of evening bright light to phase delay rhythms should improve sleep. There appear to be just two research groups that have explored this possibility. Consistent with the finding that EMA insomnia is associated with phase-advanced circadian rhythms (91), the group in Australia showed that EMA insomnia could benefit from evening bright light therapy (92). Nine EMA insomnia sufferers were exposed to 2,500 lux intensity white light from 8 P.M. to 12 midnight on two successive evenings. Constant routine evaluations of circadian rhythms before and immediately after bright white light treatment showed two-hour delays in both core temperature and melatonin rhythms. Their sleep, which was evaluated for the week following the light treatment, showed no change of sleep onset time but showed more than an hour's delay of final wake-up time and an hour's increase of total sleep time.

This pilot study was then followed by a larger ($n = 22$) and longer placebo-controlled study (93–94). The active treatment group ($n = 11$) received 2,500 lux white light while the placebo control ($n = 11$) received dim (200 lux) red light from 9 P.M. to 1 A.M. on two consecutive nights. Again, constant routines used to evaluate the endogenous circadian rhythms pre- and posttreatment showed significant circadian rhythm phase delays of two to three hours while the dim light procedure produced no phase change. Follow-up of the melatonin rhythm and sleep continued over a four-week period. Although the initial phase delay in the active group showed some regression toward the baseline phase, the active group maintained later melatonin rhythms than the control group for the entire period. As in the earlier study, bedtimes and sleep latencies did not change for either group after treatment. However, for the active group, a combination of delayed final wake-up time and reduced amount of nocturnal wake time resulted in a significantly greater increase of total sleep time (100 minutes) than the control group (24 minutes). This improvement in the bright light group was accompanied by a significant reduction of subjective anxiety as to the ability to reinitiate sleep after a nocturnal awakening. In summary, evening bright light therapy appears to be an effective treatment for insomnia marked by premature spontaneous termination of sleep.

The other group assessing this potential therapy at about the same time was at the Cornell Medical Center in New York. Their first study was a randomized placebo control trial comparing evening bright white light ($n = 8$ at 4,000 lux) with dim red light ($n = 6$ at 50 lux) for sleep maintenance insomnia (95). Although their participants were selected for sleep maintenance insomnia, they also met the criteria for advanced sleep phase syndrome (ASPS). Pretreatment evaluation of sleep and circadian temperature rhythms showed considerably more sleep disturbance in the last third of the sleep period, total sleep time of less than six hours, and early timed CTmin. Therefore, the sleep characteristics of their participants were similar to the early morning awakening insomnia groups in Australia.

The treatment protocol consisted of 12 consecutive nights of two hours of light within the time window of 8 P.M. to 11 P.M. each night. The temperature rhythm showed a two-hour greater phase delay in the bright light group with CTmin changing from 3:11 A.M. to 5:37 A.M. compared with 3:17 A.M. to 3:35 A.M. for the control group. Bedtimes and sleep latency did not change for the two groups. In this study, final wake-up times also did not vary. However, compared to the control group, the active group showed a 60-minute decrease of nocturnal wake time, decreased stage 1 sleep, and number of sleep stage changes. As a result, the bright light treatment group showed consistent increases of sleep efficiency from an average 78% to 90%. Of particular interest was that the typical increase of disturbed sleep in the last third of the night, seen in the control group pre- and posttreatment and active group pretreatment, was ameliorated following bright light treatment such that the amount of wake time during the night stayed at a low value across the total sleep period.

The Cornell group's second study extended the evaluation of evening bright light therapy to its possible benefits on daytime performance over an extended maintenance therapy period (96). Sixteen elderly with sleep maintenance insomnia initially received the same 12 nights of light treatment as in the earlier study's active group. The average sleep efficiency increased 6% to a value of 84%, and CTmin delayed 73 minutes to 4:25 A.M. Although the increase of sleep efficiency was half that of the earlier study, the phase delay was also just half that of the earlier study. Because the treatment was at home and unmonitored, there may have been less compliance in the acute treatment phase of this second study. Nevertheless, there were significant increases on three of the four cognitive performance tests following this treatment, which were generally positively correlated with the increase of sleep efficiency and circadian phase delay.

During the following three-month maintenance phase of this study, seven patients received periodic evening bright light exposure while six placebo controls received periodic bright light exposure only during the day, which was predicted to have no circadian phase-delaying effect. The active group maintained a later circadian phase while the control group showed a regression toward the pretreatment circadian phase. Similarly, the active treatment group maintained a higher sleep efficiency measure and significantly better cognitive performance on three of the four tasks. Therefore, this study was consistent with their earlier study and showed that evening bright light therapy can be therapeutic for sleep maintenance insomnia as well as daytime functioning. It also showed that the gains from acute treatment can be maintained with periodic evening bright light treatment.

A recent third study of the Cornell group (97) described patients treated to a similar protocol as the second study (96). Despite a significant delay of temperature rhythm and improvement of subjective sleep quality, there were no significant improvements in objective sleep measures in this study. The authors suggest that because the patients' sleep onset and wake-up times also delayed, the circadian phase delay with respect to sleep period may not have been great enough to generate an improved sleep efficiency in this study. The earlier studies of this same group and the Australian group produced circadian phase delays without changes in sleep onset time, thus greater circadian phase delays relative to sleep period than in this last study. This difference may account for the difference in the extent of sleep improvements between the studies. In summary, five studies have treated early awakening and sleep maintenance insomnia with evening bright light. All studies have resulted in circadian phase delays with general improvement in objective and subjective sleep, which were also related to improvements in daytime functioning.

Some question remains as to the direct role of phase delay in the sustained sleep improvement. It may be that learned or psychophysiological insomnia as well as phase advance had contributed to the pretreatment poor sleep. If this is true, extinction of this learned insomnia may contribute to the sleep improvement.

Although this putative extinction process may initially be facilitated by a relative circadian phase delay, further extinction of this learned insomnia may also be dependent on psychological variables rather than circadian phase. For example, individuals with greater sleep-associated anxiety (98) or more dysfunctional beliefs and attitudes about sleep (99) may benefit less than average from the phase delay produced by evening bright light treatment. The involvement of such psychological variables may explain the low variance accounted for by the circadian phase delay in the cognitive performance improvement.

Another issue is the apparent need to use periodic evening bright light treatment (about twice a week or more) to maintain the initial gains of circadian phase delay following the acute treatment phase. Without this periodic evening bright light, all studies have found a regression of circadian phase toward the original phase position as well as, in one of the studies, the loss of therapeutic gains to sleep and cognitive functioning (96). As suggested earlier, a possible explanation of this, as well as an initially phase-advanced circadian rhythm, is that this insomnia is associated with an intrinsic circadian period length less than 24 hours (100–101). Thus, in the absence of sufficiently bright evening light to maintain the phase delay, they would have a natural tendency to phase advance.

Does Aging Lead to Early Morning Insomnia because of Phase Advance?

It has long been known that the sleep of the aged is more fragmented, particularly in the latter half of the night, and sleep onset and wake are timed earlier (102). This led to the suggestion that the sleep maintenance problems of the elderly may be due to a phase-advanced circadian rhythm. More recently, with the use of the constant routine methodology, it was established that aging is, in fact, associated with a phase-advanced core body temperature rhythm (103). However, the advance of sleep onset and wake time was greater than the advance of their temperature rhythm. Another recent study found equal phase advances of temperature rhythm and habitual wake-up time in healthy elderly (104). For both of these studies, the CTmin time occurred about 70% through the bed period, which is the same phase position as in young, healthy good sleepers. If the wake-up zone follows CTmin after the same elapsed time in the young and elderly, these results would suggest that the early awakening of the healthy elderly is not being driven by the circadian phase advance. Instead, it is suggested that the diminished strength of Process S produces the greater sleep fragmentation and earlier awakening of the elderly (104–105).

However, there is some recent evidence that this zone of increasing alertness may be timed earlier following CTmin for the elderly than for young, good sleepers (103, 106). Therefore, aging may contribute to greater sleep fragmentation and early awakening both through a diminished strength of Process S and an earlier wake-up zone relative to CTmin. In any case, the early awakening could then result in some exposure to early light, which, in turn, would exacerbate the phase advance of the endogenous circadian system.

It must be remembered that these latter studies were of healthy, good-sleeping elderly, not of those with chronic insomnia. In fact, the CTmin times of the healthy elderly in these two studies were 5:15 A.M. and 4:18 A.M., respectively (103–104). In contrast, the temperature minimum times for the Australian early morning awakening insomnia groups were 2:31 A.M., 3:12 A.M., and 12:20 A.M. (91–93) and for the Cornell studies with the ASPS and sleep maintenance insomnia groups were 3:13 A.M., 3:12 A.M., and 2:59 A.M. (95–97). For these chronic insomnia groups, the CTmin occurred at a relatively earlier phase, about 50% through the bed period. Therefore, in chronic early morning insomnia, the circadian phase is relatively phase advanced compared to young and elderly healthy good sleepers; this relative phase advance could well be contributing to the insomnia. This would be particularly true if, in the elderly who show the greatest prevalence of early morning awakening insomnia, the wake-up zone followed CTmin sooner than it does in the young.

Considering specifically the endogenous period length, there is no evidence that it is any shorter for the average healthy elderly than in healthy young adults (107). The endogenous period length mean (s.d.) of a group of healthy, good-sleeping elderly was 24.18 (0.13) hours, which was no different from young, good sleepers (108). Nevertheless, in a group of healthy elderly, if there is a normal distribution of period lengths, approximately 8% would have an endogenous period length less than 24 hours and, therefore, be susceptible to a tendency to phase advance in the absence of entraining stimuli. The question is whether those with chronic early morning insomnia have period lengths less than 24 hours associated with their relatively phase-advanced circadian rhythms. Only one of the studies of early morning awakening insomnia has reported estimated period lengths of temperature rhythms (92). Period lengths were estimated from a least-squares best-fit two component (24 h plus 12 h) cosine function in which the 24 h component was allowed to vary around 24 hours. The mean period estimates before and after two nights of evening bright light treatment were 22.6 and 22.4 hours ($t = 0.09$, ns). These estimates based on only one completed circadian period are likely to have low reliability and must be treated cautiously. Nevertheless, they provide some tentative support for the possibility that individuals with period lengths shorter than 24 hours will be susceptible to developing early morning insomnia, particularly with the decline of the strength of Process S because of aging.

Other Possible Zeitgebers for Changing Circadian Phase

Two other nonpharmacological tools have been recently suggested as possible Zeitgebers for the treatment of circadian phase problems such as sleep onset and early morning awakening insomnia. Daily aerobic physical exercise has been suggested as therapeutic for abnormal or disrupted circadian rhythms (109–111). Physical exercise seems to act similarly to the administration of bright light (87, 112–115). Exercise in the morning, independent of light exposure, phase advances rhythms and exercise in the evening phase delays.

Passive body heating has also been suggested to affect circadian phase. Passive heating in the evening can cause immediate phase delays in the temperature rhythm as well as increase the amount of slow wave deep sleep in the early part of the sleep period (116–117). However, whether this is only an acute effect or a longer lasting phase change of the endogenous circadian rhythm was not clear from these studies. Passive body heating effects in the morning have yet to be investigated. Because the effects of physical exercise appear to be similar to passive body heating, it could be the elevated core temperature usually resulting from physical exercise that is the critical Zeitgeber. Moreover, because the effect of bright light during the dark period is to block the decrease of core temperature because of its inhibition of melatonin and the effect of melatonin administration is a decrease of core temperature, it may be that all these Zeitgeber effects operate through either direct or indirect effects on core temperature (118). If that is true, their effects may not be additive. There is some evidence to support this notion. Youngstedt et al. (119) found that the combination of evening bright light and physical exercise produced no greater phase delay than bright light alone. These questions still need considerable research.

There have been other Zeitgebers suggested, such as some benzodiazepine hypnotics (120–122). However, there is some question as to whether these drugs act directly to reset the SCN or if the phase shift results from the light/dark altering effects of helping to induce sleep at a phase-shifted time. There is some suggestion that caffeine may act similarly to the phase-shifting effects of light but with reduced strength of effect (123). Numerous Zeitgebers may eventuate with further research, which begs to be done. However, this research needs to take care to separate the acute effects of treatment on physiological measures from the longer term circadian phase-shifting effects. Furthermore, it is not only of theoretical interest but also of longer term clinical importance to determine if treatments are acting directly on the SCN to effect phase shifts or indirectly through an intervening variable such as alteration of light/dark timing.

In summary, although visual light stimulation, particularly bright blue light, is considered the most potent Zeitgeber for humans, there appear to be several others that can change human circadian phase and, therefore, potentially be useful for treating sleep onset and early morning awakening insomnia. A phase delay for treating early morning insomnia can be produced by evening bright light, passive body heating, aerobic physical exercise, and morning darkness with melatonin administration. A phase advance to treat sleep onset insomnia can be produced by morning bright light, aerobic exercise, and evening melatonin administration in darkness. Whether combinations of these Zeitgebers can produce greater phase changes than one alone is yet to be investigated.

CIRCADIAN RHYTHM AMPLITUDE EFFECTS

Although most research attention has been directed to circadian rhythm phase effects on sleep, there has been some recent discussion about the involvement of other dimensions of circadian rhythms in sleep-wake disorders. One suggestion is that a reduced amplitude of circadian rhythms (i.e., a reduction of the difference between peak and trough values) may lead to sleep difficulties at night as well as impaired functioning during the day (e.g., reduced alertness, motivation, productivity). The reduced amplitude may arise from a higher trough (nadir) value during the night, such as higher nocturnal core temperature, higher metabolic rate, and so on, resulting in higher overall nervous system activation and more sleep difficulties. Thus, if sleep quantity and quality is chronically lower, this by itself will produce negative consequences for daytime functioning and mood.

However, in addition to the possibility of lowered daytime functioning following sleep disruption, a reduced amplitude of circadian rhythm may also arise from lower endogenous rhythm peak values during the day. This would also contribute to lower daytime functioning. Just as the nighttime functioning and daytime sleep of a night shift worker are considerably impaired by a reversed circadian rhythm amplitude relative to the shift work sleep-wake timing, it is felt that even a reduction of the normal amplitude can impair both sleep and wakeful functioning.

There is some evidence of a positive correlation between CT rhythm amplitude and total sleep time (124). Furthermore, a phase advance manipulation in elderly good sleepers resulted in correlated decreases of CT rhythm amplitude and sleep efficiency (125). The fact that aging is associated with a general decrease of circadian rhythm amplitudes and sleep efficiency also suggests a possible involvement of decreased amplitude in insomnia (107, 126–127). Based on this assumption, it has been suggested that treatments to enhance circadian rhythm amplitude such as increased daytime activity and bright light exposure may enhance amplitude and improve the quality of nighttime sleep and daytime functioning (111, 128–129).

However, not all studies have found a decrease of amplitude with age (130), and the earlier evidence directly relating a reduced amplitude to insomnia has not been consistent (58–59, 124). Because these earlier studies measured core temperature during ad lib wake and sleep, it could not be determined if the elevated nocturnal temperatures of the insomniacs contributed to the poor sleep or if the poor sleep with extended wakeful periods produced the elevated nocturnal core temperatures. To resolve this issue, a recent study used a constant routine to compare the endogenous core temperature rhythms of objectively confirmed good and poor sleepers (131). The poor sleepers with sleep maintenance insomnia had a higher mean and reduced amplitude compared to age-matched good sleepers. This arose, not from a difference in daytime temperature, but from significantly elevated nighttime temperature. It appears that in sleep maintenance insomnia, there is a deficiency in the endogenous down regulation of core body temperature at night as well as a reduced sleep-evoked down regulation (131). A nonpharmacological treatment suggested to improve core temperature down regulation is skin temperature (particularly of palmar hand or feet surfaces) biofeedback training to enable skin warming control at bedtime (132).

CHANGES IN THE MEAN CIRCADIAN RHYTHM LEVEL

Accumulating evidence supports the notion that chronic psychophysiological insomnia is a condition of chronic hyperarousal. This could be conceptualized in terms of circadian rhythms as a raised overall mean arousal level. In terms of physiological indicators, this may be measured as a chronically elevated core body temperature or metabolic rate in which all values, including peak, trough, and all intermediate times, are elevated a constant amount. Even though the amplitude and phase may be normal, the chronic hyperarousal can result in disrupted nocturnal sleep. This in turn can lead to negative daytime consequences such as fatigue, irritability, and dysphoria despite the hyperarousal during the daytime hours as evidenced by longer than normal sleep latencies in the Multiple Sleep Latency Test (MSLT; 133), pupillary dilation (134), subjective alertness, and cortical evoked responses (135).

The hyperarousal model has been illustrated in the caffeine model of insomnia in which chronic high consumption of caffeine across several days in normally good sleepers resulted in insomnia and the typical daytime dysphoric reports of chronic insomnia sufferers (136). The daytime caffeine tended to counteract sleepiness (sleep latencies were not shortened despite the sleep loss) but did not counteract fatigue, irritability, and so on. It is possible that this type of chronically elevated arousal may, in fact, contribute to these daytime symptoms through chronic activation and subsequent depletion of the hypothalamic-pituitary-adrenal axis (137–138).

Parenthetically, the opposite possibility should probably be mentioned, that is, a chronically decreased 24-hour mean level of circadian rhythm indicators of arousal. This may be relevant to the condition of idiopathic hypersomnia, which is marked by excessive daytime sleepiness despite an elevated amount of nocturnal sleep. This is a condition of chronic hypoarousal (139) and may be conceptualized as a circadian rhythm with lower overall mean circadian arousal without abnormalities of phase or amplitude. However, there appears to be little empirical exploration of this possibility apart from some evidence of increased melatonin secretion at nighttime (140).

CONCLUSION

In summary, the circadian rhythm model can suggest several ways in which the sleep-wake functioning can be disrupted. If the circadian rhythm is phase delayed with respect to the desired sleep period, sleep onset can be delayed, total sleep time can be reduced, and daytime functioning can be impaired, especially in the early part of the waking period. If the circadian rhythm is phase advanced with respect to the desired sleep period, early spontaneous termination of sleep will reduce total sleep time and impair daytime functioning, especially in the latter part of the wake period. If circadian amplitude is reduced, higher nocturnal arousal will disrupt sleep and lower diurnal arousal will impair daytime alertness. If, instead, the mean 24-hour level of the circadian rhythm is elevated, the result may be chronic sleep onset and maintenance insomnia resulting from chronic hyperarousal. Alternatively, if the mean level is decreased indicating chronic hypoarousal, idiopathic hypersomnia may be the result.

Whether the circadian rhythm model is appropriate for these sleep-wake disorders can be tested by the more important clinical question, "Are treatments that address the circadian rhythm abnormality therapeutic?" As to the disorders that can be conceptualized as an overall increased or decreased mean of the rhythm (chronic hyper- and hypoarousal, respectively), most suggested treatments have been pharmacological. Sedation is the most common treatment for the presumed chronic hyperarousal of combined sleep onset and sleep maintenance insomnia. However, it could be argued that the attempt to mask chronic hyperarousal with superimposed drug sedation will be less effective and less healthy than removing the source of the hyperarousal. For example, in the caffeine model of insomnia, it would be healthier in the long term to reduce the caffeine consumption than to add hypnotic drug sedation at night in an attempt to counteract the caffeine effect. Cognitive-behavioral therapies for insomnia are aimed at reducing the source of this hyperarousal. Earlier chapters showed the effectiveness of cognitive-behavioral therapies in the treatment of chronic insomnia. It would be interesting now to see a comprehensive assessment of physiological and cognitive arousal before and after successful treatment.

For those suffering from sleep maintenance insomnia alone with indications of physiological hyperarousal only at night (131), in addition to cognitive-behavioral therapies, it is suggested the finger temperature biofeedback may be an effective behavioral treatment. This may enable the insomniac to enhance finger warming at night. A rapid rise of finger temperature occurs with the attempt to fall asleep and appears to be associated with more rapid sleep onsets and greater down regulation of core body temperature (141–142).

Idiopathic hypersomnolence and narcolepsy can be conceptualized as chronic hypoarousal and are most commonly treated with pharmacological stimulants. Because the source of the hypoarousal is presumed or suspected to be some neurological abnormality, pharmacological treatment is seen as most appropriate.

As to sleep-wake disorders associated with phase abnormalities such as sleep onset insomnia, DSPS, early morning awakening insomnia, and ASPS, the phase-shifting effects of bright light have been shown to be therapeutic. Whether the use of additional Zeitgebers such as melatonin and physical exercise can enhance the therapeutic benefits is yet to be tested. As mentioned earlier, a circadian phase abnormality, if it has been a long-term problem, is most likely to coexist with some degree of psychophysiological or learned insomnia. The question of the "original cause" is often unresolvable and, in any case, a moot question as suggested at the beginning of this chapter. The main point is that the cognitive-behavioral therapies as well as circadian phase therapies are appropriate for insomnias associated with circadian abnormalities. Whether a combination of circadian and cognitive-behavioral therapy will be more effective than either alone needs to be evaluated more comprehensively. Whatever the case, circadian rhythm treatments play an important new role in the nondrug treatments of insomnia.

REFERENCES

1. Borbely, A. A. Sleep: Circadian rhythm versus recovery process. In M. Koukkou et al., ed. *Functional States of the Brain: Their Determinants.* Amsterdam: Elsevier/ North-Holland. 1980: 151–161.

2. Jewett, M. E., J. K. Wyatt, A. Ritz-De Cecco, S. B. Khalsa, D. J. Dijk, and C. A. Czeisler. Time course of sleep inertia dissipation in human performance and alertness. *Journal of Sleep Research* 8(1): 1–8, 1999.

3. Aschoff, J. Features of circadian rhythms relevant for the design of shift schedules. In J. Colquhoun, ed. *Studies of Shiftwork*. London, England: Taylor & Francis. 1980: 19–34.

4. Strogatz, S. H. *The Mathematical Structure of the Human Sleep-Wake Cycle* (Volume 69). Berlin, Germany: Springer-Verlag. 1986.

5. Strogatz, S. H. and R. E. Kronauer. Circadian wake maintenance zones and insomnia in man. *Sleep Research* 14: 219, 1985.

6. Weitzman, E. D., C. Nogeire, M. Perlow, D. Fukushima, J. Sassin, P. McGregor, et al. Effects of a prolonged 3-hour sleep-wake cycle on sleep stages, plasma cortisol, growth hormone, and body temperature in man. *Journal of Clinical Endocrinology and Metabolism* 38: 1018–1030, 1974.

7. Carskadon, M. A. and W. C. Dement. Sleepiness and sleep state on a 90-minute schedule. *Psychophysiology* 14: 127–133, 1977.

8. Gander, P. H. G. and L. J. Connell. Masking of the circadian rhythms of heart rate and core temperature by the rest/activity rhythm in man. *Sleep Research* 14: 298, 1985.

9. Stefikova, H., E. Sovcikova, and M. Bronis. The circadian rhythm of selected parameters of heart rate variability. *Physiologia Bohemoslovaca* 35(3): 227–232, 1986.

10. Barrett, J., L. Lack, and M. Morris. The sleep-evoked decrease of body temperature. *Sleep* 16(2): 93–99, 1993.

11. Lavie, P. Ultrashort sleep-waking schedule. III: 'Gates' and 'forbidden zones' for sleep. *Electroencephalography Clinical Neurophysiology* 63(5): 414–425, 1986.

12. Lack, L. C. and K. Lushington. The rhythms of human sleep propensity and core body temperature. *Journal of Sleep Research* 5(1): 1–11, 1996.

13. Dijk, D. J. and C. A. Czeisler. Paradoxical timing of the circadian rhythm of sleep propensity serves to consolidate sleep and wakefulness in humans. *Neuroscience Letters* 166: 63–68, 1994.

14. Dijk, D. J., D. F. Duffy, E. Riel, T. L. Shanahan, and C. A. Czeisler. Aging and the circadian and homeostatic regulation of human sleep during forced desynchrony of rest, melatonin and temperature rhythms. *Journal of Physiology* 516(Pt 2): 611–627, 1999.

15. Luce, G. G. *Biological Rhythms in Human and Animal Physiology*. New York, NY: Dover. 1971.

16. Arand, D. M. Self-assessed circadian rhythms in individuals with sleep complaints. *Sleep Research* 7: 301, 1978.

17. Cleghorn, J. M., A. Bellissimo, R. D. Kaplan, and P. Szatmari. Insomnia. II: Assessment and treatment of chronic insomnia *Canadian Journal of Psychiatry* 28(5): 347–353, 1983.

18. Fookson, J. E., R. E. Kronauer, E. D. Weitzman, T. H. Monk, M. Moline, and E. Hoey. Induction of insomnia on non-24 hour sleep-wake schedules. *Sleep Research* 13: 220, 1984.

19. Guilleminault, C., C. Czeisler, R. Coleman, and L. Miles. Circadian rhythm disturbances and sleep disorders in shift workers. *Electroencephalography Clinical Neurophysiology* 36(Suppl.): 709–714, 1982.

20. Lewy, A., R. Sack, and C. Singer. Assessment and treatment of chronobiologic disorders using plasma melatonin levels and bright light exposure: The clock-gate model and the phase response curve. *Psychopharmacology Bulletin* 20(3): 561–565, 1984.

21. Minors, D. S. Chronobiology: Its importance in clinical medicine. *Clinical Science* 69: 364–376, 1985.

22. Moore-Ede, M. C., C. A. Czeisler, and G. S. Richardson. Circadian timekeeping in health and disease. Part 1: Basic properties of circadian pacemakers. *New England Journal of Medicine* 309(8): 469–476, 1983.

23. Strogatz, S. H., R. E. Kronauer, and C. A. Czeisler. Circadian pacemaker interferes with sleep onset at specific times each day: Role in insomnia. *American Journal of Physiology* 253(1 Pt 2): R172–R178, 1987.

24. Winfree, A. I. Circadian timing of sleepiness in man and woman. *American Journal of Physiology* 243(3): R193–R204, 1982.

25. Weitzman, E. D., C. Czeisler, R. Coleman, W. Dement, G. Richardson, and C. P. Pollack. Delayed sleep phase syndrome: A biological rhythm disorder. *Sleep Research* 8: 221, 1979.

26. Weitzman, E. D., C. A. Czeisler, R. M. Coleman, A. J. Spielman, J. C. Zimmerman, and W. C. Dement. Delayed sleep phase syndrome: A chronobiological disorder with sleep-onset insomnia. *Archives of General Psychiatry* 38: 137–146, 1981.

27. Czeisler, C. A. and K. R. Wright. Influence of light on circadian rhythmicity in humans. In F. W. Turek and P. C. Zee, eds. *Regulation of Sleep and Circadian Rhythms*. New York, NY: Marcel Dekker, Inc. 1999: 149–180.

28. Brainard, G. C., J. P. Hanifin, J. M. Greeson, B. Byrne, G. Glickman, E. Gerner, et al. Action spectrum for melatonin regulation in humans: Evidence for a novel circadian photoreceptor. *Journal of Neuroscience* 21(16): 6405–6412, 2001.

29. Thapan, K., J. Arendt, and D. J. Skene. An action spectrum for melatonin suppression: Evidence for a novel non-rod, noncone photoreceptor system in humans. *Journal of Physiology* 535(Pt 1): 261–267, 2001.

30. Wright, H. R. and L. C. Lack. Effect of light wavelength on suppression and phase delay of the melatonin rhythm. *Chronobiology International* 18(5): 801–808, 2001.

31. Wright, H. R. and L. C. Lack. Effect of wavelength on phase advance of the melatonin rhythm. *Sleep* 25(Abstract Suppl.): A124–A125, 2002.

32. Czeisler, C. A., J. S. Allan, S. H. Strogatz, J. M. Ronda, R. Sanchez, C. D. Rios et al. Bright light resets the human circadian pacemaker independent of the timing of the sleep-wake cycle. *Science* 233(4764): 667–671, 1986.

33. Dawson, D., M. Morris, and L. Lack. The phase shifting effects of a single 4h exposure to bright morning light in normals and DSPS subjects. *Sleep Research* 18: 415, 1989.

34. Drennan, M., D. Kripke, and J. Gillin. Bright light can delay human temperature rhythm independent of sleep. *American Journal of Physiology* 25: R136–R141, 1989.

35. Shanahan, T. L. and C. A. Czeisler. Light exposure induces equivalent phase shifts of the endogenous circadian rhythms of circulating plasma melatonin and core body temperature in men. *Journal of Clinical Endocrinology and Metabolism* 73(2): 227–235, 1991.

36. Boivin, D. B., J. F. Duffy, R. E. Kronauer, and C. A. Czeisler. Sensitivity of the human circadian pacemaker to moderately bright light. *Journal of Biological Rhythms* 9(3–4): 315–331, 1994.

37. Zeitzer, J. M., D. J. Dijk, R. Kronauer, E. Brown, and C. Czeisler. Sensitivity of the human circadian pacemaker to nocturnal light: Melatonin phase resetting and suppression. *Journal of Physiology* 526(Pt 3): 695–702, 2002.

38. Boivin, D. B. and F. O. James. Phase-dependent effect of room light exposure in a 5-h advance of the sleep-wake cycle: Implications for jet lag. *Journal of Biological Rhythms* 17(3): 266–276, 2002.

39. Czeisler, C. A., R. E. Kronauer, J. S. Allan, J. F. Duffy, M. E. Jewett, E. N. Brown, et al. Bright light induction of strong (type 0) resetting of the human circadian pacemaker. *Science* 244(4910): 1328–1333, 1989.

40. Jewett, M. E., D. W. Rimmer, E. B. Klerman, R. E. Kronauer, and C. A. Czeisler. Human circadian pacemaker is sensitive to light throughout subjective day without evidence of transients. *American Journal of Physiology* 273(5 Pt 2): R1800–R1809, 1997.

41. Minors, D. S., J. M. Waterhouse, and A. Wirz-Justice. A human phase-response curve to light. *Neuroscience Letter* 133(1): 36–40, 1991.

42. Duffy, J. F., R. E. Kronauer, and C. A. Czeisler. Phase-shifting human circadian rhythms: Influence of sleep timing, social contact and light exposure. *Journal of Physiology* 495(1): 289–297, 1996.

43. Yang, C. M., A. J. Spielman, P. D'Ambrosio, S. Serizawa, I. Nunes, and J. Birnbaum. A single dose of melatonin prevents the phase delay associated with a delayed weekend sleep pattern. *Sleep* 24(3): 272–281, 2001.

44. Lack, L. C. Delayed sleep and sleep loss in university students. *Journal of American College Health* 35(3): 105–110, 1986.

45. Valdez, P., C. Ramirez, and A. Garcia. Delaying and extending sleep during weekends: Sleep recovery or circadian effect? *Chronobiology International* 13(3): 191–198, 1996.

46. Wolfson, A. R. and M. A. Carskadon. Sleep schedules and daytime functioning in adolescents. *Child Development* 69(4): 875–887, 1998.

47. Allen, R. P. Social factors associated with the amount of school week sleep lag for seniors in an early starting suburban high school. *Sleep Research* 21: 114, 1992.

48. Henschel, A. and L. Lack. Do many adolescents sleep poorly or just too late? *Sleep Research* 16: 354, 1987.

49. Larsen, R. J. and M. Kasimatis. Individual differences in entrainment of mood to the weekly calendar. *Journal of Personality and Social Psychology* 58(1): 164–171, 1990.

50. Lewy, A. J. Using melatonin to chase away the Monday morning blues. *Sleep* 24(3): 271, 2001.

51. Haimov, I. and J. Arendt. The prevention and treatment of jet lag. *Sleep Medicine Reviews* 3(3): 229–240, 1999.

52. Monk, T., D. Buysse, J. Carrier, and D. Kupfer. Inducing jet-lag in older people: Directional asymmetry. *Journal of Sleep Research* 9: 101–116, 2000.

53. Monk, T. H. Spring and Autumn daylight saving time changes: Studies of adjustment in sleep timings, mood and efficiency. *Ergonomics* 23: 167–178, 1980.

54. Sack, R. L., A. J. Lewy, M. L. Blood, L. D. Keith, and H. Nakagawa. Circadian rhythm abnormalities in totally blind people: Incidence and clinical significance. *Journal of Clinical Endocrinology and Metabolism* 75(1): 127–134, 1992.

55. Klein, T., H. Martens, D. J. Dijk, R. E. Dronauer, E. W. Seely, and C. A. Czeisler. Circadian sleep regulation in the absence of light perception: Chronic non-24-hour circadian rhythm sleep disorder in a blind man with a regular 24-hour sleep-wake schedule. *Sleep* 16(4): 333–343, 1993.

56. Czeisler, C. A., T. L. Shanahan, E. B. Klerman, H. Martens, D. J. Brotman, J. S. Emans, et al. Suppression of melatonin secretion in some blind patients by exposure to bright light. *New England Journal of Medicine* 332(1): 6–11, 1995.

57. Monroe, L. J. Psychological and physiological differences between good and poor sleepers. *Journal of Abnormal Psychology* 72: 255–264, 1967.

58. Lack, L. The circadian rhythm of body temperature in poor sleepers. *Sleep Research* 14: 301, 1985.

59. MacFarlane, J., J. M. Cleghorn, G. M. Brown, R. Kaplan, P. Brown, and J. Mitton. Circadian rhythms in chronic insomnia. *Sleep Research* 13: 223, 1984.

60. Morris, M., L. Lack, and D. Dawson. Sleep-onset insomniacs have delayed temperature rhythms. *Sleep* 13(1): 1–14, 1990.

61. Kerkhof, G. and B. Van Vianen. Circadian phase estimation of chronic insomniacs relates to their sleep characteristics. *Archives of Physiology and Biochemistry* 107(5): 383–392, 1999.

62. American Sleep Disorders Association. *The International Classification of Sleep Disorders: Diagnostic and Coding Manual.* Rochester, MN: American Sleep Disorders Association. 1990.

63. Regestein, Q. R. and T. H. Monk. Delayed sleep phase syndrome: A review of its clinical aspects. *American Journal of Psychiatry* 152(4): 602–608, 1995.

64. Schrader, H. [Delayed sleep phase syndrome. The most frequent cause of primary chronic insomnia?]. *Tidsskr Nor Laegeforen* 110(30): 3851–3853, 1990.

65. Wagner, D. R., M. L. Moline, C. P. Pollack, and C. A. Czeisler. Entrained sleep and temperature rhythms in delayed sleep phase syndrome. *Sleep Research* 15: 179, 1986.

66. Nagtegaal, J. E., G. A. Kerkhof, M. G. Smits, A. C. Swart, and Y. G. Van der Meer. Delayed sleep phase syndrome: A placebo-controlled cross-over study on the effects of melatonin administered five hours before the individual dim light melatonin onset. *Journal of Sleep Research* 7(2): 135–143, 1998.

67. Oren, D. A., E. H. Turner, and T. A. Wehr. Abnormal circadian rhythms of plasma melatonin and body temperature in the delayed sleep phase syndrome. *Journal of Neurology, Neurosurgery, and Psychiatry* 58(3): 379, 1995.

68. Ozaki, S., M. Uchiyama, S. Shirakawa, and M. Okawa. Prolonged interval from body temperature nadir to sleep offset in patients with delayed sleep phase syndrome. *Sleep* 19(1): 36–40, 1996.

69. Rosenthal, N. E., J. R. Joseph-Vanderpool, A. A. Levendosky, S. H. Johnston, R. Allen, K. A. Kelly, et al. Phase-shifting effects of bright morning light as treatment for delayed sleep phase syndrome. *Sleep* 13(4): 354–361, 1990.

70. Shibui, K., M. Uchiyama, and M. Okawa. Melatonin rhythms in delayed sleep phase syndrome. *Journal of Biological Rhythms* 14(1): 72–76, 1999.

71. Uchiyama, M., M. Okawa, K. Shibui, X. Liu, T. Hayakawa, Y. Kamei, et al. Poor compensatory function for sleep loss as a pathogenic factor in patients with delayed sleep phase syndrome. *Sleep* 23(4): 553–558, 2000.

72. Hansen, T., T. Bratlid, O. Lingjarde, and T. Brenn. Midwinter insomnia in the subarctic region: Evening levels of serum melatonin and cortisol before and after treatment with bright artificial light. *Acta Psychiatrica Scandinavica* 75(4): 428–434, 1987.

73. Lack, L., H. Wright, and D. Paynter. The treatment of sleep onset insomnia with morning bright light. *Sleep Research* 24A: 338, 1995.

74. Bootzin, R. R., L. Lack, and H. Wright. Efficacy of bright light and stimulus control instructions for sleep onset insomnia. *Sleep* 22(1 Suppl.): 153, 1999.

75. Chesson, A. L., Jr., M. Littner, D. Davila, W. M. Anderson, M. Grigg-Damberger, K. Hartse, et al. Practice parameters for the use of light therapy in the treatment of sleep disorders. Standards of Practice Committee, American Academy of Sleep Medicine. *Sleep* 22(5): 641–660, 1999.

76. Dawson, D. and S. M. Armstrong. Chronobiotics—Drugs that shift rhythms. *Pharmacology and Therapeutics* 69(1): 15–36, 1996.

77. Skene, D. J., S. W. Lockley, and J. Arendt. Use of melatonin in the treatment of phase shift and sleep disorders. *Advances in Experimental Medicine and Biology* 467: 79–84, 1999.

78. Terman, M., A. Lewy, D. J. Dijk, Z. Boulus, C. Eastman, and S. Campbell. Light treatment for sleep disorders: Consensus report. IV: Sleep phase and duration disturbances. *Journal of Biological Rhythms* 10(2): 135–147, 1995.

79. Cole, R. J., J. S. Smith, Y. C. Alcala, J. A. Elliott, and D. F. Kripke. Bright-light mask treatment of delayed sleep phase syndrome. *Journal of Biological Rhythms* 17(1): 89, 2002.

80. Lewy, A. and R. Sack. Exogenous melatonin's phase-shifting effects on the endogenous melatonin profile in sighted humans: A brief review and critique of the literature. *Journal of Biological Rhythms* 12(6): 588–594, 1997.

81. Lewy, A. J., S. Ahmed, J. M. Jackson, and R. L. Sack. Melatonin shifts human circadian rhythms according to a phase-response curve. *Chronobiology International* 9(5): 380–392, 1992.

82. Lewy, A. J., V. K. Bauer, S. Ahmed, K. H. Thomas, N. L. Cutler, C. M. Singer, et al. The human phase response curve (PRC) to melatonin is about 12 hours out of phase with the PRC to light. *Chronobiology International* 15(1): 71–83, 1998.

83. Armstrong, S. M., O. M. McNulty, B. Guardiola-Lemaitre, and J. R. Redman. Successful use of S20098 and melatonin in an animal model of delayed sleep-phase syndrome (DSPS). *Pharmacology, Biochemistry, and Behavior* 46(1): 45–49, 1993.

84. Dagan, Y., I. Yovel, D. Hallis, M. Eisenstein, and I. Raichik. Evaluating the role of melatonin in the long-term treatment of delayed sleep phase syndrome (DSPS). *Chronobiology International* 15(2): 181–190, 1998.

85. Dahlitz, M., B. Alvarez, J. Vignau, J. English, J. Arendt, and J. D. Parkes. Delayed sleep phase syndrome response to melatonin. *Lancet* 337(8750): 1121–1124, 1991.

86. Buxton, O. M., M. L'Hermite-Baleriaux, F. W. Turek, and E. Van Cauter. Daytime naps in darkness phase shift the human circadian rhythms of melatonin and thyrotropin secretion. *American Journal of Physiology: Regulatory, Integrative and Comparative Physiology* 278(2): R373–R382, 2000.

87. Van Cauter, E., J. Sturis, M. M. Byrne, J. D. Blackman, N. H. Scherberg, R. Leproult, et al. Preliminary studies on the immediate phase-shifting effects of light and exercise on the human circadian clock. *Journal of Biological Rhythms* 8(Suppl.): S99–S108, 1993.

88. Cajochen, C., K. Krauchi, K. V. Danilenko, and A. Wirz-Justice. Evening administration of melatonin and bright light: Interactions on the EEG during sleep and wakefulness. *Journal of Sleep Research* 7(3): 145–157, 1998.

89. Krauchi, K., C. Cajochen, K. Danilenko, and A. Wirz-Justice. The hypothermic effect of late evening melatonin does not block the phase delay induced by concurrent bright light in human subjects. *Neuroscience Letters* 232: 57–61, 1997.

90. Dijk, D. J. and C. A. Czeisler. Contribution of the circadian pacemaker and the sleep homeostat to sleep propensity, sleep structure, electroencephalographic slow waves, and sleep spindle activity in humans. *Journal of Neuroscience* 15(5 Pt 1): 3526–3538, 1995.

91. Lack, L. C., J. D. Mercer, and H. Wright. Circadian rhythms of early morning awakening insomniacs. *Journal of Sleep Research* 5(4): 211–219, 1996.

92. Lack, L. and H. Wright. The effect of evening bright light in delaying the circadian rhythms and lengthening the sleep of early morning awakening insomniacs. *Sleep* 16(5): 436–443, 1993.

93. Lack, L. C., S. Gibbon, K. Schumacher, and H. Wright. Comparison of bright and placebo light treatment for morning insomnia. *Sleep Research* 23: 278, 1994.

94. Lack, L. C., H. Wright, K. Lushington, G. Zimmermann, J. Mercer, and K. Schumacher. The use of bright light therapy for insomnia. In E. G. Jung and M. F. Holick, eds. *Biologic Effects of Light 1993*. Basel, Switzerland: Walter de Gruyter. 1994: 228–240.

95. Campbell, S. S., D. Dawson, and M. W. Anderson. Alleviation of sleep maintenance insomnia with timed exposure to bright light. *Journal of the American Geriatrics Society* 41(8): 829–836, 1993.

96. Murphy, P. J. and S. S. Campbell. Enhanced performance in elderly subjects following bright light treatment of sleep maintenance insomnia. *Journal of Sleep Research* 5(3): 165–172, 1996.

97. Suhner, A. G., P. J. Murphy, and S. S. Campbell. Failure of timed bright light exposure to alleviate age-related sleep maintenance insomnia. *Journal of the American Geriatrics Society* 50(4): 617–623, 2002.

98. Bootzin, R. R., V. Shogam, and T. F. Kuo. Sleep anticipatory anxiety question naire: A measure of anxiety about sleep. *Sleep Research* 23: 188, 1994.

99. Morin, C. M., J. Stone, D. Trinkle, J. Mercer, and S. Remsberg. Dysfunctional beliefs and attitudes about sleep among older adults with and without insomnia complaints. *Psychology and Aging* 8(3): 463–467, 1993.

100. Campbell, S. S. Intrinsic disruption of normal sleep and circadian patterns. In F. W. Turek and P. C. Zee, eds. *Regulation of Sleep and Circadian Rhythms* (Volume 133). New York, NY: Marcel Dekker, Inc. 1999: 465–486.

101. Moldofsky, H., S. Musisi, and E. A. Phillipson. Treatment of a case of advanced sleep phase syndrome by phase advance chronotherapy. *Sleep* 9(1): 61–65, 1986.

102. Miles, L. E. and W. C. Dement. Sleep and aging. *Sleep* 3(2): 1–220, 1980.

103. Duffy, J. F., D. J. Dijk, E. B. Klerman, and C. A. Czeisler. Later endogenous circadian temperature nadir relative to an earlier wake time in older people. *American Journal of Physiology* 275(2/5): R1478–R1487, 1998.

104. Carrier, J., T. H. Monk, C. F. Reynolds, D. J. Buysse, and D. J. Kupfer. Are age differences in sleep due to phase differences in the output of the circadian timing system? *Chronobiology International* 16(1): 79–91, 1999.

105. Monk, T. H. Intrinsic circadian rhythm sleep disorders. *Sleep Medicine Reviews* 3(3): 177–178, 1999.

106. Duffy, J., D. Dijk, and C. Czeisler. Circadian and homeostatic modulation of cognitive throughput in older subjects. *Sleep* 21(3 Suppl): 301, 1998.

107. Dijk, D. J., J. F. Duffy, and C. A. Czeisler. Contribution of circadian physiology and sleep homeostasis to age-related changes in human sleep. *Chronobiology International* 17(3): 285–311, 2000.

108. Czeisler, C. A., J. F. Duffy, T. L. Shanahan, E. N. Brown, J. F. Mitchell, D. W. Rimmer, et al. Stability, precision, and near-24-hour period of the human circadian pacemaker. *Science* 284(5423): 2177–2181, 1999.

109. Copinschi, G., K. Spiegel, R. Leproult, and E. Van Cauter. Pathophysiology of human circadian rhythms. *Novartis Foundation Symposium* 227: 143–157, 2001.

110. Van Someren, E. J., C. Lijzenga, M. Mirmiran, and D. F. Swabb. Long-term fitness training improves the circadian rest-activity rhythm in healthy elderly males. *Journal of Biological Rhythms* 12(2): 146–156, 1997.

111. Weinert, D. Age-dependent changes of the circadian system. *Chronobiology International* 17(3): 261–283, 2000.

112. Buxton, O. M., S. A. Frank, M. L'Hermite-Baleriaux, R. Leproult, F. W. Turek, and E. Van Cauter. Roles of intensity and duration of nocturnal exercise in causing phase delays of human circadian rhythms. *American Journal of Physiology* 273(3 Pt 1): E536–E542, 1997.

113. Miyazaki, T., S. Hashimoto, S. Masubuchi, S. Honma, and K. I. Honma. Phase-advance shifts of human circadian pacemaker are accelerated by daytime physical exercise. *American Journal of Physiology: Regulatory, Integrative and Comparative Physiology* 281(1): R197–R205, 2001.

114. Piercy, J. and L. Lack. Daily exercise can shift the endogenous circadian phase. *Sleep Research* 17: 393, 1988.

115. Van Reeth, O., J. Sturis, M. M. Byrne, J. D. Blackman, M. L'Hermite-Baleriaux, R. Leproult, et al. Nocturnal exercise phase delays circadian rhythms of melatonin and thyrotropin secretion in normal men. *American Journal of Physiology* 266(6 Pt 1): E964–E974, 1994.

116. Dorsey, C. M., S. E. Lukas, M. H. Teicher, D. Harper, J. W. Winkelman, S. L. Cunningham, et al. Effects of passive body heating on the sleep of older female insomniacs. *Journal of Geriatric Psychiatry and Neurology* 9(2): 83–90, 1996.

117. Dorsey, C. M., M. H. Teicher, M. Cohen-Zion, L. Stefanovic, A. Satlin, W. Tartarini, et al. Core body temperature and sleep of older female insomniacs before and after passive body heating. *Sleep* 22(7): 891–898, 1999.

118. Van Someren, E. J. More than a marker: Interaction between the circadian regulation of temperature and sleep, age-related changes, and treatment possibilities. *Chronobiology International* 17(3): 313–354, 2000.

119. Youngstedt, S. D., D. F. Kripke, and J. A. Elliott. Circadian phase-delaying effects of bright light alone and combined with exercise in humans. *American Journal of Physiology: Regulatory, Integrative and Comparative Physiology* 282(1): R259–R266, 2002.

120. Buxton, O. M., G. Copinschi, A. Van Onderbergen, T. G. Karrison, and E. Van Cauter. A benzodiazepine hypnotic facilitates adaptation of circadian rhythms and sleep-wake homeostasis to an eight hour delay shift simulating westward jet lag. *Sleep* 23(7): 915–927, 2000.

121. Mistlberger, R. E., T. A. Houpt, and M. C. Moore-Ede. The benzodiazepine triazolam phase-shifts circadian activity rhythms in a diurnal primate, the squirrel monkey (Saimiri sciureus). *Neuroscience Letters* 124(1): 27–30, 1991.

122. Turek, F. W. Manipulation of a central circadian clock regulating behavioral and endocrine rhythms with a short-acting benzodiazepine used in the treatment of insomnia. *Psychoneuroendocrinology* 13(3): 217–232, 1988.

123. Pelissier, A. L., M. Gantenbein, and B. Bruguerolle. Caffeine-induced modifications of heart rate, temperature, and motor activity circadian rhythms in rats. *Physiology and Behavior* 67(1): 81–88, 1999.

124. Campbell, S. S. and P. J. Murphy. When sleep goes bad: Relationships between sleep and body temperature in middle-aged and older subjects. *Sleep Research* 25: 120, 1996.

125. Carrier, J., T. H. Monk, D. J. Buysse, and D. J. Kupfer. Amplitude reduction of the circadian temperature and sleep rhythms in the elderly. *Chronobiology International* 13(5): 373–386, 1996.

126. Copinschi, G. and E. Van Cauter. Effects of aging on modulation of hormonal secretions by sleep and circadian rhythmicity. *Hormone Research* 43(1–3): 20–24, 1995.

127. Czeisler, C. A., M. Dumont, J. F. Duffy, J. D. Steinberg, G. S. Richardson, and E. N. Brown. Association of sleep-wake habits in older people with changes in output of circadian pacemaker. *Lancet* 340(8825): 933–936, 1992.

128. Mishima, K., M. Okawa, S. Hozumi, and Y. Hishikawa. Supplementary administration of artificial bright light and melatonin as potent treatment for disorganized circadian rest-activity and dysfunctional autonomic and neuroendocrine systems in institutionalized demented elderly persons. *Chronobiology International* 17(3): 419–432, 2000.

129. Mouton, A., P. D. Penev, A. Ruth, I. Janssen, M. Keng, S. Finkel, et al. The effects of timed bright light exposure on temperature, mood and performance rhythms in the elderly. *Sleep Research* 25: 564, 1996.

130. Monk, T. H., D. J. Buysse, C. F. Reynolds, J. Kupfer, and P. R. Houck. Circadian temperature rhythms of older people. *Experimental Gerontology* 30(5): 455–474, 1995.

131. Lushington, K., D. Dawson, and L. Lack. Core body temperature is elevated during constant wakefulness in elderly poor sleepers. *Sleep* 23(4): 504–510, 2000.

132. De Koninck, J., P. G. Swingle, M. Hebert, C. Couture-Cote, and Y. Cote. Self-regulation of core body temperature and sleep. *Sleep Research* 22: 399, 1993.

133. Stepanski, E., F. Zorick, J. Sicklesteel, D. Young, and T. Roth. Daytime alertness-sleepiness in patients with chronic insomnia. *Sleep Research* 15: 174, 1986.

134. Lichstein, K. L., R. S. Johnson, S. Sen Gupta, D. L. O'Laughlin, and T. A. Dykstra. Are insomniacs sleepy during the day? A pupillometric assessment. *Behavioural Research and Therapy* 30(3): 283–292, 1992.

135. Regestein, Q. R., J. Dambrosia, M. Hallett, B. Murawski, and M. Paine. Daytime alertness in patients with primary insomnia. *American Journal of Psychiatry* 150(10): 1529–1534, 1993.

136. Bonnet, M. H. and D. L. Arand. Caffeine use as a model of acute and chronic insomnia. *Sleep* 15(6): 526–536, 1992.

137. Rodenbeck, A. and G. Hajak. Neuroendocrine dysregulation in primary insomnia. *Revue Neurologique* 157(11 Pt 2): S57–S61, 2001.

138. Rodenbeck, A., G. Huether, E. Ruther, and G. Hajak. Interactions between evening and nocturnal cortisol secretion and sleep parameters in patients with severe chronic primary insomnia. *Neuroscience Letters* 324(2): 159–163, 2002.

139. Vgontzas, A. N., E. O. Bixler, A. Kales, C. Criley, and A. Vela-Bueno. Differences in nocturnal and daytime sleep between primary and psychiatric hypersomnia: Diagnostic and treatment implications. *Psychosomatic Medicine* 62(2): 220–226, 2000.

140. Blazejova, K., S. Nevsimalova, H. Illnerova, I. Hajek, and K. Sonka. [Sleep disorders and the 24-hour profile of melatonin and cortisol]. *Sbornik Lekarsky* 101(4): 347–351, 2000.

141. Krauchi, K., C. Cajochen, E. Werth, and A. Wirz-Justice. Functional link between distal vasodilation and sleep-onset latency? *American Journal of Physiology: Regulatory, Integrative and Comparative Physiology* 278(3): R741–R748, 2000.

142. Lack, L. and M. Gradisar. Acute finger temperature changes preceding sleep onsets over a 45-h period. *Journal of Sleep Research* 11: 275–282, 2002.

Chapter 13 ————————————————————————————

CLINICAL ASSESSMENT OF PEDIATRIC SLEEP DISORDERS

AVI SADEH

Assessing pediatric sleep problems is a complex task. In addition to having extensive knowledge of sleep disorders and their clinical manifestations, clinicians need to employ a developmental perspective and to consider relevant psychosocial factors that are less pertinent in assessing adults. Developmental issues include the following:

- How many night wakings constitute a sleep problem at a given age?
- Should we assess only the objective nature of the problem or the degree of disruption these problems present to the family as well?
- What is the natural developmental course of a specific problem, and how does it relate to treatment decisions?

To answer these and similar questions, clinicians need solid normative data on the natural course of the development of various sleep-related phenomena such as night wakings, parasomnias, and sleep needs. The development of the required normative database is dependent on establishing standard assessment tools. The focus of this chapter is to provide working schemata for diagnosing pediatric sleep problems using scientifically based procedures and instruments in the field. The first section describes the most common pediatric sleep disorders according to the presented complaint. The second section reviews scientifically based instruments and procedures for clinical diagnosis and research.

DIAGNOSTIC GUIDELINES

Commonly presented complaints or reasons for referral can be divided into five main areas:

1. Difficulty falling asleep
2. Difficulty maintaining sleep: multiple and/or extended night wakings
3. Breathing-related sleep disorders
4. Excessive fatigue and sleepiness
5. Special phenomena during sleep or sleep-wake transitions

There can be much overlap among these presented problem areas, but for the purpose of clarity, they are discussed separately with the related diagnostic issues.

Difficulty Falling Asleep

Difficulties falling asleep in children are usually related to one or more of the following factors:

1. Lack of self-soothing capacities, excessive reliance on parental help, and difficulties of the parents in setting limits
2. Stress, fears, and anxiety in the child
3. Sleep schedule-related problems

Self-soothing and the capacity to fall asleep alone is an acquired ability that usually develops during infancy (1–2). Difficulties in falling asleep and maintaining sleep have often been associated with dependence on parental help in this process (3). Often, the process of falling asleep with parental presence is extended because of the rewarding quality of extra interaction with the parents, particularly if a specific parent's availability is limited and the extra time serves the emotional needs of both parent and child (4–5). A very common problem in this area is parental difficulties in setting limits. Confronting a child and conveying a clear message that it is time to go to sleep and discouraging any other demands is a very difficult task for many parents. The child's protests and crying often trigger unbearable fears and anxieties in the parent, the parent yields, and falling asleep becomes an endless process. These issues can be identified and clarified during the clinical interview and by using specific questionnaires.

In young children, separation anxiety can become a major issue interfering with going to sleep and falling asleep. In older children, fear of darkness and other fears related to monsters, bad dreams, and so on can peak at bedtime and become much more intense when the child is expected to disengage from social stimuli and fall asleep (6). An evaluation of the child's fears and anxiety is, therefore, needed when assessing difficulty falling asleep.

Another factor that may play a role in difficulty falling asleep is related to sleep hygiene and sleep schedule-related problems. A child may have difficulties falling asleep because of an erratic sleep schedule such as a late-afternoon nap or delayed sleep-phase tendencies that reduce the likelihood of being sleepy at a reasonable bedtime. Assessing such sleep schedule-related problems could be conducted by experimental manipulations of bedtime and the sleep schedule to test the effects of such manipulations on the child's difficulty falling asleep.

Other factors should be considered when assessing difficulty falling asleep. Among these factors are the consumption of stimulating substances (e.g., caffeine), stimulating activities before bedtime, and special motivating factors such as late night TV shows or Internet activities that older children may find very rewarding. Maturational factors and psychiatric disorders could also play a role in determining sleep schedule and difficulty falling asleep (7–11).

Difficulty Maintaining Sleep—Multiple and/or Extended Night Wakings

Difficulties in maintaining sleep or sleep fragmentation is the most common complaint in early childhood (3, 12–17). It has recently been demonstrated that these problems are still very common in older children (10, 18). Because of the lack of a standard definition for sleep fragmentation, we have proposed that criteria for such a definition, based on actigraphy (see later discussion), would be based on three or more night wakings on average or sleep efficiency that is below 90% (10, 18). These criteria should not serve as definite clinical criteria because other considerations (e.g., distress to child and family, effects on daytime functioning) should also be taken into account. However, in school-age children, such sleep fragmentation has been associated with compromised neurobehavioral functioning and behavior problems (19).

The main factors that should be assessed when sleep fragmentation is involved include:

1. Medical and physiological factors
2. Maturational and psychosocial behavioral factors
3. Sleep schedule-related problems

Many potential medical and physiological factors can lead to sleep fragmentation. Breathing-related problems are among the common factors discussed in the following sections. Other medical factors include allergies, such as colic (20), cow milk allergy (21–22), dermatitis (23–26), gastroesophageal reflux, and ear infections. The contribution of these physiological factors as well as the consumption of stimulants should be assessed in the clinical interview and sometimes by further medical examination or by exploratory trials (e.g., cow milk replacement diet trial). The role of other "popular" factors such as food composition and teething in persistent night-waking problems has not been supported (27–29).

Sleep consolidation for one main nocturnal episode is a result of a rapid maturational process that occurs during the first year of life (1–2, 30). However, many infants fail to develop consolidated sleep because of psychosocial and behavioral factors. Parental involvement in the soothing and falling asleep process plays a major role, similar to the role it plays in problems associated with sleep onset. Actually, there is much overlap between these two problem areas and their underlying biobehavioral causes. Sleep fragmentation has also been associated with stress and anxiety in children (31).

Sleep fragmentation, particularly when it involves very long bouts of wakefulness with no apparent behavioral maintaining system, can be related to sleep schedule problems. Sleep fragmentation has been associated with immature melatonin secretion patterns in young infants (32). It has been shown that some children, particularly blind children and children with severe neurological problems, suffer from sleep schedule disorders. These disorders, such as delayed sleep-phase and free-running clock, have clinical presentations that include difficulty falling asleep or awakening in the middle of the night with an inability to resume sleep (33–38).

Breathing-Related Sleep Problems

The breathing system is very sensitive during sleep. Arousal is the survival response of the brain to low oxygen level. In severe cases, hundreds of brief arousals and very shallow sleep have been documented. Sleep apnea is the most severe form of a breathing-related sleep problem (39–42). The most common causes for sleep apnea in children are airway obstructions due to enlarged tonsils or adenoids and other anatomical defects. The full diagnosis of sleep apnea requires polysomnographic study and complementary assessment by experts in the areas of ear, nose, and throat and respiratory disorders. Snoring is often associated with sleep apnea, although snoring is prevalent in many children without sleep apnea.

In recent years, snoring, even in the absence of other breathing problems, has been associated with excessive sleepiness, learning attention difficulties, and behavior problems in children (43–47). Children with asthma, another common breathing problem, are also characterized by poorer sleep patterns and increased daytime sleepiness (48–50).

Because of the high prevalence of breathing disorders in children, it is essential to include a thorough inquiry of this health issue in any assessment of a sleep problem. When a breathing problem during sleep is suspected, it should be further assessed by experts in the related fields.

Excessive Fatigue and Sleepiness

Excessive fatigue and sleepiness can result from many potential factors including:

1. Insufficient sleep
2. Specific sleep disorders
3. Psychiatric disorders and stress
4. Other medical disorders

Any assessment of excessive sleepiness should cover these areas, according to their relevance and prevalence.

Insufficient sleep appears to be a major health problem. Studies suggest that sleep time of both adults and children has been decreasing over the past few decades (51). These studies are often accompanied by increased reports of daytime sleepiness. Research has shown that adolescents are particularly prone to sleep deprivation and excessive sleepiness (8, 52–53). Because sleep needs vary significantly among individuals, it is very difficult to determine how much sleep is necessary for a specific child at a specific age. However, clinical "experiments" that include extending the child's sleep and monitoring his or her daytime behavior and alertness could help in determining whether the child receives adequate sleep.

Any of the specific sleep disorders listed in previous sections can lead to excessive daytime sleepiness. In addition, specific neurological sleep disorders such as restless legs syndrome (RLS) or periodic limb movement disorder (PLMD) and narcolepsy have been associated with increased daytime sleepiness in children (45, 54–56).

Psychiatric disorders such as mood disorders and, particularly, major depression can be associated with increased fatigue. Fatigue is also a major sign of stress, particularly chronic stress. Almost any medical disorders, transient or chronic, can lead to fatigue and excessive sleepiness. Chronic fatigue syndrome has also been identified in adolescents (57). It is beyond the scope of this chapter to review all links between medical disorders and excessive fatigue. Any complaint about fatigue and excessive sleepiness without an identifiable sleep-related problem should be subjected to broad medical and psychiatric evaluation.

Special Phenomena during Sleep or Sleep-Wake Transitions

Special phenomena occurring during sleep or sleep-wake transitions elicit concern in many parents. Common events such as night terrors, sleepwalking, teeth-grinding, intense body rocking, and head banging (also referred to as the *parasomnias*) trigger alarm because of their unique manifestations. Many of these phenomena are transitional, occur at a specific developmental phase or for a short transitional period, and disappear with no definable causes or consequences. However, the parasomnias are more prevalent in children suffering from neurological-developmental disorders.

Night terrors may appear during the first year of life. Parents may become very concerned when the infant wakes up with a piercing scream, cries his lungs out inconsolably, and resists parental soothing efforts. Night terrors, as isolated episodes, are very common in early childhood and usually require no professional intervention. If these events become very intense and frequent or if seizures are suspected, a more thorough evaluation is needed.

Body rocking and head banging are common self-soothing techniques that usually disappear with age. It is often sufficient to recommend that parents protect their child from possible injury rather than interfere with this self-soothing activity. Similarly, isolated episodes of sleepwalking and other forms of confusional arousals are also very common in children. When isolated episodes are involved, the main concern should be to the child's safety during the episodes.

However, when any of the phenomena described in this section become very intense or persistent, a more thorough evaluation is needed. The parasomnias are often linked to stress or insufficient sleep, and these issues should be further explored. It is also important to emphasize that although the systematic research on behavioral interventions for the parasomnias in children is limited, behavioral interventions appear to be effective in many cases (58–60).

INSTRUMENTS FOR ASSESSING SLEEP IN CHILDREN

Clinical Interview

The clinical interview is aimed at collecting information on the presented problem and understanding the history of the problem and its various manifestations, possible medical, psychosocial, and behavioral causes or contributing factors (5, 61–63). In addition to the assessment of the presented sleep problem, it is often important to assess the family dynamics, the parental and child's interpretation, attitudes, and motivation for change. These factors may play a major role in determining specific intervention and tailoring it to the actual characteristics of the child and his or her parents and to their real needs.

Questionnaires

Sleep-related questionnaires include:

1. Questionnaires that address general sleep patterns and include probes to specific sleep problems (e.g., difficulty falling asleep, night wakings, parasomnia, snoring)
2. Questionnaires that address daytime sleepiness or alertness
3. Questionnaires that address bedtime interactions, bedtime fears, and other issues related to sleep

An important feature that distinguishes between questionnaires is who completes them. Most studies with infants and young children are based on parental reports, whereas in older children (from school age), the tendency is to rely on self-reports.

Among the instruments developed for parental reports are instruments for assessing infant sleep (3, 12, 16, 64–67) and that of children and adolescents (6, 45, 66, 68–76). These instruments are generally used for surveys assessing the prevalence of sleep problems and links to other factors. However, they can be used for screening purposes and for comparing to normal samples. Self-report instruments have been used in older children and adolescents (53, 74, 77–80).

The validity of parental- and self-reports on children's sleep has never been strongly supported. Systematic clinical use of state-of-the-art questionnaires has never been established. Therefore, the diversity of existing questionnaires delays the creation of a sound normative database and the development of questionnaires for efficient clinical use. In spite of these limitations, sleep questionnaires can be used for screening purposes and for identifying specific areas of difficulties in clinical settings.

Sleep Diary

Sleep diaries or daily sleep logs are widely used in clinical settings for assessment and research purposes. These instruments are particularly useful when there is a need for more detailed information on a specific phenomenon (e.g., night wakings) or when longitudinal follow-up is needed, as in intervention follow-up studies (18, 81–86).

Studies comparing sleep diaries to objective measures of sleep suggest that parents are good reporters of their children's sleep-wake schedule (e.g., sleep onset time, sleep duration), but their accuracy drops dramatically when it comes to sleep quality measures (e.g., number of night wakings, sleep efficiency; 18, 84–85). One explanation for such discrepancies is that parents are aware of their child's nocturnal behavior mostly when their child requires intervention but may be totally unaware of night wakings if the child is a self-soother (1–2, 18, 85). Another possible explanation is that parents fail to report night wakings for extended periods because of lapses in attention or because they become weary of repeating this task every night (84–85). It has been demonstrated that if a clinical decision is to be made on the basis of a specific criterion for reported night wakings, the results would be totally different from those based on objective recordings of night wakings (85).

The importance of sleep diaries should not be undermined by their methodological limitations. Sleep diaries provide valuable information beyond the specific sleep characteristics. When assessing night wakings, essential information can be obtained vis-à-vis parental interventions and their effects on the child's sleep. This is a valuable part of the behavioral assessment of the sleep problem because it provides clues to behavioral mechanisms sustaining the disruption. Important topics include:

1. Who intervenes (e.g., father or mother)
2. What kind of intervention is provided (e.g., feeding, rocking, joining parental bed, car ride)
3. Child's specific response to each intervention (e.g., continued crying, sleep resumption, quiet wakefulness)
4. Parental cognitions and feelings (e.g., "I enjoyed nursing her in my bed," "I can't tolerate abandoning her when she cries her heart out")

It is often surprising how large the gaps are between parents' reports during the initial intake interview and the information they provide in their sleep diaries or in response to issues elicited by information included in the diaries (5).

Ambulatory Sleep Monitoring

A number of home-monitoring methods that can provide objective information as to children's sleep-wake patterns have been developed over the years. Unfortunately, these methods have mostly been adopted by researchers and, with some exceptions, not by clinicians for clinical practice.

Direct observations (87–88) and *pressure sensitive mattresses* (89–90) are methods that have been developed, validated, and used in sleep research. A special sleep-wake state taxonomy was developed for the infancy period (87, 91–92). However, these methods are probably too complex to apply for clinical purposes.

Video recordings have been used for research purposes with infants and young children (1–2, 43, 93–97). Video recordings in infants enable reliable sleep-wake scoring. In addition to documenting sleep-wake patterns, video recordings provide information on bedtime interactions and parental interventions. Furthermore, video recordings enable documenting special phenomenon during sleep (25, 43, 98–100). For instance, video recordings have been used to document scratching during sleep in children with atopic dermatitis (25). Similarly, parents can use a video camera to document parasomnia-related behaviors such as head banging, sleepwalking, night terrors, and so forth. Such home monitoring can often provide sufficient information for clinical diagnosis.

Although video recordings have demonstrated reliability and validity for sleep-wake scoring and for documenting special phenomena during sleep, it appears that the use of home video monitoring has not become a practical tool in the clinical practice of sleep medicine. The requirements of home installation of recording equipment and the demanding task of video reviewing and scoring may have deterred clinicians from adopting the method for clinical practice.

Actigraphy is based on a wristwatch-like device that can be used to collect activity data for extended periods. Actigraphy has been established as a reliable and valid method to document sleep in infants, children, and adults (101–103). A number of studies have validated actigraphy against the gold standard of polysomnography in infants and young children (15, 104) and in older children (105–106). Good night-to-night reliability indexes have been reported for actigraphic measures for various age groups during childhood (10, 18, 107). See Figures 13.1 and 13.2 for sample sleep records.

Normative data, or at least data that represent large samples of normal children, have been collected for various age groups (10, 18, 108–110). Furthermore, pediatric studies have demonstrated the informative value of using actigraphy in clinical settings for both phases of assessment (15, 85) and intervention (84, 111–114).

Polysomnography

Polysomnography (PSG) is the traditional gold-standard method for assessing sleep for clinical and research purposes (115). PSG is usually based on a laboratory study (although ambulatory studies have gained popularity in recent years) for a single night. PSG provides information about the EEG, the electro-oculogram

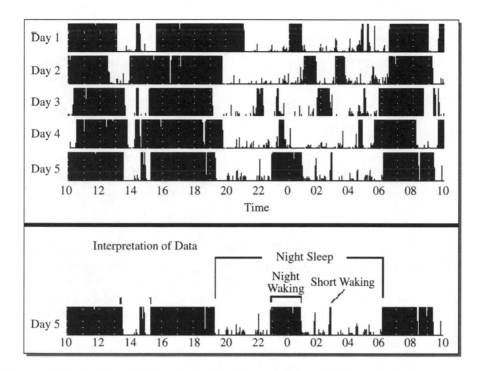

Figure 13.1   A Sample Record of a One-Year-Old Baby's Sleep-Wake Patterns over the Course of Five Consecutive 24-Hour Periods. The detailed explanation in the lower frame represents the last night of the diagram. From *Sleeping Like a Baby: A Sensitive and Sensible Approach to Solving Your Child's Sleep Problems,* by A. Sadeh, New Haven, CT: Yale University Press, 2001. Reprinted with permission.

(eye movements), the electromyogram (muscle tone), and respiratory signals during sleep. These data enable assessment of sleep structure, sleep stages, and specific disturbances during sleep such as those related to disordered breathing. A normative database for PSG in children has been developed as well as significant understanding of developmental processes (116–120). However, in assessing nonmedical sleep disorders, PSG provides very limited, but costly, information. EEG and other physiological data may not be clinically informative in many common clinical problems such as night wakings, difficulty falling asleep, schedule disorders, and some parasomnias. The information collected at the sleep lab is not only redundant but often distorted because it usually represents only a single night of the child's sleep patterns, under very unusual conditions. PSG should, therefore, be recommended when a medical or physiological disorder is suspected or when excessive and unexplained daytime sleepiness exists (61–63).

Sleep apnea, seizure disorders, and restless leg movements are the most common pediatric medical sleep disorders that should be ruled out. The Multiple

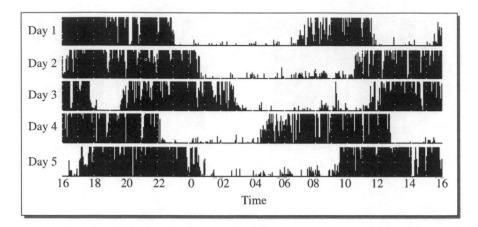

Figure 13.2   Sleep Record of a 3.5-Year-Old Girl with Pervasive Developmental Disorder. The child presents a sleep-schedule disorder while the original complaint was related to difficulty falling asleep and maintaining sleep. From *Sleeping Like a Baby: A Sensitive and Sensible Approach to Solving Your Child's Sleep Problems*, by A. Sadeh, New Haven, CT: Yale University Press, 2001. Reprinted with permission.

Sleep Latency Test (121), which is based on repeated PSG studies, can be used to verify the existence of excessive daytime sleepiness.

COMPLEMENTARY ASSESSMENT INSTRUMENTS

A comprehensive assessment of a sleep problem entails much more than assessing sleep itself. Assessment should not only address sleep but also include an evaluation of potential causes or exacerbating factors because sleep problems have multiple sources. For instance, allergies, esophageal reflux, and breathing difficulties have been associated with persistent sleep problems in infants and children (21, 23, 25–26, 43, 45, 49–50, 122). Medical and physical problems identified as potential sources for sleep problems in children should be addressed in the clinical interview or by a screening questionnaire (61–63).

Often, sleep problems in young children involve inappropriate and/or anxious parenting. Major themes are related to parental anxieties and limit setting. These issues that entail parental feelings, beliefs, or cognitions related to children's sleep can be addressed in the clinical interview, but they can also be assessed with standardized tools (123–124). This topic is particularly important when intervention is aimed at behavioral change that engages parental cognitions and fears (5, 125–127).

Stress and behavior or emotional problems are highly correlated with pediatric sleep problems (128–130). When relevant, clinical assessment should include evaluation sources of stress and psychopathology in the child or in the family. Such assessment can be facilitated by standardized instruments such as the Child Behavior Checklist (131–132), Parenting Stress Index (133), and adult psychopathology scales.

LIMITATIONS AND FUTURE DIRECTIONS

The good news is that sleep is a measurable phenomenon that can be quantified subjectively and objectively. The bad news is that:

1. We still do not have good normative databases for sleep measures across development.
2. Individual variability in sleep needs and patterns is so large that it is difficult to determine how much sleep is needed or how many night wakings should be considered as a sleep problem.

Extensive efforts have led to the creation of a normative database for PSG and actigraphy measures during childhood. Such efforts should be pursued with other scientifically based sleep assessment methods.

Because large variability exists in sleep patterns in children, future clinical research should be focused on these individual differences and on how to assess the match between the sleep needs and the actual sleep patterns of an individual child. Research on the effects of sleep duration and sleep disruptions on children's functioning and well being can lead to better knowledge on where to draw the line between normal variations in sleep and sleep disorders.

The limitations of covering this broad topic in a single chapter are obvious. Thorough reviews on many of the topics discussed in this chapter and other relevant topics that were not covered are recommended (5, 61–63, 92, 134–141).

REFERENCES

1. Anders, T. F., L. F. Halpern, and J. Hua. Sleeping through the night: A developmental perspective. *Pediatrics* 90(4): 554–560, 1992.
2. Goodlin-Jones, B. L., M. M. Burnham, E. E. Gaylor, and T. F. Anders. Night waking, sleep-wake organization, and self-soothing in the first year of life. *Journal of Developmental and Behavioral Pediatrics* 22(4): 226–233, 2001.

3. Adair, R., H. Bauchner, B. Philipp, S. Levenson, and B. Zuckerman. Night waking during infancy: Role of parental presence at bedtime. *Pediatrics* 87(4): 500–504, 1991.

4. Daws, D. *Through the Night: Helping Parents and Sleepless Infants.* London, England: Free Association Books. 1989: 274.

5. Sadeh, A. *Sleeping like a Baby: A Sensitive and Sensible Approach to Solving Your Child's Sleep Problems.* New York, NY: Yale University Press. 2001.

6. Blader, J. C., H. S. Koplewicz, H. Abikoff, and C. Foley. Sleep problems of elementary school children: A community survey. *Archives of Pediatrics and Adolescent Medicine* 151(5): 473–480, 1997.

7. Alvarez, B., M. J. Dahlitz, J. Vignau, and J. D. Parkes. The delayed sleep phase syndrome: Clinical and investigative findings in 14 subjects. *Journal of Neurology, Neurosurgery and Psychiatry* 55(8): 665–670, 1992.

8. Carskadon, M. A., C. Vieira, and C. Acebo. Association between puberty and delayed phase preference. *Sleep* 16(3): 258–262, 1993.

9. Gruber, R., A. Sadeh, and A. Raviv. Instability of sleep patterns in children with attention-deficit/hyperactivity disorder. *Journal of the American Academy of Child and Adolescent Psychiatry* 39(4): 495–501, 2000.

10. Sadeh, A., A. Raviv, and R. Gruber. Sleep patterns and sleep disruptions in school-age children. *Developmental Psychology* 36(3): 291–301, 2000.

11. Thorpy, M. J., E. Korman, A. J. Spielman, and P. B. Glovinsky. Delayed sleep phase syndrome in adolescents. *Journal of Adolescent Health Care* 9(1): 22–27, 1988.

12. Armstrong, K. L., R. A. Quinn, and M. R. Dadds. The sleep patterns of normal children. *Medical Journal of Australia* 161(3): 202–206, 1994.

13. Beltramini, A. U. and M. E. Hertzig. Sleep and bedtime behavior in preschool-aged children. *Pediatrics* 71(2): 153–158, 1983.

14. Moore, T. and L. E. Ucko. Night waking in early infancy. *Archives of Diseases in Childhood* 32: 333–342, 1957.

15. Sadeh, A., P. Lavie, A. Scher, E. Tirosh, and R. Epstein. Actigraphic home-monitoring sleep-disturbed and control infants and young children: A new method for pediatric assessment of sleep-wake patterns. *Pediatrics* 87(4): 494–499, 1991.

16. Scher, A., E. Tirosh, M. Jaffe, L. Rubin, A. Sadeh, and P. Lavie. Sleep patterns of infants and young children in Israel. *International Journal of Behavioral Development* 18(4): 701–711, 1995.

17. Zuckerman, B., J. Stevenson, and V. Bailey. Sleep problems in early childhood: Continuities, predictive factors, and behavioral correlates. *Pediatrics* 80(5): 664–671, 1987.

18. Tikotzky, L. and A. Sadeh. Sleep patterns and sleep disruptions in kindergarten children. *Journal of Clinical Child Psychology* 30(4): 579–589, 2001.

19. Sadeh, A., R. Gruber, and A. Raviv. Sleep, neurobehavioral functioning and behavior problems in school-age children. *Child Development* 73(2): 405–417, 2002.

20. White, B. P., M. R. Gunnar, M. C. Larson, B. Donzella, and R. G. Barr. Behavioral and physiological responsivity, sleep, and patterns of daily cortisol production in infants with and without colic. *Child Development* 71(4): 862–877, 2000.

21. Kahn, A., M. J. Mozin, E. Rebuffat, M. Sottiaux, and M. F. Muller. Milk intolerance in children with persistent sleeplessness: A prospective double-blind crossover evaluation. *Pediatrics* 84(4): 595–603, 1989.

22. Kahn, A., E. Rebuffat, D. Blum, G. Casimir, J. Duchateau, M. J. Mozin, et al. Difficulty in initiating and maintaining sleep associated with cow's milk allergy in infants. *Sleep* 10(2): 116–121, 1987.

23. Dahl, R. E., J. Bernhisel-Broadbent, S. Scanlon-Holdford, H. A. Sampson, and M. Lupo. Sleep disturbances in children with atopic-dermatitis. *Archives of Pediatrics and Adolescent Medicine* 149(8): 856–860, 1995.

24. Reid, P. and M. S. Lewis-Jones. Sleep difficulties and their management in preschoolers with atopic eczema. *Clinical and Experimental Dermatology* 20(1): 38–41, 1995.

25. Reuveni, H., G. Chapnick, A. Tal, and A. Tarasiuk. Sleep fragmentation in children with atopic dermatitis. *Archives of Pediatrics and Adolescent Medicine* 153(3): 249–253, 1999.

26. Stores, G., A. Burrows, and C. Crawford. Physiological sleep disturbance in children with atopic dermatitis: A case control study. *Pediatric Dermatology* 15(4): 264–268, 1998.

27. Macknin, M. L., S. V. Medendorp, and M. C. Maier. Infant sleep and bedtime cereal. *American Journal of Diseases of Children* 143(9): 1066–1068, 1989.

28. Macknin, M. L., M. Piedmonte, J. Jacobs, and C. Skibinski. Symptoms associated with infant teething: A prospective study. *Pediatrics* 105(4 Pt 1): 747–752, 2000.

29. Wake, M., K. Hesketh, and J. Lucas. Teething and tooth eruption in infants: A cohort study. *Pediatrics* 106(6): 1374–1379, 2000.

30. Anders, T. F. and M. Keener. Developmental course of nighttime sleep-wake patterns in full-term and premature infants during the first year of life. I. *Sleep* 8(3): 173–192, 1985.

31. Sadeh, A. Stress, trauma, and sleep in children. *Child and Adolescent Psychiatric Clinics of North America* 5(3): 685–700, 1996.

32. Sadeh, A. Sleep and melatonin in infants: A preliminary study. *Sleep* 20(3): 185–191, 1997.

33. Hering, E., R. Epstein, S. Elroy, D. R. Iancu, and N. Zelnik. Sleep patterns in autistic children. *Journal of Autism and Developmental Disorders* 29(2): 143–147, 1999.

34. Mindell, J. A. and C. M. De Marco. Sleep problems of young blind children. *Journal of Visual Impairment and Blindness* 91(1): 33–39, 1997.

35. Richdale, A. L. Sleep problems in autism: Prevalence, cause, and intervention. *Developmental Medicine and Child Neurology* 41(1): 60–66, 1999.

36. Sadeh, A., M. Klitzke, T. F. Anders, and C. Acebo. Case study: Sleep and aggressive behavior in a blind, retarded adolescent. A concomitant schedule disorder? *Journal of the American Academy of Child and Adolescent Psychiatry* 34(6): 820–824, 1995.

37. Schreck, K. A. and J. A. Mulick. Parental report of sleep problems in children with autism. *Journal of Autism and Developmental Disorders* 30(2): 127–135, 2000.

38. Tzischinsky, O., D. Skene, R. Epstein, and P. Lavie. Circadian rhythms in 6-sulphatoxymelatonin and nocturnal sleep in blind children. *Chronobiology International* 8(3): 168–175, 1991.

39. Bendell, R. D., J. L. Culbertson, T. L. Shelton, and B. D. Carter. Interrupted infantile apnea: Impact on early development, temperament, and maternal stress. *Journal of Clinical Child Psychology* 15(4): 304–310, 1986.

40. Brouilette, R., D. Hanson, R. David, L. Klemka, A. Szatkowski, S. Fernbach, et al. A diagnostic approach to suspected obstructive sleep apnea in children. *Journal of Pediatrics* 105(1): 10–14, 1984.

41. Carrol, J. L. and G. M. Louglin. Obstructive sleep apnea syndrome in infants and children: Diagnosis and management. In R. Ferber and M. Kryger, eds. *Principles and Practice of Sleep Medicine in the Child.* Philadelphia, PA: W.B. Saunders Company. 1995: 136–191.

42. Gaultier, C. Sleep apnea in infants. *Sleep Medicine Reviews* 3(4): 303–312, 1999.

43. Ali, N. J., D. J. Pitson, and J. R. Stradling. Snoring, sleep disturbance, and behavior in 4–5 year olds. *Archives of Disease in Childhood* 68(3): 360–366, 1993.

44. Blunden, S., K. Lushington, D. Kennedy, J. Martin, and D. Dawson. Behavior and neurocognitive performance in children aged 5–10 years who snore compared to controls. *Journal of Clinical and Experimental Neuropsychology* 22(5): 554–568, 2000.

45. Chervin, R. D., J. E. Dillon, C. Bassetti, D. A. Ganoczy, and K. J. Pituch. Symptoms of sleep disorders, inattention, and hyperactivity in children. *Sleep* 20(12): 1185–1192, 1997.

46. Ferreira, A. M., V. Clemente, D. Gozal, A. Gomes, C. Pissarra, H. Cesar, et al. Snoring in Portuguese primary school children. *Pediatrics* 106(5): U24–U29, 2000.

47. Gozal, D. and D. W. Pope. Snoring during early childhood and academic performance at ages thirteen to fourteen years. *Pediatrics* 107(6): 1394–1399, 2001.

48. Avital, A., D. G. Steljes, H. Pasterkamp, M. Kryger, I. Sanchez, and V. Chernick. Sleep quality in children with asthma treated with theophylline or cromolyn sodium. *Journal of Pediatrics* 119(6): 979–984, 1991.

49. Sadeh, A., I. Horowitz, L. Wolach-Benodis, and B. Wolach. Sleep and pulmonary function in children with well-controlled, stable asthma. *Sleep* 21(4): 379–384, 1998.

50. Stores, G., A. J. Ellis, L. Wiggs, C. Crawford, and A. Thomson. Sleep and psychological disturbance in nocturnal asthma. *Archives of Disease in Childhood* 78(5): 413–419, 1998.

51. Ferrara, M. and L. De Gennaro. How much sleep do we need? *Sleep Medicine Reviews* 5(2): 155–179, 2001.

52. Carskadon, M. A. Patterns of sleep and sleepiness in adolescents. *Pediatrician* 17(1): 5–12, 1990.

53. Wolfson, A. R. and M. A. Carskadon. Sleep schedules and daytime functioning in adolescents. *Child Development* 69(4): 875–887, 1998.

54. Picchietti, D. L., S. J. England, A. S. Walters, K. Willis, and T. Verrico. Periodic limb movement disorder and restless legs syndrome in children with attention-deficit hyperactivity disorder. *Journal of Child Neurology* 13(12): 588–594, 1998.

55. Picchietti, D. L. and A. S. Walters. Moderate to severe periodic limb movement disorder in childhood and adolescence. *Sleep* 22(3): 297–300, 1999.

56. Picchietti, D. L. and A. S. Walters. Restless legs syndrome and periodic limb movement disorder in children and adolescents—Comorbidity with attention-deficit hyperactivity disorder. *Child and Adolescent Psychiatric Clinics of North America* 5(3): 729, 1996.

57. Smith, M. S., J. Mitchell, L. Corey, D. Gold, E. A. McCauley, D. Glover, et al. Chronic fatigue in adolescents. *Pediatrics* 88(2): 195–202, 1991.

58. Frank, N. C., A. Spirito, L. Stark, and J. Owens-Stively. The use of scheduled awakenings to eliminate childhood sleepwalking. *Journal of Pediatric Psychology* 22(3): 345–353, 1997.

59. Golding, K. Nocturnal headbanging as a settling habit: The behavioral treatment of a 4-year-old boy. *Clinical Child Psychology and Psychiatry* 3(1): 25–30, 1998.

60. Thompson, B. A., B. W. Blount, and T. S. Krumholz. Treatment approaches to bruxism. *American Family Physician* 49(7): 1617–1622, 1994.

61. Ferber, R. Assessment of sleep disorders in the child. In R. Ferber and M. Kryger, eds. *Principles and Practice of Sleep Medicine in the Child*. Philadelphia, PA: W.B. Saunders Company. 1995: 45–53.

62. Ferber, R. Clinical Assessment of Child and Adolescent Sleep Disorders. *Child and Adolescent Psychiatric Clinics of North America* 5(3): 569–579, 1996.

63. Sheldon, S. H., J. P. Spire, and H. B. Levy. *Pediatric Sleep Medicine*. Philadelphia, PA: W.B. Saunders Company, 1992.

64. Hiscock, H. and M. Wake. Infant sleep problems and postnatal depression: A community-based study. *Pediatrics* 107(6): 1317–1322, 2001.

65. Johnson, C. M. Infant and toddler sleep: A telephone survey of parents in one community. *Journal of Developmental and Behavioral Pediatrics* 12(2): 108–114, 1991.

66. Ottaviano, S., F. Giannotti, F. Cortesi, O. Bruni, and C. Ottaviano. Sleep characteristics in healthy children from birth to 6 years of age in the urban area of Rome. *Sleep* 19(1): 1–3, 1996.

67. Thunstrom, M. Severe sleep problems among infants in a normal population in Sweden: Prevalence, severity and correlates. *Acta Paediatrica* 88(12): 1356–1363, 1999.

68. Bruni, O., S. Ottaviano, V. Guidetti, M. Romoli, M. Innocenzi, F. Cortesi, et al. The Sleep Disturbance Scale for Children (SDSC). Construction and validation of an instrument to evaluate sleep disturbances in childhood and adolescence. *Journal of Sleep Research* 5(4): 251–261, 1996.

69. Chervin, R. D., K. H. Archbold, P. Panahi, and K. J. Pituch. Sleep problems seldom addressed at two general pediatric clinics. *Pediatrics* 107(6): 1375–1380, 2001.

70. Fisher, B. E., C. Pauley, and K. McGuire. Children's Sleep Behavior Scale: Normative data on 870 children in grades 1 to 6. *Perceptual and Motor Skills* 68(1): 227–236, 1989.

71. Kahn, A., C. Van de Merckt, E. Rebuffat, M. J. Mozin, M. Sottiaux, D. Blum, et al. Sleep problems in healthy preadolescents. *Pediatrics* 84(3): 542–546, 1989.

72. Laberge, L., D. Petit, C. Simard, F. Vitaro, R. E. Tremblay, and J. Montplaisir. Development of sleep patterns in early adolescence. *Journal of Sleep Research* 10(1): 59–67, 2001.

73. Owens, J., R. Maxim, M. McGuinn, C. Nobile, M. Msall, and A. Alario. Television-viewing habits and sleep disturbance in school children. *Pediatrics* 104(3): E27, 1999.

74. Owens, J. A., A. Spirito, M. McGuinn, and C. Nobile. Sleep habits and sleep disturbance in elementary school-aged children. *Journal of Developmental and Behavioral Pediatrics* 21(1): 27–36, 2000.

75. Seifer, R., A. J. Sameroff, S. Dickstein, and L. C. Hayden. Parental psychopathology and sleep variation in children. *Child and Adolescent Psychiatric Clinics of North America* 5(3): 715–727, 1996.

76. Stein, M. A., J. Mendelsohn, W. H. Obermeyer, J. Amromin, and R. Benca. Sleep and behavior problems in school-aged children. *Pediatrics* 107(4): U102–U110, 2001.

77. Kirmil-Gray, K., J. R. Eagleston, E. Gibson, and C. E. Thoresen. Sleep disturbance in adolescents: Sleep quality, sleep habits, beliefs about sleep, and daytime functioning. *Journal of Youth and Adolescence* 13(5): 375–384, 1984.

78. Mercer, P. W., S. L. Merritt, and J. M. Cowell. Differences in reported sleep need among adolescents. *Journal of Adolescent Health* 23(5): 259–263, 1998.

79. Morrison, D. N., R. McGee, and W. R. Stanton. Sleep problems in adolescence. *Journal of the American Academy of Child and Adolescent Psychiatry* 31(1): 94–99, 1992.

80. Tynjaelae, J., L. Kannas, and R. Vaelimaa. How young Europeans sleep. *Health Education Research* 8(1): 69–80, 1993.

81. Corkum, P., R. Tannock, H. Moldofsky, S. Hogg-Johnson, and T. Humphries. Actigraphy and parental ratings of sleep in children with attention-deficit-hyperactivity disorder (ADHD). *Sleep* 24(3): 303–312, 2001.

82. France, K. G., N. M. Blampied, and P. Wilkinson. Treatment of infant sleep disturbance by trimeprazine in combination with extinction. *Journal of Developmental and Behavioral Pediatrics* 12(5): 308–314, 1991.

83. Kirjavainen, J., T. Kirjavainen, V. Huhtala, L. Lehtonen, H. Korvenranta, and P. Kero. Infants with colic have a normal sleep structure at 2 and 7 months of age. *Journal of Pediatrics* 138(2): 218–223, 2001.

84. Sadeh, A. Assessment of intervention for infant night waking: Parental reports and activity-based home monitoring. *Journal of Consulting and Clinical Psychology* 62(1): 63–68, 1994.

85. Sadeh, A. Evaluating night wakings in sleep-disturbed infants: A methodological study of parental reports and actigraphy. *Sleep* 19(10): 757–762, 1996.

86. Wolfson, A., P. Lacks, and A. Futterman. Effects of parent training on infant sleeping patterns, parents' stress, and perceived parental competence. *Journal of Consulting and Clinical Psychology* 60(1): 41–48, 1992.

87. Thoman, E. B. Sleep and wake behaviors in neonates: Consistencies and consequences. *Merrill Palmer Quarterly* 21(4): 295–314, 1975.

88. Thoman, E. B., V. H. Denenberg, J. Sievel, L. P. Zeidner, and P. Becker. State organization in neonates: Developmental inconsistency indicates risk for developmental dysfunction. *Neuropediatrics* 12(1): 45–54, 1981.

89. Freudigman, K. A. and E. B. Thoman. Infant sleep during the first postnatal day: An opportunity for assessment of vulnerability. *Pediatrics* 92(3): 373–379, 1993.

90. Thoman, E. B. and R. C. Glazier. Computer scoring of motility patterns for states of sleep and wakefulness: Human infants. *Sleep* 10(2): 122–129, 1987.

91. Thoman, E. B. Sleeping and waking states in infants: A functional perspective. *Neuroscience and Biobehavioral Reviews* 14(1): 93–107, 1990.

92. Thoman, E. B. and C. Acebo. Monitoring of sleep in neonates and young children. In R. Ferber and M. Kryger, eds. *Principles and Practice of Sleep Medicine in the Child.* Philadelphia, PA: W.B. Saunders Company. 1995: 55–68.

93. Anders, T. F. Night-waking in infants during the first year of life. *Pediatrics* 63(6): 860–864, 1979.

94. Anders, T. F. and A. M. Sostek. The use of time lapse video recording of sleep-wake behavior in human infants. *Psychophysiology* 13(2): 155–158, 1976.

95. Gaylor, E. E., B. L. Goodlin-Jones, and T. F. Anders. Classification of young children's sleep problems: A pilot study. *Journal of the American Academy of Child and Adolescent Psychiatry* 40(1): 61–67, 2001.

96. Ingersoll, E. W. and E. B. Thoman. Sleep/wake states of preterm infants: Stability, developmental change, diurnal variation, and relation with caregiving activity. *Child Development* 70(1): 1–10, 1999.

97. Morielli, A., S. Ladan, F. M. Ducharme, and R. Brouilette. Can sleep and wakefulness be distinguished in children by cardiorespiratory and videotape recordings? *Chest* 109(3): 680–687, 1996.

98. Hayes, M. J. and D. Mitchell. Spontaneous movements during sleep in children: Temporal organization and changes with age. *Developmental Psychobiology* 32(1): 13–21, 1998.

99. Konofal, E., M. Lecendreux, M. P. Bouvard, and M. C. Mouren-Simeoni. High levels of nocturnal activity in children with attention-deficit hyperactivity disorder: A video analysis. *Psychiatry and Clinical Neurosciences* 55(2): 97–103, 2001.

100. Sivan, Y., A. Kornecki, and T. Schonfeld. Screening obstructive sleep apnoea syndrome by home videotape recording in children. *European Respiratory Journal* 9(10): 2127–2131, 1996.

101. American Sleep Disorders Association. Practice parameters for the use of actigraphy in the clinical assessment of sleep disorders. American Sleep Disorders Association. *Sleep* 18(4): 285–287, 1995.

102. Sadeh, A. and C. Acebo. The role of actigraphy in sleep medicine. *Sleep Medicine Reviews* 6(2): 113–124, 2002.

103. Sadeh, A., P. J. Hauri, D. F. Kripke, and P. Lavie. The role of actigraphy in the evaluation of sleep disorders. *Sleep* 18(4): 288–302, 1995.

104. Sadeh, A., C. Acebo, R. Seifer, S. Aytur, and M. A. Carskadon. Activity-based assessment of sleep-wake patterns during the 1st year of life. *Infant Behavior and Development* 18(3): 329–337, 1995.

105. Sadeh, A., J. Alster, D. Urbach, and P. Lavie. Actigraphically based automatic bedtime sleep-wake scoring: Validity and clinical applications. *Journal of Ambulatory Monitoring* 2(3): 209–216, 1989.

106. Sadeh, A., K. M. Sharkey, and M. A. Carskadon. Activity-based sleep-wake identification: An empirical test of methodological issues. *Sleep* 17(3): 201–207, 1994.

107. Acebo, C., A. Sadeh, R. Seifer, O. Tzischinsky, A. R. Wolfson, A. Hafer, et al. Estimating sleep patterns with activity monitoring in children and adolescents: How many nights are necessary for reliable measures? *Sleep* 22(1): 95–103, 1999.

108. Acebo, C., A. Sadeh, R. Seifer, O. Tzischinsky, and M. A. Carskadon. Sleep/ wake patterns in one to five year old children from activity monitoring and maternal reports. *Sleep* 23: A30–A31, 2000.

109. Carskadon, M. A., A. R. Wolfson, C. Acebo, O. Tzischinsky, and R. Seifer. Adolescent sleep patterns, circadian timing, and sleepiness at a transition to early school days. *Sleep* 21(8): 871–881, 1998.

110. Sadeh, A., I. Dark, and B. R. Vohr. Newborns' sleep-wake patterns: The role of maternal, delivery and infant factors. *Early Human Development* 44(2): 113–126, 1996.

111. McArthur, A. J. and S. S. Budden. Sleep dysfunction in Rett syndrome: A trial of exogenous melatonin treatment. *Developmental Medicine and Child Neurology* 40(3): 186–192, 1998.

112. Pillar, G., E. Shahar, N. Peled, S. Ravid, P. Lavie, and A. Etzioni. Melatonin improves sleep-wake patterns in psychomotor retarded children. *Pediatric Neurology* 23(3): 225–228, 2000.

113. Smits, M. G., E. E. Nagtegaal, J. van der Heijden, A. M. L. Coenen, and G. A. Kerkhof. Melatonin for chronic sleep onset insomnia in children: A randomized placebo-controlled trial. *Journal of Child Neurology* 16(2): 86–92, 2001.

114. Zhdanova, I. V., R. J. Wurtman, and J. Wagstaff. Effects of a low dose of melatonin on sleep in children with Angelman syndrome. *Journal of Pediatric Endocrinology and Metabolism* 12(1): 57–67, 1999.

115. Anders, T. F., R. N. Emde, and A. A. Parmelee. *A Manual of Standardized Terminology, Techniques and Criteria for the Scoring of States of Sleep and Wakefulness in Newborn Infants.* Los Angeles: UCLA Brain information Service. 1971.

116. Acebo, C., R. P. Millman, C. Rosenberg, A. Cavallo, and M. A. Carskadon. Sleep, breathing, and cephalometrics in older children and young adults. Part I: Normative values. *Chest* 109(3): 664–672, 1996.

117. Coble, P. A., D. J. Kupfer, L. S. Taska, and J. Kane. EEG sleep of normal healthy children. Part I: Findings using standard measurement methods. *Sleep* 7(4): 289–303, 1984.

118. Erler, T. and E. Wischniewski. Sleep medicine in infants—practicability and limitations. *Early Human Development* 63(1): 23–35, 2001.

119. Hoppenbrouwers, T., J. Hodgman, K. Arakawa, S. A. Geidel, and M. B. Sterman. Sleep and waking states in infancy: Normative studies. *Sleep* 11(4): 387–401, 1988.

120. Kahn, A., B. Dan, J. Groswasser, P. Franco, and M. Sottiaux. Normal sleep architecture in infants and children. *Journal of Clinical Neurophysiology* 13(3): 184–197, 1996.

121. Carskadon, M. A., W. C. Dement, M. M. Mitler, T. Roth, P. R. Westbrook, and S. Keenan. Guidelines for the multiple sleep latency test (MSLT): A standard measure of sleepiness. *Sleep* 9(4): 519–524, 1986.

122. Kahn, A., M. Sottiaux, J. Appelboom-Fondu, D. Blum, E. Rebuffat, and J. Levitt. Long-term development of children monitored as infants for an apparent life-threatening event during sleep: A 10-year follow-up study. *Pediatrics* 83(5): 668–673, 1989.

123. Hock, E., S. McBride, and M. T. Gnezda. Maternal separation anxiety: Mother-infant separation from the maternal perspective. *Child Development* 60(4): 793–802, 1989.

124. Morrell, J. M. The role of maternal cognitions in infant sleep problems as assessed by a new instrument, the maternal cognitions about infant sleep questionnaire. *Journal of Child Psychology and Psychiatry* 40(2): 247–258, 1999.

125. Mindell, J. A. Empirically supported treatments in pediatric psychology: Bedtime refusal and night wakings in young children. *Journal of Pediatric Psychology* 24(6): 465–481, 1999

126. Owens, J. L., K. G. France, and L. Wiggs. Behavioral and cognitive-behavioral interventions for sleep disorders in infants and children: A review. *Sleep Medicine Reviews* 3(4): 281–302, 1999.

127. Ramchandani, P., L. Wiggs, V. Webb, and G. Stores. A systematic review of treatments for settling problems and night waking in young children. *British Medical Journal* 320(7229): 209–213, 2000.

128. Dahl, R. E. The regulation of sleep and arousal: Development and psychopathology. *Development and Psychopathology* 8(1): 3–27, 1996.

129. Dahl, R. E. and J. Puig-Antich. Sleep disturbances in child and adolescent psychiatric disorders. *Pediatrician* 17(1): 32–37, 1990.

130. Sadeh, A. Sleep and trauma in children. In G. Stores and L. Wiggs, eds. *Sleep Disturbances in Children and Adolescents with Disorders of Development: Its Significance and Management.* London, England: MacKeith Press. 2001: 169–173.

131. Achenbach, T. M. and C. S. Edelbrock. The classification of child psychopathology: A review and analysis of empirical efforts. *Psychological Bulletin* 85(6): 1275–1301, 1978.

132. Achenbach, T. M. and C. S. Edelbrock. *Manual for the Child Behavior Checklist and Revised Child Behavior Profile.* Burlington: University of Vermont, Department of Psychiatry. 1983.

133. Abidin, R. R. *Parenting Stress Index—Manual.* Charlottesville, VA: Pediatric Psychology Press. 1983.

134. Anders, T., B. Goodlin-Jones, and A. Sadeh. Sleep disorders. In C. H. Zeanah, ed. *Handbook of Infant Mental Health* (2nd Edition). New York, NY: Guilford Press. 2000: 236–338.

135. Anders, T. F. and L. A. Eiben. Pediatric sleep disorders: A review of the past 10 years. *Journal of the American Academy of Child and Adolescent Psychiatry* 36(1): 9–20, 1997.

136. Ferber, R. *Solve Your Child's Sleep Problems.* New York, NY: Simon & Schuster, 1985.

137. Kuhn, B. R., J. W. Mayfield, and R. H. Kuhn. Clinical assessment of child and adolescent sleep disturbance. *Journal of Counseling and Development* 77(3): 359–368, 1999.

138. Mindell, J. A. Sleep disorders in children. *Health Psychology* 12(2): 151–162, 1993.

139. Mindell, J. A., J. A. Owens, and M. A. Carskadon. Developmental features of sleep. *Child and Adolescent Psychiatric Clinics of North America* 8(4): 695–725, 1999.

140. Sadeh, A. and R. Gruber. Sleep disorders. In T. Ollendick, ed. *Comprehensive Clinical Psychology* (Volume 5). Oxford, England: Pergamon/Elsevier Science. 1998: 629–653.

141. Stores, G. Practitioner review: Assessment and treatment of sleep disorders in children and adolescents. *Journal of Child Psychology and Psychiatry* 37(8): 907–925, 1996.

Chapter 14

BEHAVIORAL INSOMNIAS OF CHILDHOOD—LIMIT SETTING AND SLEEP ONSET ASSOCIATION DISORDER: DIAGNOSTIC ISSUES, BEHAVIORAL TREATMENT, AND FUTURE DIRECTIONS

DANIEL S. LEWIN

Sleep onset, sleep maintenance, and bedtime behavior problems are particularly common among children. As many as 30% of parents address the problems with primary care pediatricians (1–4). Five percent to 10% of patients are referred for evaluation to a sleep specialist (5), and as many as 50% of children may have at least transient sleep-related behavior problems that are not brought to the attention of a health care provider. An even higher percentage of sleep disorders is found among children who have psychiatric disorders (e.g., attention-deficit hyperactivity disorder and affective disorders; 6–8) medical problems (9–10), developmental disabilities (11–12), or daytime behavior or learning problems (13–15). While only a handful of studies (16–18) have investigated the sequelae of childhood sleep problems, extensive anecdotal evidence from child clinicians and published reports from adult studies suggest that insufficient sleep interferes with the regulation of attention and affective states and cognitive processes (19–26). When sleep problems are chronic, they may affect the course of normal development. Children's sleep problems also disturb their parents' sleep. Sleep-deprived parents who also have economic, occupational, or medical problems may have difficulty meeting the needs of their child because of their own impaired coping abilities and lower frustration tolerance.

Difficulty initiating and maintaining sleep are problems that affect children as well as adults, although the etiology and manifestation of the problems differ in important respects across the life span. The most common childhood dyssomnias defined in the *International Classification of Sleep Disorders* (27) are categorized as dyssomnias, extrinsic type, sleep onset association disorder (307.42-5), and limit setting sleep disorder (307.42-4). Psychophysiological insomnia (307.42-0), adjustment sleep disorder (307.41-0), and insufficient sleep disorder (307.49-4) also occur in children and adolescents; in most cases, the causes and treatments do not differ greatly from those in adults (1). This chapter focuses on sleep onset association disorder, limit setting sleep disorder, and several child-specific issues that are important to consider in the treatment of psychophysiologic insomnia. A brief definition of these disorders is provided and is followed by a theoretical discussion of their etiology couched in an evolutionary and developmental context. The second half of the chapter is an in-depth review of behaviorally based treatment strategies. The chapter closes with a discussion of future research priorities.

DEFINITIONS

Sleep onset association disorder is defined as impairment in sleep onset as a result of the absence of certain objects or circumstances (27; see Table 14.1 for specific criteria outlined in the *International Classification of Sleep Disorders*).

Table 14.1   ISCD-R Criteria for Sleep Onset Association Disorder

A. The patient has a complaint of insomnia.
B. The complaint is temporally associated with absence of certain conditions (e.g., being held, rocked, or nursed; listening to the radio; or watching television, etc).
C. The disorder has been present for at least three weeks.
D. With the particular association present, sleep is normal in onset, duration, and quality.
E. Polysomnographic monitoring demonstrates:
    1. Normal timing, duration, and quality of the sleep period when the associations are present.
    2. Sleep latency and the duration or number of awakenings can be increased when the associations are absent.
F. No significant underlying mental or medical disorder accounts for the compliant.
G. The symptoms do not meet the criteria for any other sleep disorder causing difficulty in initiating sleep (e.g., limit setting sleep disorder).

Minimal Criteria: A plus B plus D plus F plus G.

Source: From *The International Classification of Sleep Disorders Diagnostic and Coding Manual, Revised,* by The American Sleep Disorders Association, Rochester, MN: American Sleep Disorders Association, 1997.

A typical example of this disorder is an infant who always falls asleep while nursing or using a pacifier and has significant difficulty falling asleep when the breast or pacifier is not present. This problem is generally diagnosed in infants and young children between 4 months and 3 years of age and is associated with significant difficulty initiating sleep and multiple extended nighttime awakenings that require parental intervention. Crying spells at bedtime and in the middle of the night may persist for two to three hours, placing a significant burden on parents and resulting in shorter sleep duration and poor sleep quality for the infant. The disorder may occur even after an infant has established a relatively well-consolidated nighttime sleep.

Limit setting sleep disorder is defined as delayed sleep onset resulting from "inadequate enforcement of bedtime" by caregivers (27; see Table 14.2 for specific criteria outlined in the *International Classification of Sleep Disorders*). Once the child falls asleep, the remainder of the sleep period tends to be normal. A typical example of this disorder is a 3- to 8-year-old child who attempts to engage a parent multiple times following bedtime. Bids for attention include requests for water or food, another story or kiss goodnight, tantrums, and expression of fears. Parents typically give in to their children's requests on a variable reinforcement schedule and increase the frequency of bids for attention.

ETIOLOGY

The etiology of these two sleep disorders is heterogeneous. Occasional and short-term difficulty settling and bedtime resistance may be considered a variant of

Table 14.2   ISCD-R Criteria for Limit Setting Sleep Disorder

A. The patient has difficulty in initiating sleep.

B. The patient stalls or refuses to go to bed at an appropriate time.

C. Once the sleep period is initiated, sleep is of normal quality and duration.

D. Polysomnographic monitoring demonstrates normal timing, quality, and duration of the sleep period.

E. No significant underlying mental or medical disorder accounts for the complaint.

F. The symptoms do not meet criteria for any other sleep disorder causing difficulty in initiating sleep (e.g., sleep onset association disorder).

Minimal Criteria: B plus C.

Source: From *The International Classification of Sleep Disorders Diagnostic and Coding Manual, Revised,* by The American Sleep Disorders Association, Rochester, MN: American Sleep Disorders Association, 1997.

normal development. This is based on the assumption that the behavior (mental and physical relaxation and self-soothing) that facilitates the transition from wake to sleep is learned or developed. When sleep-related behavior problems persist and are refractory to parents' attempts to modify their children's behavior, a host of etiological or moderating factors need to be considered. For example, child temperament and psychopathology (28–31), parent psychopathology (including transient problems such as postpartum depression; 32), inconsistent limit setting, irregular bedtime activities, and a history of feeding or health problems (e.g., otitis media or gastroesophageal reflux; 33–35) are all possible complicating factors. Trauma and chronic stressors can initiate a course of psychophysiologic insomnia in both adults and children (36–38). Children with developmental disabilities may have a higher prevalence of childhood insomnias and are often referred to sleep specialists given the persistence and tenacity of their sleep onset and maintenance problems (11–12).

AN EVOLUTIONARY PERSPECTIVE

Under normal conditions, the transition from wake to a sleep state requires physical and mental relaxation and the letting down of vigilance. However, turning off vigilance has a potentially high cost for all animals (22, 39). For our ancestors, who had no electricity and inadequate domiciles, turning off vigilance made them susceptible to myriad threats from the elements, predators, and opportunistic fellow hominids. Increasing the threshold of vigilance has a potentially high cost as the network of neurophysiological systems supporting the maintenance of vigilance, attention, and the response to threat is magnificently complex and plays a critical role in protecting the organism.

For at least the past century, our species has developed far more control over our environment. Even so, sleep-related ritual and diverse behavioral repertoires are pervasive. They may be necessary to cue sympathetic and parasympathetic mechanisms responsible for the shift in conscious and behavioral states. A perceived or actual threat calls these systems into action, increases vigilance, and may prevent the transition to sleep. Chronic sleep problems may ensue when the organism is repeatedly at risk or has an abnormally low threshold for responsiveness to environmental stimuli. While it is not currently known how these hypothesized mechanisms function in children, learned rituals, control of affective states, and developing cognitive abilities (e.g., self-soothing, distraction through independent play) gradually play a more central role in facilitating a smooth transition to sleep after 6 months of age (40).

In summary, feeling safe, comfortable, and secure facilitates the letting down of vigilance and an easy transition to sleep. Problems with the wake-to-sleep transition may be caused by hypervigilance for real or imagined threats or the absence of ritual, habit, and features of the environment that represent safety, security, and comfort. The extent to which making the transition to sleep involves a series of learned behaviors is debatable. However, it is most certainly the case that the factors that mediate a smooth wake-to-sleep transition in children parallel developmental changes.

A DEVELOPMENTAL PERSPECTIVE

Normal and pathological developmental changes in cognition, the control of affect and attention, and social interactions, as well as sleep architecture, can be important precipitants for childhood insomnias. There are several critical periods during the first six years of life in which specific complications may arise in the wake-to-sleep transition. The transition from wake to sleep is complicated by numerous and sometimes competing factors, most notably a high level of dependence on parents and a high sleep drive. In the remainder of this section, developmental achievements and links to specific sleep problems are described. The following lists of developmental achievements are not comprehensive, and their role in perpetuating sleep problems has not been rigorously established.

Birth to Six Months of Age

Developmental Achievements

Between birth and 6 months of age, there are dramatic changes in the organization of infants' sleep, wake, and feeding schedules. Other changes include gradual recognition of parents as primary caregivers, development of increasingly powerful emotional bonds with parents, fear of strangers and threatening situations, observation of simple cause and effect relationships, and increased mobility.

Developmental Changes and Associated Sleep Problems

While it is likely that attachment to parents is well under way as early as 1 to 2 months, it is around 6 months that it is a measurable and robust phenomena (41). At this stage, infants become distressed when separated from parents for short intervals during the day. Bedtime may also become particularly difficult for both parents and infants. The infant who has already developed an attachment to a transitional object (e.g., a soft blanket or stuffed animal) or who can self-soothe (e.g., a physically self-stimulating behavior or vocalizing) will likely make a relatively smooth transition from wake to sleep.

Parents feel varying amounts of ambivalence about being separated from their infant and may experience a great deal of distress when their child protests being left alone. Infants and children of all ages are sensitive to parents' affective state and may become more upset, thus setting off a vicious cycle. If difficulty settling extends beyond a couple of weeks, the crib may become a noxious stimulus, making interventions even more difficult to implement. Patterns of interaction at bedtime at this stage of development can set the tone for months and sometimes years to come.

Infants who are temperamentally reactive (42), who have not been able to form productive attachments to parents, or who will not tolerate being separated from a parent for even short periods during the day may have greater difficulty with the transition to sleep. Each of these infants may have a lower threshold for arousability, which results in reactivity to both internal and external stimuli and a generally higher level of vigilance. High arousability and high vigilance are not compatible with a smooth transition from wake to sleep.

Four to Eight Months of Age

Developmental Achievements

Between 4 and 8 months of age, feeding patterns optimally shift from feeds every 2 hours (sometimes more often for breast milk-only babies) to increasingly longer intervals during the day. During this period, the infant can also achieve a consolidated 8 to 12 hours of uninterrupted sleep at night (28, 43–47).

Developmental Changes and Associated Sleep Problems

Even in healthy infants, these changes in feeding and sleep can be difficult to manage. It may be the first time that the infant's hunger has not been satisfied immediately on demand and spells of intense crying may ensue. Parents may feel ambivalent about a marked decrease in intimate time with their infant and that they are depriving their infant or causing the distress. The naturally occurring increase in intervals between feeds can result in better consolidated nighttime sleep and an increase in the duration of the sleep period. For the infant, a well-consolidated and long nighttime sleep period may result in longer and better quality waking periods during the day (i.e., being well rested, less irritable, ability to focus for longer periods; 18, 48–50). For the first time in many months, the parents may have uninterrupted sleep, and there is no question that the infant will benefit from interactions with well-rested parents.

Twelve to Thirty-Six Months of Age

Developmental Achievements

The next critical phase of development is between 12 and 36 months of age when the older infant is mobile, can climb out of a crib independently, experiment with longer periods of separation from parents, test limits set by parents. During this period, the child is moved from a crib to a toddler bed. Learning about the internal control of emotional states and the firmness of external limits (e.g., the boundaries of the bedroom and the security of the home) occurs concurrently. Testing cause and effect relationships and attempts to exert control over the environment are also hallmarks of this period.

Development Changes and Associated Sleep Problems

Ferber (51) addresses the anxiety some children experience when the secure limits of the crib rails are no longer present. For many young children, exploration of these limits involves calling out or leaving the bedroom to find parents. Inconsistent limit setting at bedtime, highly charged affective responses, and ambivalence on the part of parents are powerful reinforcers that maintain or increase the frequency of the child's attention-seeking behaviors.

Children who are anxious, overly reactive, or who have difficulty regulating thoughts and feelings can have a particularly hard time at this stage. Increased anxiety and fearful thoughts, heightened arousal, and vigilance can be magnified by separation from parents, being alone in a dimly lit room, and being tired. The birth of a sibling is a common event during this period and can cause sleep disturbance in even the best sleeper as a result of excitement, parental stress, and less time with a parent.

Five to Seven Years of Age

Developmental Achievements and Associated Sleep Problems

A final critical period falls between 5 and 7 years of age as the child develops a more complex concept of self and others. During this period, abstract thinking comes on line, and the child has the ability to think through real or imagined scenarios.

Developmental Changes and Associated Sleep Problems

Worry about school performance and relationships with peers may interfere with mental relaxation and the letting down of vigilance that is critical for sleep onset to occur. Integration of knowledge about local and world events, greater imaginative abilities, as well as more exposure to the media may further exacerbate bedtime fears. Parents' interactions with children may need to strike a delicate balance. Too much attention can undermine the child's independence and reinforce fears and attention-seeking behavior, while too little can leave the child to cope with issues that are overwhelming and deserve some intervention. Children's verbal ability and developing insight can be used to effectively draw the parent back into the room. While seemingly manipulative, the fears that the child describes in very vivid and frightening terms to the parent are based in the child's emotional discomfort about being alone. The bed and the bedtime routine may become the conditioned stimuli for fears and affective arousal.

DEVELOPMENTAL CHANGES IN SLEEP

Until about three months of age, there are three sleep stages—active sleep, quiet sleep, and indeterminate sleep. These stages are roughly analogous to rapid eye movement sleep (REM), non-REM (nREM), stages 3 and 4, and nREM (stages 1 and 2) that emerge after three months and remain relatively stable in form and definition throughout the life span. These stages can be reliably identified on polysomnographic records (see Chapter 2 in this volume for a more in-depth review of measurement). Polysomnography (PSG) is the gold standard for the measurement of sleep and involves electrophysiological recordings of brain activity, muscle tone, and eye movements. REM sleep is defined as an active mind in a paralyzed body and repeated conjugal movements of the eyes under closed lids. During REM, the majority of long narrative dreams occur. During nREM stages 3 and 4, brain activity is characterized as high voltage, highly synchronized, large slow waves (called delta) that are prominent during more than 20% of a 30-second epoch. There is thought to be minimal mental activity during nREM stages 3 and 4, and when aroused from these stages, the individual is groggy and disoriented. The greatest percentage of the night is generally spent in nREM stage 2, which is lighter than stages 3 and 4 (i.e., there is a lower arousal threshold), and a very small percentage of the night is spent in nREM stage 1, which is a very light transitional stage. Several measures of sleep disruption and sleep continuity can be derived from PSG and from sleep logs and questionnaires: sleep latency, the time between lights out and sleep onset, wake time after sleep onset, and total sleep time. Sleep efficiency is a composite and useful ratio of the sleep time to the duration of the sleep period.

The sleep drive in children is particularly strong and appears to decrease gradually during the first two decades (40, 52). There is a good deal of evidence that documents the developmental trajectory of the sleep drive. Average total sleep time ranges from 16 to 18 hours during the first few months of life, 12 to 14 hours in infants 6 to 24 months of age, 11 to 12 hours in children 24 months to 6 years of age, 10 to 11 hours in children 7 to 10 years of age, and 9 to 10 hours during adolescence (53–56). The amplitude of delta waves during nREM stages 3 and 4 (44, 57) and the common anecdotal experience of the child who can be carried from the car to bed without waking are further evidence of the depth of sleep and high sleep drive. During the first two to three months of life, infants transition from a wake state to lighter stages of nREM and then relatively quickly to active sleep which is comparable to REM sleep (44). After about three months, infants transition quickly from lighter stages of nREM sleep to a 60- to 90-minute period of deep nREM (delta, stages 3 and 4) sleep characterized by high amplitude delta. As with adults, children have partial or complete arousals multiple times throughout the night at the transition between sleep stages. The nighttime arousals can become long periods of wakefulness, particularly when a child has been unable to fall asleep independently at the beginning of the night.

During the first three months of life, many infants fall asleep in their parents' arms and are then put down in a crib or bassinet shortly after sleep onset. Because infants enter the sleep cycle through REM or active sleep, their arousal threshold is lower and they are more likely to have a brief arousal when the parent puts them down. If the arousal leads to a full awakening and protest, the process may become particularly frustrating for parents who do not understand the underlying cause.

ENVIRONMENTAL, PSYCHIATRIC, AND MEDICAL CONTRIBUTORS

Parents' contributions to sleep problems must also be considered. While cosleeping is preferred by some parents, it becomes problematic when it results in a shorter sleep duration or inadequate sleep quality for parents and/or children or a significant curtailment of adult activities in the period between the child's and parents' bedtime (39). Parental conflict about sleeping arrangements may be a sign of underlying marital problems, and if there is disagreement about a preferred approach and the child may receive a confusing and convoluted message from parents. Parental psychopathology, for example, postpartum depression, a particularly common problem (57–59), can result in a wide range of daytime behavior problems that for some children may also be prominent at night. The problems can include parental sleep deprivation persisting beyond the first few postpartum months. Sleep deprivation and psychiatric symptoms are a particularly problematic combination and may result in more reactivity in response to stressors, passivity, inconsistent limit setting, or anger and frustration directed at a demanding child. The potential for a vicious cycle of problematic behavior patterns ensuing between a parent and a child may be particularly problematic at night when both are tired.

Several studies have indicated that children with developmental disabilities have significantly more sleep-related behavior problems than normally developing children (11). There are several possible causes of the increased prevalence of problems in these populations. Entrainment to social and environmental cues may be impaired as a result of underlying neurophysiological anomalies, and cognitive limitations may interfere with the perception of environmental sleep cues (e.g., light and dark, changing to pajamas, quiet time with parents). Because the transition to sleep is facilitated by learned behaviors, impairment and delays in the ability to learn new behavior may interfere with the establishment of bedtime rituals, self-soothing, and attachment to a transitional object. In children with autism and profound developmental delays, parents and health care providers may have more difficulty identifying signs of anxiety and sadness. These emotional disturbances can manifest in many ways (for example, compulsive behaviors and agitation). Safety is always a primary concern because poor judgment and unpredictable behavior can place a child and family members at significant risk of injury in the middle of the night. Getting up with their child multiple times during the night, sometimes for extended periods, can result in a significant sleep debt and place a tremendous burden on parents who are already challenged by a child with exceptional needs.

Current and past medical problems and birth complications can all have an impact on a child's sleep. Particularly common problems that sometimes remain untreated in otherwise healthy children are gastroesophageal reflux, recurrent abdominal pain, and headaches (34–35, 60). Each of these disorders can cause increased arousal because of pain and physical discomfort, and their symptoms can actually cause decrements in sleep quality. Children who have had significant postnatal complications or multiple hospitalizations and medical procedures may also have a higher incidence of sleep problems. While the specific mechanisms of these effects have not been clearly identified, they may include increased arousal and vigilance for returning symptoms, cognitive fears about sickness and death, and a learned pattern of sleep disruption. Par ents of children who have had significant health problems may have a particularly hard time setting bedtime limits or allowing their children to cry for any length of time. These parents may have spent the first three months of their infant's life listening for an apnea monitor alarm or may have listened helplessly to hours of crying because of pain or colic. The result may be a very powerfully conditioned insomnia for parents.

Several miscellaneous etiological factors should also be noted. Ruling out the presence of other sleep disorders is of key importance. Sleep-disordered breathing, restless legs syndrome, and periodic limb movement disorders may all be associated with bedtime behavior problems (21, 31, 61–62). Environmental noise, a chaotic home, inconsistent bedtime routines, and variable bedtimes impact some children but not others. Aside from the factors discussed previously and temperamental factors, there appears to be no way to predict which child will fall into a regular schedule and sleep through any disturbance and which will never be able to achieve a good night's sleep.

ASSESSMENT

Measures and Instruments

The primary assessment techniques for childhood sleep problems are subjective parent report measures. During the past several years, the psychometric properties of a few bedtime questionnaires have been evaluated. Chervin's Pediatric Sleep Questionnaire (63) and Owens' Children's Sleep Habits Questionnaire (64) are parent report instruments that are useful in guiding clinical assessments of specific sleep disorders and the identification of behaviors associated with sleep. These instruments identify problem areas related to bedtime behaviors (tantrums, multiple bids for parents' attention, etc.), sleep schedule irregularities, and the subject's sleep quality and quantity. Daytime tiredness and symptoms of other sleep disorders (e.g., snoring, restlessness, repetitive movements) are often included in these questionnaires. While useful as adjuncts to a thorough assessment of sleep problems, there is an inverse association between the child's age and the amount of time that the parents observe the child's sleep. Additionally, children's self-reports of their own sleep quality and daytime somnolence are unreliable until they reach early adolescence.

Daily sleep logs provide invaluable information on the night-to-night variability of children's sleep schedules. A more objective measure of sleep and wake periods, wrist actigraphy, is an excellent adjunct to sleep logs and questionnaires

(65). Wrist actigraphy and sleep logs provide important data on patients' progress and compliance with treatment protocols.

Clinical History

A thorough clinical history is vital and should include an in-depth assessment of sleep, health and psychiatric problems, current developmental status, and the regularity and nature of activities leading up to bedtime (34, 66). Carefully defining the child's sleep-related behavior problem is critical for the implementation of a treatment plan. Identifying reinforcers, the extent of the parents' involvement, consistency of the sleep schedule and rituals, fears, disruptors in the bedroom (noise, too much or too little light, temperature extremes), and media use (television, Internet, music, etc.) are critical. The child's age, developmental status, and temperament will determine the extent to which the child will participate and respond to specific interventions. The sleep problems must be understood in the context of other problems, such as psychiatric disorders, effects of arousing or sedating medications, medical problems, and chronic fears associated with recent stressors or trauma. The parents of a child who has had multiple medical procedures since birth may have realistic fears about leaving the child alone or may need to adjust these concerns and acknowledge their own feelings of fear, separation, and guilt before making changes. Identification and treatment of other sleep disorders, such as sleep-disordered breathing and periodic limb movement disorder, is key because they may disrupt sleep, cause nighttime arousals, and increase tiredness.

As previously noted, understanding the cause of the sleep disturbance is critical and may guide the pace and order of interventions. In some cases, it is appropriate to institute a treatment plan immediately, and in other cases, stabilizing the child's comorbid condition is a first step and, in some cases, may be sufficient to solve the sleep problem. For example, treating a child's gastroesophageal reflux should invariably begin before most aspects of a treatment plan are implemented.

Observation of Behavior

The child's and the parents' interactions in the examination room may provide a wealth of information. For example, an informal observation of the child's ability to play independently and control negative affective states and bids for parental attention, comfort, and intimacy can highlight problem areas. Observations of parents' responses to their children's positive and negative bids for attention can be useful in guiding the choice of techniques the parent will be able to apply at home. A more formal assessment of the child's behavior problems and the parents' ability to identify and respond to problematic behavior is indicated in some cases, particularly with children who have severe behavior problems, and development delays. Functional behavioral analysis (11) is one such method; it identifies environmental reinforcers that maintain both positive and negative patterns of behavior.

Miscellaneous Assessment Issues

Differentiating full awakenings from parasomnias in infants and young children can be difficult. Helping parents to differentiate partial and complete arousals will help guide their response to their child during a nighttime awakening. Failure to differentiate a night terror from a full agitated awakening can be particularly frustrating for parents who may assume that they are not capable of calming their child or that the awakenings are uncontrollable.

Evaluating a particular family's ability to comprehend and implement a plan is critical. While there is no formal method of evaluating the potential for compliance with sleep interventions, attention to the parents' thoroughness in completing paperwork, compliance with prior interventions, number of children in the home, and number of parents should provide guidance on the practicality of implementing interventions.

Several additional factors are important to evaluate before implementing a treatment plan. First, parents' treatment goals differ both within and between families. Attitudes toward cosleeping or allowing a child to cry for more than five minutes can vary greatly as can less complex issues such as sleeping with a nightlight. Evaluating both parents' goals and attitudes before implementation of a treatment plan will sometimes head off problems. When there is a disagreement, helping parents negotiate an acceptable middle ground is critical. In some cases, these disagreements are signs of marital problems, which may be a cause of the child's sleep problem. For example, a child's sleep problems may be a convenient way for parents to avoid facing relationship or sexual problems. Parental disagreement may result in inconsistent rituals and an increase in emotional lability at bedtime, and a vicious cycle of negative interactions may take hold at a relatively fragile time in the child's day.

TARGETS AND TECHNIQUES OF BEHAVIORAL INTERVENTIONS FOR CHILDHOOD INSOMNIAS

Over the past 50 years, approximately 100 published reports of studies have evaluated the efficacy of interventions for childhood insomnias. Mindell (3) and

Ramchandani et al. (67) reviewed this literature and provided very thorough in-depth summaries of intervention strategies. While there are numerous variations, there are seven basic categories of intervention, each of which is discussed in detail later. A combination of a few techniques in both clinical practice and research is most commonly used. All of these interventions rest on three assumptions or principles:

Principle 1. Infants and children learn to fall asleep at the beginning of the night under specific conditions. To fall back to sleep after normal awakenings that occur throughout the night, the same conditions must exist. Teaching a child to fall asleep independently at the beginning of the night is usually sufficient to correct sleep maintenance problems. Falling asleep at the breast while being held by a parent or while using a pacifier are conditions that are not replicable in the middle of the night unless a parent wakes up and responds to the child.

Principle 2. An overtired infant or young child does not transition to sleep or sleep as well as a child who is not tired. Therefore, increasing the sleep drive by delaying sleep onset and setting a rigid morning wake-up time (a common intervention for adults with psychophysiological insomnia) can worsen an infant's or young child's transition to sleep. The assumption underlying this principle is that tiredness leads to disregulation of affective states. An overtired child is often overactive, irritable, and demanding, and this elevated level of arousal is incompatible with a smooth wake-to-sleep transition. Falling asleep in an aroused state may also lower the threshold for parasomnias and nightmares as well as cause some decrement in sleep quality. When this pattern exists for weeks and months at a time, the bedroom, the bed, and bedtime rituals may be classically conditioned stimuli for increased vigilance and arousal. Parents may learn to dread bedtimes, and their anxiety and frustration can worsen their child's mood.

Principle 3. Finding the optimal bedtime can be difficult because it varies by age and from child to child. There is assumed to be a window of time during which infants or young children are not overtired and their sleep drive is sufficiently high. Within two hours of bedtime, there is a period of activation called the *danger zone* when a child is wide awake and highly activated. Putting a child down during this period can lead to conflict and frustration for the parent and child. As previously noted, an overtired child also has a hard time making a smooth transition to sleep. Identifying an optimal bedtime is not essential, but it goes a long way toward facilitating a smooth wake-to-sleep transition.

Education

An introduction to normal sleep patterns and good sleep habits is an essential component of all interventions. Several studies have demonstrated that education alone is an effective intervention (3, 68) and that prenatal education can also help parents anticipate the types of problems that may arise (69). At minimum, there are three topics that should be covered with parents:

1. Basic information about the duration of day and nighttime sleep patterns and expectations about the occurrence of multiple nighttime awakenings
2. The importance of consistent bedtimes, wake-up times, nighttime activities preceding bedtime, and bedtime rituals
3. The optimal sleep environment (i.e., temperature, noise, light)

Establishing Appropriate Bedtime Routines

A careful analysis of the activities and rituals that lead up to bedtime helps to identify several categories of activities that require adjustment. Activities that may exacerbate sleep problems include watching television and movies, playing video games, excessive exercise, rough play, conflict with siblings and parents, and large meals. Frightening images abound in today's media, and a surprisingly large number of children have televisions, VCRs, and Internet access in their rooms. Moreover (70), in some homes, there is little or no monitoring of material that is viewed. Strict limitations on scary and violent books, movies, and television programming is critical. Mediation of the child's exposure to media and a debriefing period within a couple of hours of bedtime are critical.

Consistency in schedule and routine is probably the most important issue while sometimes the most difficult to implement. A child's tantrums and parents' frustration can derail attempts to establish a routine as can variable employment schedules and chaos due to limited resources. Teaching parents basic limit setting skills, changing bedrooms, modifying bedtimes of siblings, and identifying responsibilities of different caretakers may be necessary first steps.

Another challenge involves identifying an optimal lights-out time. While circadian abnormalities are relatively uncommon in young children, they must be ruled out as a cause of sleep problems. A mismatch between the child's and parents' schedules may not have an optimal solution. For example, parents who are phase delayed and an infant or young child who by comparison is phase advanced may remain incompatible. When feasible, two parents can trade off spending early waking hours with the infant.

Work and day care schedules represent common and sometimes irresolvable problems. Typically, most children ages 6 months to 6 years are able to go to sleep between 7 and 8 P.M. and wake up between 6 and 8 A.M. A 60- to 120-minute morning nap and a shorter afternoon nap of 30 to 90 minutes are also typical of infants until 18 to 24 months of age when there tends to be one 60- to 120-minute nap in the early afternoon. By 6 years of age, a child might have a slightly later bedtime and they have eliminated their daytime nap.

From the age of 3 on, differentiating between bedtime and lights-out time can be useful with children who lie in bed awake and ruminate for long periods of time. Allowing children to read or play quietly in their room until they are tired and decide independently to go to bed is a version of stimulus control, which is an effective intervention for adults with insomnia.

For an anxious, traumatized, or reactive child who is 3 years of age and older, a worry check with parents can both be rewarding and diminish bedtime worries. This check-in should optimally occur between 90 and 120 minutes before bedtime (a review of worries and fears immediately before bedtime may be overly activating). Teaching parents to avoid open-ended questions and to ask specific questions about important topics (e.g., conflicts with friends, fears of separation and illness, disturbing media images), is more likely to elicit the child's fears and concerns, which the parent can then help to resolve.

During the hour before bedtime, a gradual decrease in stimulating physical and mental activity helps to prepare the child for a smooth transition to sleep. The optimal activities involve mild effort and focus (reading, drawing, solving puzzles) rather than arousing and passive activities (watching television and movies and playing video games). When possible, time with one or both parents reading together, talking, or cuddling can be rewarding for everyone. Consistency in the order of other routines, such as bathing, putting on pajamas, or saying a prayer is important. A "monster" and "shadow" and "under-the-bed check" can be conducted just before lights out and may help to put the child at ease. Although excessive attention to frightening areas of the bedroom may reinforce fears. Specific methods of addressing behavioral problems that interfere with a positive and consistent bedtime routine are described later.

Education about feeding and sleep patterns is relevant for parents of young infants. The infant who is older than 6 months and has always had a bottle at bedtime and multiple times during the night or who has access to the breast throughout the night may have significant difficulty breaking the association between feeding and sleep (33). Gradual extinction and fading procedures discussed later are effective methods of eliminating bedtime and middle-of-the-night feeds. For breast-fed children, nighttime weaning can be facilitated by allowing a second parent to take on night duty for a couple of weeks.

A transitional object is a carefully chosen, soft, huggable item such as a stuffed animal, blanket, or small pillow that provides comfort and a sense of security. In the attachment literature, a transitional object temporarily represents the parent (51–52, 60). An object may be introduced at any time, but 3 to 6 months may be best because it may be a critical period for the development of attachments, and it is the period when the first major challenge in making an independent wake-to-sleep transition usually occurs. A transitional object should not have a noise maker or solid part that could wake the infant when he or she rolls or lies on top of it. Introducing the object into the bedtime ritual and using it exclusively for sleep time can make it a very potent cue for the process of letting down vigilance. The object should be introduced at least one to two weeks before the commencement of an extinction procedure.

Extinction Techniques

Extinction techniques are the most effective and expedient method of eliminating an infant's or child's dependence on parents to help them transition from awake to sleep (2, 51, 71–73). These techniques involve fast or gradual systematic ignoring of the child's bids for attention. The fast approach, also called the *cold-turkey* or *cry it out* approach, is effective (3) and generally resolves the problem within one week. However, parents often have difficulty tolerating long periods of crying. Other parents do not even consider the approach to be acceptable because of the perceived distress that it causes. If medical and psychiatric histories have not revealed significant problems, extinction techniques are appropriate for use with infants and children who have sleep onset association disorder and limit setting sleep disorder. However, the acceptability of these approaches may be generally low despite their being highly effective.

The *fast approach* involves the parent's putting the child in the crib, leaving the room, and not returning until morning. While the procedure is essentially the same with older children, the parent must set a limit that the child is not allowed out of the bed or bedroom (methods of using the bedroom door to set limits is discussed later) and must not call out to the parent. Several brief checks may be scheduled to ensure that the child is all right. While difficult to implement, the parent can be instructed to check on the child when there is a pause or decrease in the intensity of the crying to reinforce the infant's calmer and more controlled states. There should be little or no physical contact with the child during the check-ins. A brief calming verbal comment can be reassuring to both the child and parent. Within 3 days, most children will have learned to settle on their own. Parents must be told to expect an extinction burst (an increase in the attention-seeking behavior that is more persistent and dramatic than the behavior that occurred at baseline) within 5 to 10 nights of the implementation of the plan. A period of spontaneous recovery (a mild increase in problem behaviors) may occur between days 15 and 30 (2). Differentiating these phenomena from relapse is critical because parents may give in and feel significant disappointment.

The *gradual approach* involves a scheduled fading of parents' involvement in the wake-to-sleep transition. There are unlimited variations on this approach, allowing it to be adapted to the specific needs and preferences of different families. There are four general categories of variables that can be faded:

1. The amount of physical contact the parent has with the child (i.e., hugging, holding, patting on the back, and so on)
2. The proximity of the parent to the child (e.g., ignoring the child while sitting or lying in the child's bedroom)
3. The duration of intervals between check-ins
4. The duration of the check-in

Dr. Richard Ferber's well-known approach (33) involves a fading of check-ins over the course of a seven-day period (i.e., day 1, 2 minutes; day 2, 5 minutes; day 3, 7 minutes), a fixed amount of physical contact (minimal, patting the back), and a fixed duration of check-ins (maximum, 2 minutes). The duration of the program can vary from a couple of weeks to a few months depending on the parents' preference. An extinction burst and a period of spontaneous recovery should also be expected with the gradual approach although it is often less pronounced (2).

Relapses also occur and are often associated with developmental changes, teething, illnesses, and stressful events. During these events, children need increased attention and may be taken into the parents' bed for a couple of nights. Parents should be reassured that the setback is only temporary and that they have the skill and ability to help their child get right back to the improved schedule.

Daytime behavior may also be affected, particularly during the first phase of these systematic ignoring techniques. In addition to being overtired, the child may feel anxious because of the newly enforced nighttime independence. Tolerating some irritability and increasing supportive nurturing interactions during the day can help to decrease nighttime anxiety. However, if the child has day- and nighttime separation problems, a consistent response to the child both during the day and at night is important.

Parents' affective state plays a critical role during the implementation of these behavior modification procedures. Frustrated and irritable parents and parents who are ambivalent about leaving their child often send confusing and contradictory messages to a child. Parents who have a child with medical complications may have a particularly hard time with these procedures because they go against all of the impulses that have played a vital role in the past Teaching parents to monitor their own emotions and to model the type of emotional state that their child should assume increases their effectiveness in helping their child transition to sleep.

The child's bedroom door is a potentially powerful tool that can be used when a child has moved from a crib to a toddler bed and is not compliant with the parents' request that he or she stay in his or her bedroom. Closing the door may help to establish a firm and supportive "passive limit" (51) but should not be used in an angry manner or as a punishment. It is recommended that a parent monitor a child very closely when the door is closed and keep it closed for a specified period of time. For anxious or fearful children, being in their bedroom with the door closed can intensify their negative feelings and state of arousal and have a long-term negative effect on their ability to settle. Differentiating anxiety from the testing of limits is critical. Using a gate in the doorway is comparable to the use of the door but is more tolerable. Care must be taken to ensure that children will not injure themselves if they try to climb or remove the gate.

Several factors can increase the ease of implementation and the probability of success of an extinction program. As noted previously, a well-established transitional object can be very comforting to an infant. The parents can introduce a self-soothing behavior derived from observations of the child's daytime activities (sucking on fingers, caressing the face, playing with hair; 74). During the week preceding the extinction intervention, the parent can model or teach the child repetitive behaviors that are associated with a calm and relaxed state. Choosing an optimal time to intervene can be critical. Incorporating a weekend into the plan or, even better, a vacation will allow the parents time to recover from several days of stress and sleep deprivation that may be associated with an intervention. Assigning parents specific duties or having them alternate "on-call nights" can be a very good use of available resources. Having one parent implement the program or alternating trips to the child's room during a single night can be burdensome and decrease the probability of success.

Children who are verbal can be prepared for the implementation of the plan during the preceding weeks, which allows them control and an important role (35). A more tangible reward program, such as a star or a sticker chart, can also increase compliance and motivation to fix the problem. For example, a child can be told that part of being a big boy is learning to sleep alone in a bed. Once a goal is achieved (e.g., three stars for three consecutive nights of staying in bed the whole night), the child's compliance and success can be rewarded with a special activity for all family members or extra solo time with one parent. While more tangible material rewards can be given to a child, their use may set an expensive precedent for future behavior modification programs.

Scheduled Awakenings

Waking the child briefly before the usual middle-of-the-night awakening is an approach that has been shown to have moderate efficacy (3, 75). This approach has been used with infants as young as 3 months and children up to 4 years of age. Based on careful logging of the timing of the child's nighttime awakenings, the parent can wake the child within 15 minutes of his or her usual wake-up time. Over the course of a few weeks, the child's awakenings and callouts generally decrease in frequency and duration.

The rationale for this approach is that the parent is present for a brief awakening and the child is likely to transition back to sleep quickly and never reach a level of arousal that will result in a full awakening. Drawbacks to the approach include the difficulty of implementing the plan for parents. Children's awakenings are not always predictable. Finally, the impact of waking a child from a deep sleep should not be problematic but in some children may cause a parasomnia.

Medications

Use of medication to treat children's sleep problems is somewhat controversial and has not been shown to be particularly effective, particularly in the long term. Two studies in the United Kingdom (76–77) have evaluated Trimeprazine, a relatively long-acting phenothiazine-derived antihistamine, which is approved for use outside the United States for children older than 6 months of age. Some positive results were noted when children were at relatively high doses, and the medication may be effective when combined with systematic ignoring interventions. Both prescription (chloral hydrate, clonodine) and over-the-counter medications (antihistamines) that are approved for children are used on a relatively frequent basis to treat children's sleep problems; however, their efficacy has not been demonstrated. While in the short-term, sedative hypnotics and other medications may improve sleep quality, their long-term usage may cause complications, such as increased tolerance and changes in sleep architecture (78). The half-life of these medications (some are more effective for sleep onset problems, but not sleep maintenance problems) and carryover effects that result in daytime somnolence are also important to consider. Use of medication as an adjunct to behavioral interventions may be helpful, but rebound insomnia following the withdrawal of the medication can undo many of the gains achieved during active treatment. It is also not clear how sedative hypnotics interact with behavioral interventions.

Melatonin has recently been shown to be of some utility as an adjunct to other treatments in adults with psychophysiological insomnia. When administered in doses of 1 to 3 mg two to three hours before bedtime, it may advance sleep onset. A recent report of a study of 40 children ages 6 to 12 years reported beneficial effects of melatonin when compared to placebo (79). No adverse side effects were noted. More research is needed to replicate these results, and some caution must be exercised because adequate dosing of melatonin has yet to be established and there is little control over the quality of melatonin that is sold over the counter in a variety of stores. Melatonin is also reported to have some impact on the regulation of estrogen, and it causes vasoconstriction. The effects of exogenous melatonin in children are not known. Use of melatonin in children with developmental disabilities or visual impairment may be relatively common and helpful when typical environmental cues are not effective in entraining the circadian pacemaker.

Trazadone, a sedating antidepressant that differs from serotonin reuptake inhibitors and tricyclic antidepressants, is commonly used with adults who have psychophysiologic insomnia, particularly when sedative hypnotics are not a good option (patients with sleep-disordered breathing or a history of substance abuse). A few studies have evaluated the efficacy of Trazadone for treating child and adolescent depression, but no studies have evaluated its impact on children's sleep problems.

PSYCHOPHYSIOLOGIC INSOMNIA IN CHILDREN— TREATMENT CONSIDERATIONS

While less common in children ages 6 to 12 years of age, psychophysiologic insomnia can occur in this age group. As in adult populations (refer to Chapter 9), insomnia in children can be associated with affective disorders, trauma, significant stressors, illness, and medication side effects. Treatment approaches for adults and children are also comparable. Sleep hygiene training and general information about the sleep-wake cycle is important for both parents and children. Relaxation and stimulus control techniques are somewhat harder to implement in young children. Parents must play a key role guiding their child's relaxation exercises and monitoring compliance with stimulus control. The worry check discussed previously is also a key component so that by the time bedtime comes, the child has already put aside his or her worries.

Sleep-related behavior problems are common among children with developmental disabilities. As previously noted, safety is a primary concern, and monitoring a child during nighttime awakenings is necessary. This places a significant burden on parents who already have many extraordinary challenges. Most of the principles that apply to young children also apply to these populations. Implementation of extinction procedures must be more gradual and can be expected to take months, depending on the type of problem. Rigid adherence to schedules and routines is particularly important, and experimentation with various types of cues may be necessary. For example, children with autism may respond to a series of visual prompts better than to verbal prompts. Anxiety and fear can be more difficult to detect in these populations, but they are probably just as pervasive as in normally developing children. Given the tremendous challenges of modifying behavior in these populations and the burden on parents, sedative hypnotics are commonly used. It is important to determine the extent to which these medications have morning carryover effects. Additionally, long-term use of benzodiazepines can result in tolerance and abnormalities in sleep architecture (78). A change in medication or a brief cessation can result in significant rebound insomnia, which may cause significant setbacks in any gains that have been made with behavioral programs.

FUTURE DIRECTIONS

Pediatric sleep medicine is a very young field, and there are many research agendas. While numerous studies have demonstrated the efficacy of education, extinction, and bedtime routine modification, there are no guidelines for choosing the type of program and the variables that are appropriate for different age groups. For example, Mindell (3) points out that the graduated visits to the child's bedroom function as an intermittent reinforcement schedule for some children, particularly infants and toddlers whose internal sense of time is relatively undeveloped. Understanding the impact of insufficient sleep on daytime and bedtime behavior is a relatively new area of investigation and, based on some initial reports (24, 61), may provide valuable information. Clarifying the role and safety of medications (sedative hypnotics, antidepressants, beta blockers, and melatonin) as an adjunct to behavior interventions will help to resolve longstanding controversy and guide primary care pediatricians who see distressed parents desperate for a quick fix. Understanding the nature of sleep problems and developing interventions for special populations (e.g., children with medical and psychiatric problems) is a grossly understudied area. Several recent studies have examined the impact of parental psychopathology and postpartum depression on children's behavior and sleep. Finally, during the past two decades, there have been drastic changes in use of infant and child care as there has been a sharp increase in the number of homes in which both parents are employed full time. Evaluating sleep practices in child care settings and the impact of significant reductions in the amount of time that parents spend with children is challenging, but these are important areas of investigation.

CONCLUSION

Sleep-related behavior problems are very common in children, cause decrements in daytime behavioral control, and place a significant burden on parents. There are various well-tested interventions available for these problems. Self-help books abound, and each provides a unique twist on established interventions. Relatively few clinicians are trained to implement the interventions (80–81), and parents who have a child with a particularly tenacious problem may be confused by the great variety of options. Careful assessment is critical because sleep-related behavior problems may be caused by other sleep disorders, medical and psychiatric problems, and relational problems in a home. Diagnosing and treating sleep problems in healthy and medically ill populations may have a long-term impact on developmental trajectories because these problems appear to affect both children and families. Education of health providers and research initiates in these areas have increased 10-fold over the past two decades.

REFERENCES

1. Ferber, R. Sleeplessness in children. In R. Ferber and M. Kryger, eds. *Principles and Practice of Sleep Medicine in the Child.* Philadelphia, PA: W.B. Saunders Company. 1995: 79–89.
2. France, K., J. Henderson, and S. Hudson. Fact, act, and tact: A three-stage approach to treating the sleep problems of infants and young children. In M. Lewis and R. Dahl, eds. *Child and Adolescent Psychiatric Clinics of North America: Sleep Disorder.* Philadelphia, PA: W.B. Saunders Company. 1996: 581–600.
3. Mindell, J. A. Empirically supported treatments in pediatric psychology: Bedtime refusal and night wakings in young children. *Journal of Pediatric Psychology* 24(6): 465–481, 1999.
4. Mindell, J. A., J. A. Owens, and M. A. Carskadon. Developmental features of sleep. *Child and Adolescent Psychiatric Clinics of North America* 8(4): 695–725, 1999.
5. Stein, M. A., J. Mendelsohn, W. H. Obermeyer, J. Amromin, and R. Benca. Sleep and behavior problems in school-aged children. *Pediatrics* 107(4): E60, 2001.
6. Dahl, R. E., W. E. Pelham, and M. Wierson. The role of sleep disturbances in attention deficit disorder symptoms: A case study. *Journal of Pediatric Psychology* 16(2): 229–239, 1991.
7. Dahl, R. E., N. D. Ryan, M. K. Matty, B. Birmaher, M. al-Shabbout, D. E. Williamson, et al. Sleep onset abnormalities in depressed adolescents. *Biological Psychiatry* 39(6): 400–410, 1996.
8. Pichietti, D. L., D. J. Underwood, W. A. Farris, A. S. Walters, M. M. Shah, R. E. Dahl, et al. Further studies on periodic limb movement disorder and restless legs

syndrome in children with attention-deficit hyperactivity disorder. *Movement Disorders* 14(6): 1000–1007, 1999.

9. Lewin, D. and R. Dahl. Importance of sleep in the management of pediatric pain. *Developmental and Behavioral Pediatrics* 20(4): 244–252, 1999.

10. Rose, M., A. Sanford, C. Thomas, and M. R. Opp. Factors altering the sleep of burned children. *Sleep* 24(1): 45–51, 2001.

11. Johnson, C. Sleep problems in children with mental retardation and autism. In M. Lewis and R. Dahl, eds. *Child and Adolescent Psychiatric Clinics of North America: Sleep Disorder.* Philadelphia, PA: W.B. Saunders Company. 1996: 673–683.

12. Piazza, C. C., W. W. Fisher, and S. W. Kahng. Sleep patterns in children and young adults with mental retardation and severe behavior disorders. *Developmental Medicine and Child Neurology* 38(4): 335–344, 1996.

13. Gozal, D. *Learning Deficits Associated with OSAS in Children.* Paper presented at the Association of Professional Sleep Societies, Orlando, FL. 1999.

14. Lewin, D. S., R. C. Rosen, S. E. England, and R. E. Dahl. Preliminary evidence of behavioral and cognitive sequelae of obstructive sleep apnea in children. *Sleep Medicine* 3: 5–13, 2002.

15. Owens, J., A. Spirito, A. Marcotte, M. McQuinn, and L. Berkelhammer. Neuropsychological and behavioral correlates of obstructive sleep apnea syndrome in children: A preliminary study. *Sleep and Breathing* 4(2): 67-78, 2000.

16. Fallone, G., C. Acebo, J. T. Arnedt, R. Seifer, and M. A. Carskadon. Effects of acute sleep restriction on behavior, sustained attention, and response inhibition in children. *Perceptual and Motor Skills* 93(1): 213–229, 2001.

17. Marcotte, A. C., P. V. Thacher, M. Butters, J. Bortz, C. Acebo, and M. A. Carskadon. Parental report of sleep problems in children with attentional and learning disorders. *Journal of Developmental and Behavioral Pediatrics* 19(3): 178–186, 1998.

18. Minde, K., A. Faucon, and S. Falkner. Sleep problems in toddlers: Effects of treatment on their daytime behavior. *Journal of the American Academy of Child and Adolescent Psychiatry* 33(8): 1114–1121, 1994.

19. Bliwise, D. L. Sleep apnea and cognitive function: Where do we stand now? *Sleep* 16(8 Suppl.): S72–S73, 1993.

20. Bonnet, M. H. Cognitive effects of sleep and sleep fragmentation. *Sleep* 16(8 Suppl.): S65–S67, 1993.

21. Chervin, R. D. and K. H. Archbold. Hyperactivity and polysomnographic findings in children evaluated for sleep-disordered breathing. *Sleep* 24(3): 313–320, 2001.

22. Dahl, R. E. The regulation of sleep and arousal: Development and psychopathology. *Development and Psychopathology* 8: 3–27, 1996.

23. Dahl, R. E. The impact of inadequate sleep on children's daytime cognitive function. *Seminars in Pediatric Neurology* 3(1): 44–50, 1996.

24. Dahl, R. E. The consequences of insufficient sleep for adolescents: Links between sleep and emotional regulation. *Phi Delta Kappan* January: 354–359, 1999.

25. Dinges, D. F., F. Pack, K. Williams, K. A. Gillen, J. W. Powell, G. E. Ott, et al. Cumulative sleepiness, mood disturbance, and psychomotor vigilance performance decrements during a week of sleep restricted to 4–5 hours per night. *Sleep* 20(4): 267–267, 1997.

26. Drummond, S. A., G. G. Brown, J. C. Gillin, J. L. Stricker, E. C. Wong, and R. B. Buxton. Altered brain response to verbal learning following sleep deprivation. *Nature* 403(10): 655–657, 2000.

27. American Sleep Disorders Association. *The International Classification of Sleep Disorders Diagnostic and Coding Manual, Revised.* Rochester, MN: American Sleep Disorders Association. 1997.

28. Anders, T. F., L. F. Halpern, and J. Hua. Sleeping through the night: A developmental perspective. *Pediatrics* 90(4): 554–560, 1992.

29. Beltramini, A. U. and M. E. Hertzig. Sleep and bedtime behavior in preschool-aged children. *Pediatrics* 71(2): 153–158, 1983.

30. Dahl, R. E. and J. Puig-Antich. Sleep disturbances in child and adolescent psychiatric disorders. *Pediatrician* 17(1): 32–37, 1990.

31. Picchietti, D. L. and A. S. Walters. Attention deficit hyperactivity disorder and periodic limb movement disorder. *Sleep Research* 23: 303, 1994.

32. Seifer, R., A. Sameroff, S. Dicksein, L. Hayden, and M. Schiller. Parental psychopathology and Sleep Variation in Children. In M. Lewis and R. Dahl, eds. *Child and Adolescent Psychiatric Clinics of North America: Sleep Disorder.* Philadelphia, PA: W.B. Saunders Company. 1996: 715–727.

33. Ferber, R. *Solve Your Child's Sleep Problems.* New York, NY: Simon & Schuster. 1985.

34. Ferber, R. Clinical assessment of child and adolescent sleep disorders. In M. Lewis and R. Dahl, eds. *Child and Adolescent Psychiatric Clinics of North America: Sleep Disorder.* Philadelphia, PA: W.B. Saunders Company. 1996: 569–580.

35. Mindell, J. *Sleeping through the Night.* New York, NY: Harper Collins Publishers. 1997.

36. Hall, M., R. E. Dahl, M. A. Dew, and C. F. Reynolds. Sleep patterns following major negative life events. *Directions in Psychiatry* 15(9): 1–7, 1995.

36. Lichstein, K. L., N. M. Wilson, and C. T. Johnson. Psychological treatment of secondary insomnia. *Psychology and Aging* 15(2): 232–240, 2000.

38. Perlis, M. L., M. Sharpe, M. T. Smith, D. Greenblatt, and D. E. Giles. Behavioral treatment of insomnia: Treatment outcome and the relevance of medical and psychiatric morbidity. *Journal of Behavioral Medicine* 24(3): 281–296, 2001.

39. McKenna, J. J. and S. S. Mosko. Sleep and arousal, synchrony and independence, among mothers and infants sleeping apart and together (same bed): An experiment in evolutionary medicine. *Acta Paediatrica* 397(Suppl.): 94–102, 1994.

40. Anders, T. F., A. Sadeh, and V. Appareddy. *Normal Sleep in Neonates and Children.* Philadelphia, PA: W.B. Saunders Company. 1995.

41. Flavel, J. H., P. H. Miller, and S. A. Miller. *Cognitive Development* (3rd Edition). Englewood Cliffs, NJ: Prentice Hall. 1993.

42. Kagan, J. Behavior, biology, and the meanings of temperamental constructs. *Pediatrics* 90(3 Pt 2): 510–513, 1992.

43. Anders, T. F. Biological rhythms in development. *Psychosomatic Medicine* 44(1): 61–72, 1982.

44. Anders, T. F. and M. Keener. Developmental course of nighttime sleep-wake patterns in full-term and premature infants during the first year of life. I. *Sleep* 8(3): 173–192, 1985.

45. Borghese, I. F., K. L. Minard, and E. B. Thoman. Sleep rhythmicity in premature infants: Implications for development status. *Sleep* 18(7): 523–530, 1995.

46. Novosad, C., K. Freudigman, and E. B. Thoman. Sleep patterns in newborns and temperament at eight months: A preliminary study. *Journal of Developmental and Behavioral Pediatrics* 20(2): 99–105, 1999.

47. Whitney, M. P. and E. B. Thoman. Early sleep patterns of premature infants are differentially related to later developmental disabilities. *Journal of Developmental and Behavioral Pediatrics* 14(2): 71–80, 1993.

48. Blampied, N. M. and K. G. France. A behavioral model of infant sleep disturbance. *Journal of Applied Behavior Analysis* 26(4): 477–492, 1993.

49. Guedeney, A. and L. Kreisler. Sleep disorders in the first 18 months of life: Hypothesis on the role of mother-child emotional exchanges. *Infant Mental Health Journal* 8(3): 307–318, 1987.

50. Zuckerman, B., J. Stevenson, and V. Bailey. Sleep problems in early childhood: Continuities, predictive factors, and behavioral correlates. *Pediatrics* 80(5): 664–671, 1987.

51. Ferber, R. Sleeplessness in the child. In M. H. Kryger, T. Roth, and W. C. Dement, eds. *Principles and Practice of Sleep Medicine.* Philadelphia, PA: W.B. Saunders Company. 1989: 633–639.

52. Wolfson, A. R. Sleeping patterns of children and adolescents: Developmental trends, disruptions, and adaptations. In M. Lewis and R. Dahl, eds. *Child and Adolescent Psychiatric Clinics of North America: Sleep Disorder.* Philadelphia, PA: W.B. Saunders Company. 1996: 549–568.

53. Cahill, L. and J. L. McGaugh. Mechanisms of emotional arousal and lasting declarative memory. *Trends Neuroscience* 21: 294–299, 1998.

54. Carskadon, M. A. Patterns of sleep and sleepiness in adolescents. *Pediatrician* 17(1): 5–12, 1990.

55. Carskadon, M. A., S. Keenan, and W. C. Dement. Nighttime sleep and daytime sleep tendency in preadolescent. In C. Guilleminault, ed. *Sleep and Its Disorders in Children.* New York, NY: Raven Press. 1987: 43–52.

56. Coble, P. A., D. J. Kupfer, L. S. Taska, and J. Kane. *EEG Sleep of Normal Healthy Children. Part I: Findings Using Standard Measurement Methods* (Volume 7). New York, NY: Raven Press. 1984.

57. Smith, J. R., I. Karacan, and M. Yang. Ontogeny of delta activity during human sleep. *Electroencephalography and Clinical Neurophysiology* 43(2): 229–237, 1977.

58. Dawson, G., L. G. Klinger, H. Panagiotides, D. Hill, and S. Spieker. Frontal lobe activity and affective behavior of infants of mothers with depressive symptoms. *Child Development* 63(3): 725–737, 1992.

59. Rosenblum, L. A. and M. W. Andrews. Influences of environmental demand on maternal behavior and infant development. *Acta Paediatrica* 397(Suppl.): 57–63, 1994.

60. Mindell, J. A. Sleep disorders in children. *Health Psychology* 12(2): 151–162, 1993.

61. Owens, J., L. Opipari, C. Nobile, and A. Spirito. Sleep and daytime behavior in children with obstructive sleep apnea and behavioral sleep disorders. *Pediatrics* 102(5): 1178–1184, 1998.

62. Owens, J. A., A. Spirito, M. McGuinn, and C. Nobile. Sleep habits and sleep disturbance in elementary school-aged children. *Journal of Developmental and Behavioral Pediatrics* 21(1): 27–36, 2000.

63. Chervin, R. D., K. Hedger, J. E. Dillon, and K. J. Pituch. Pediatric sleep questionnaire (PSQ): Validity and reliability of scales for sleep-disordered breathing, snoring, sleepiness, and behavioral problems. *Sleep Medicine Reviews* 1(1): 21–32, 2000.

64. Owens, J. A., A. Spirito, and M. McGuinn. The Children's Sleep Habits Questionnaire (CSHQ): Psychometric properties of a survey instrument for school-aged children. *Sleep* 23(8): 1043–1051, 2000.

65. Sadeh, A., J. Alster, D. Urbach, and P. Lavie. Actigraphically based automatic bedtime sleep-wake scoring: Validity and clinical applications. *Journal of Ambulatory Monitoring* 2(3): 209–216, 1989.

66. Sheldon, S. H. *Evaluating Sleep in Infants and Children.* Philadelphia, PA: Lippincott—Raven. 1996.

67. Ramchandani, P., L. Wiggs, V. Webb, and G. Stores. A systematic review of treatments for settling problems and night waking in young children. *British Medical Journal* 320(7229): 209–213, 2000.

68. Kerr, S. M., S. A. Jowett, and L. N. Smith. Preventing sleep problems in infants: A randomized controlled trial. *Journal of Advances in Nursing* 24(5): 938–942, 1996.

69. Wolfson, A., P. Lacks, and A. Futterman. Effects of parent training on infant sleeping patterns, parents' stress, and perceived parental competence. *Journal of Consulting and Clinical Psychology* 60(1): 41–48, 1992.

70. Brown, J. D. and J. Cantor. An agenda for research on youth and the media. *Journal of Adolescent Health Care* 27(2 Suppl.): 2–7, 2000.

71. Durand, V. M. and J. A. Mindell. Behavioral treatment of multiple childhood sleep disorders. Effects on child and family. *Behavior Modification* 14(1): 37–49, 1990.

72. France, K. G. and S. M. Hudson. Behavior management of infant sleep disturbance. *Journal of Applied Behavior Analysis* 23(1): 91–98, 1990.

73. Piazza, C. C., W. W. Fisher, and M. Sherer. Treatment of multiple sleep problems in children with developmental disabilities: Faded bedtime with response cost versus bedtime scheduling. *Developmental Medicine and Child Neurology* 39(6): 414–418, 1997.

74. Wolfson, A. R. Sleeping patterns of children and adolescents: Developmental trends, disruptions, and adaptations. In R. Dahl, ed. *Child and Adolescent Psychiatric Clinics of North America: Sleep Disorder.* Philadelphia, PA: W.B. Saunders Company. 1996: 549–568.

75. Rickert, V. I. and C. M. Johnson. Reducing nocturnal awakening and crying episodes in infants and young children: A comparison between scheduled awakenings and systematic ignoring. *Pediatrics* 81(2): 203–212, 1988.

76. France, K. G., N. M. Blampied, and P. Wilkinson. Treatment of infant sleep disturbance by trimeprazine in combination with extinction. *Journal of Developmental and Behavioral Pediatrics* 12(5): 308–314, 1991.

77. Simonoff, E. A. and G. Stores. Controlled trial of trimeprazine tartrate for night waking. *Archives of Disease in Childhood* 62(3): 253–257, 1987.

78. Nichollson, A. N., C. M. Bradley, and P. A. Pascoe. Medications: Effect on sleep and wakefulness. In T. Roth, M. H. Kryger, and W. C. Dement, eds. *Principles and Practice of Sleep Medicine* (2nd Edition). Philadelphia, PA: W.B. Saunders Company. 1994: 364–372.

79. Smits, M. G., E. E. Nagtegaal, J. van der Heijden, A. M. Coenen, and G. A. Kerkhof. Melatonin for chronic sleep onset insomnia in children: A randomized placebo-controlled trial. *Journal of Child Neurology* 16(2): 86–92, 2001.

80. Mindell, J. A., M. L. Moline, S. M. Zendell, L. W. Brown, and J. M. Fry. Pediatricians and sleep disorders: Training and practice. *Pediatrics* 94(2 Pt 1): 194–200, 1994.

81. Rosen, R. C., M. Rosekind, C. Rosevear, W. E. Cole, and W. C. Dement. Physician education in sleep and sleep disorders: A national survey of U.S. medical schools. *Sleep* 16(3): 249–254, 1993.

Chapter 15

PARASOMNIAS

GERALD M. ROSEN, DANIEL P. KOHEN, AND MARK W. MAHOWALD

Parasomnias are defined as a group of clinical disorders that are not abnormalities of the processes responsible for sleep and wake states per se, but rather are an undesirable phenomenon that occur predominantly during sleep (ASDA, 1990). The parasomnias of greatest interest to clinicians caring for children include disorders of arousal, rhythmic movement disorders, sleep bruxism, and sleep enuresis. Disorders of arousal and sleep enuresis are discussed in this chapter.

DISORDERS OF AROUSAL IN CHILDREN

Disorders of arousal comprise a common group of sleep disorders seen in children (1) that was first described as a distinct clinical entity by Broughton in 1968 (2). The clinical presentation varies from a child who quietly sits up in bed, mumbles briefly, and then lies back down and returns to sleep, to an arousal that begins with a sudden bloodcurdling scream, followed by headlong flight (3). The entire clinical spectrum of disorders of arousal shares a common pathophysiology, which accounts for the similarities in family history, timing, and many clinical features in all disorders of arousal.

CLINICAL DESCRIPTION

Clinical features common to most children experiencing any type of disorder of arousal from sleep include timing in the nighttime sleep cycle, misperception of and unresponsiveness to the environment, automatic behavior, a high arousal threshold, varying levels of autonomic arousal, and variable retrograde amnesia. Disorders of arousal typically begin abruptly at the transition from the first period of slow wave sleep (see Figure 15.1) of the night (nonrapid eye movement [NREM]

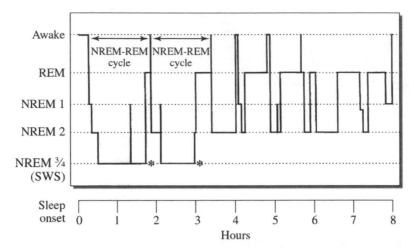

Figure 15.1   Idealized Sleep Hypnogram Showing Ultradian Rhythm through the Night. NREM-REM cycles are approximately 90 min; the majority of slow-wave sleep (SWS) occurs early in the sleep period; the majority of REM sleep occurs late in the sleep period. Disorders of arousal generally occur at the transition out of SWS (noted by asterisks).

stage 4), which accounts for the typical timing 60 to 90 minutes after sleep onset at the end of the first ultradian sleep cycle. The duration of each event can vary from a few seconds to more than 90 minutes. In most cases, the arousal will terminate with the child's returning to sleep without ever fully awakening. Although only a single event usually occurs on a given night, some children may have more. When there are multiple events, they typically will recur at 60- to 90-minute intervals during the first half of the night corresponding to subsequent transitions out of slow wave sleep at the end of each subsequent ultradian sleep cycle (see Figure 15.1). Successive events on the same night tend to be progressively milder.

The clinical manifestations of disorders of arousal occur along a spectrum, but for ease of description and to establish a common nomenclature, the diagnostic classification steering committee of the American Sleep Disorder Association (now the American Academy of Sleep Medicine) divided the spectrum into three distinct entities: sleepwalking, confusional arousals, and sleep terrors (Table 15.1). This nomenclature is used throughout this chapter unless otherwise stated.

Sleepwalking

The stereotypical behavior of sleepwalking is fairly similar at all ages. The child simply gets up and walks about. The young child may walk or crawl about in the crib. If he or she is quiet, these events often go unnoticed. An older child usually

Table 15.1   Clinical Characteristics of Disorders of Arousal

Clinical Characteristics	Quiet Sleepwalking	Confusional Arousals	Sleep Terrors
Timing in the night	First third	First third	First third
Duration	1 to 40 minutes	1 to 40 minutes	1 to 5 minutes
Agitation	None	Moderate	Severe
Age of peak incidence	School age	Early childhood	Adolescence
Amnesia	Yes	Yes	Yes
Arousal threshold	High	High	High
Family history	Positive	Positive	Positive

gets up and walks toward the light or the parents' room. He or she may be found simply standing in the living room or quietly next to the parents' bed. Some inappropriate behavior, such as urinating in the corner or next to the toilet, is common. Such a child may easily be led back to bed, perhaps with a stop at the bathroom, with little evidence of complete waking. Occasionally, the child may go to another room and return to sleep. Sleepwalking is not dangerous per se, but the child may put himself or herself in harm's way during a sleepwalking episode by climbing out a window or leaving the house.

Sleepwalking is very common. In Klackenberg's (4) longitudinal study of a group of 212 randomly selected children from Stockholm ages 6 to 16 years, the incidence of quiet sleepwalking was 40%. The yearly prevalence varied from 6% to 17%, although only 2% to 3% had more than one episode per month. The sleepwalking persisted for 5 years in 33% of the children and for more than 10 years in 12%. In Laberge's (1) longitudinal study of parasomnias in 1,353 children in Quebec, sleepwalking was present in 13.8% of all the children between ages 3 and 13 years, 9.2% of the children between ages 3 and 10 years, 7% of the children age 11 years, 6.8% of the children age 12 years, and 3.3% of the children 13 years of age. In the majority of these children, the sleepwalking began and ended between ages 3 and 10 years. Sleepwalking persisted beyond age 13 years in 24% of the sleepwalkers.

Confusional Arousals

Confusional arousals may seem bizarre and frightening to parents. The arousal usually starts with some movements and moaning, progressing to crying and perhaps calling out, often in association with intense thrashing about in the bed or crib or simply crying inconsolably. These arousals are very common in infants and toddlers. Eyes may be open or closed, a look of "terror" is not described; rather, the child is felt to look very confused, agitated, upset, or "possessed."

These events can last anywhere from minutes up to more than an hour, with 5 to 15 minutes being typical. Even if the child calls for the parents, he or she often does not recognize them and may appear to "look right through" them. Holding and cuddling usually does not provide reassurance; instead, the child often resists, twists, pushes away, and may become more agitated. Even vigorous attempts to wake the child are often unsuccessful. In Laberge's (1) longitudinal study of children in Quebec, the prevalence of confusional arousals overall was 17.3%, 15% between ages 3 and 10 years, 4% at age 11 years, 3% at age 12 years, and 1% at age 13. In this study, confusional arousals first appeared between the ages of 3 and 10 years in 85% and disappeared before age 10 years in 67%. The confusional arousals persisted beyond age 12 in 7% of the children. Sleepwalking and confusional arousals were often seen in the same child at different ages in both Laberge's and Klackenberg's studies. Laberge used the term *night terrors* in his paper to describe the events that are termed *confusional arousals* in this chapter. Confusional arousals are used here to conform to the definitions described in the *ICSD Classification of Sleep Disorders* (3).

Sleep Terrors

Sleep terrors are the most dramatic and least common of the disorders of arousal. Sleep terrors are seen more often in older children and young adults. The events usually begin precipitously with the child bolting upright with a "blood-curdling" scream. The eyes are usually wide open, the heart is racing, and there often is diaphoresis and mydriasis. The facial expression is one of intense fear. In a full-blown episode, a youngster may jump out of bed and run blindly, as if away from some unseen threat. This may be very dangerous because injury during this frenzied activity is possible. Anyone attempting to intervene may also be injured. These events are usually shorter than confusional arousals, generally terminating within a few minutes. The child may wake before the autonomic storm has died down, or the child may simply return to a quiet sleep without ever having completely awakened. The child may report some memory, but it is most often fragmented and not characteristic of imagery reported from dreams or nightmares. Anxiety, as measured by the Social Behavior Questionnaire (5), was associated with sleep terrors in Laberge's study (1) and has been noted by other authors in case reports of children and adolescents with confusional arousals and sleep terrors (4, 6–7).

PHYSIOLOGY OF SLEEP

A brief review of the basic neurophysiology of sleep is helpful in understanding disorders of arousal. First and foremost, sleep must be understood as an active, complex, highly regulated neurologic process, which involves different neuronal groups at many levels of the neuraxis (8–12). Although the exact purpose of sleep is not fully understood, it is clear that sleep is essential and that without normal sleep, there will not be normal wakefulness. Sleep is composed of two fundamentally different states: REM (rapid eye movement) sleep and NREM (nonrapid eye movement) sleep, which have some obvious, albeit superficial, similarities such as posture, unresponsiveness to the environment, reversibility, and lack of consciousness but have many more fundamental differences. During REM sleep, there are very different patterns of brain blood flow, glucose utilization, predominant neurotransmitter systems, and thalamic functioning than in NREM sleep. From the perspective of brain function, REM and NREM sleep are as different from each other as each is from wakefulness. Understood from this perspective, there are really three different states of being that humans can exist in: REM sleep, NREM sleep, and wake (10–12). State determination may be made using various criteria. Most commonly, electrographic criteria are used (electroencephalogram [EEG], electrooculogram [EOG], and chin electromyogram [EMG]) as described in the Rechtschaffen and Kales sleep stage scoring manual (13). Behavioral criteria may also be used to differentiate wake, NREM sleep, and REM sleep (14).

Each sleep state has its own unique neuroanatomic, neurophysiologic, neurochemical, and neuropharmacologic correlates. Each state consists of a number of physiologic markers, which tend to occur in concert and cycle in a predictable and uniform manner, resulting in the behavioral appearance of a single, prevailing state. There is extensive reorganization of the central nervous system as it moves across states of being (11–12, 14). Factors involved in state generation are complex and include a wide variety of neurotransmitters, neuromodulators, neurohormones, and a vast array of "sleep factors," which act on multiple neural networks. These facts lead to the conclusion that sleep is a fundamental property of numerous neuronal groups, rather than a phenomenon that requires the whole brain. Consequently, it is possible for different parts of the brain to be in different "states" at the same time. The recognition of this possibility is fundamental to the understanding of a number of sleep disorders, including disorders of arousal. If different parts of the brain can be in different states simultaneously, the physical, clinical, and polysomnographic manifestations of these states (wake, REM sleep, NREM sleep) can also occur simultaneously. When this occurs, the event can be described as a mixed or dissociated state (14).

Sleep is not a static phenomenon. There are continuous currents driving and defining the propensity toward NREM sleep, REM sleep, and wake. The most apparent biologic rhythms are the circadian and ultradian rhythms. The cyclic alternation of wake, REM sleep, and NREM sleep over the 24-hour light/dark cycle defines the circadian rhythms, while the weaving of wake, NREM sleep, and REM sleep over the sleep period defines the ultradian rhythm. Circadian cycling is controlled by a hypothalamic pacemaker located in the suprachiasmatic nucleus (SCN; 15). Virtually every aspect of mammalian life is affected by the circadian rhythm. Sleep-wake cycling is the most obvious manifestations of the circadian rhythm, but equally important are diurnal variations in body temperature, hormone secretion, drug metabolism, pulmonary function, immune response/reactivity, blood pressure, intestinal motility, gastric acid secretion, and the propensity to enter REM sleep. The ultradian rhythm as shown in the idealized hypnogram in Figure 15.1 is defined by the cycling of NREM sleep, REM sleep, and wake over the sleep period. No specific anatomic pacemaker has been identified that controls the ultradian cycling analogous to the SCN although the brainstem appears to have an important role (14). As the brain cycles among NREM sleep, REM sleep, and wake, a dynamic reorganization occurs among multiple neuronal networks and neurotransmitters at many levels of the neuraxis. A complex switching orchestrated in the midbrain and thalamus takes place (9). The transition among states usually occurs smoothly and completely and is behaviorally inapparent, but this is not always true. The transition may be gradual and incomplete, resulting in the behavioral appearance of a mixed state. This is the neurophysiologic correlate of the clinical situation that is referred to as *state dissociation.* Narcolepsy, REM sleep behavior disorder (RBD; 14), and disorders of arousal can all best be understood as clinical examples of mixed (or dissociated) states of being.

DISORDERS OF AROUSAL, A DISSOCIATED STATE

During disorders of arousal, some facets of wake appear during the transition out of slow wave sleep. As a consequence, the transition out of slow wave sleep, which normally is smooth and behaviorally inapparent, is dramatic and may be violent. The child appears caught between NREM sleep and wake. The child's behavior at this time has elements that we associate with waking (walking, talking, complex motor behaviors) and sleeping (misperception of and unresponsiveness to the environment, high arousal threshold, amnesia, automatic behavior) occurring simultaneously. The EEG during a partial arousal from sleep is typically characterized by a combination of waking and sleeping rhythms with the simultaneous occurrence of alpha, theta, and delta frequencies and likely reflects that different areas of the brain are in different states simultaneously (see Figure 15.2). This mixed state is inherently unstable and cannot persist for long, and eventually one state is fully declared. Many factors may affect the appearance of disorders of arousal. Probably the most important factor is a genetic predisposition. A positive family history in a first-degree relative is present in 60%

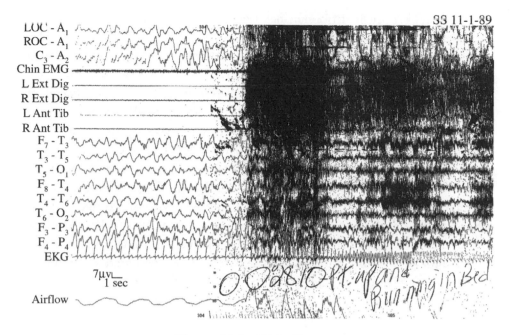

Figure 15.2   Night Terror

of children with disorders of arousal compared to 30% in the general population. Sleep state cycling and synchronization is another important factor, probably because disorders of arousal occur at the sleep state transitions. Sleep state cycling/synchronization is affected by age, homeostatic factors, circadian factors, hormones, drugs, affective disorders, anxiety, and environmental stress. These factors also may play a role in the clinical appearance of disorders of arousal, particularly in a child genetically predisposed to disorders of arousal. These associations are most likely mediated through the effect these factors have on the duration, timing, and stability of slow wave sleep. The stability of slow wave sleep has been assessed in three ways:

1. Analysis of sleep macro architecture—sleep stage percentage distribution, number of arousals per stage, sleep efficiency
2. Analysis of sleep micro architecture—delta power
3. Analysis of cyclic alternating pattern (CAP)

Three studies have evaluated sleep micro architecture and slow wave sleep stability in individuals with disorders of arousal compared with controls (16–18). The results of these studies are similar, and they are consistent with earlier studies that have looked at sleep macro architecture in disorders of arousal. These studies found very little difference between individuals with disorders of arousal and normal controls but did demonstrate an increase in the number of brief arousals from slow wave sleep during the first sleep cycle and a slight decrease in sleep efficiency in the individuals with disorders of arousal. Studies of sleep micro architecture have demonstrated more significant differences between individuals with disorders of arousals and controls. Young adults with disorders of arousal all demonstrated a lower slow wave activity (SWA) power, that is, lower delta counts during the first NREM sleep cycle, compared to controls. Individuals with disorders of arousal had normal SWA during the beginning of the first sleep cycle but not the end. This would suggest that the frequent arousals that individuals experience during slow wave sleep interfere with the normal buildup of SWA over the first sleep cycle. Two studies have looked at CAP (19–20) analysis in individuals with disorders of arousals compared with controls. Individuals with disorders of arousal have an increase in CAP rate, compared to controls. All of these lines of evidence suggest that the fundamental abnormality that underpins the disorders of arousal is instability of slow wave sleep.

Evaluation of Children with Disorders of Arousal

Children do not present to a clinician with a diagnosis but rather with a clinical problem. It is the responsibility of the clinician to arrive at the diagnosis. The children described in this chapter generally present with the complaint of unusual nocturnal awakenings. There are many causes for unusual nocturnal awakenings; the most common are listed in Table 15.2. The most powerful tool for evaluating

Table 15.2 Differential Diagnosis for Unusual Nocturnal Arousal

Nocturnal seizures
Disorders of arousal
Conditioned arousals
Nightmares
Obstructive sleep apnea
Gastroesophageal reflux
Posttraumatic stress disorder
Nocturnal dissociative state
Rhythmic sleep movement disorder
REM behavior disorder (RBD)
Nocturnal panic
Periodic movements of sleep

children with unusual nocturnal awakenings is the sleep history, which is described in Table 15.3. In most cases, this is sufficient to evaluate the problem. The history alone usually allows the clinician to distinguish among the different causes of unusual nocturnal awakenings and to formulate a treatment plan. Table 15.4 describes the key features in the clinical history of three causes of nocturnal awakenings: disorders of arousal, seizures during sleep, and nightmares.

In the evaluation and treatment of children who present with unusual nocturnal awakenings, the clinical interview serves two very important functions in addition to gathering the information necessary to establish the correct diagnosis. The interview is the mechanism whereby the clinician establishes rapport with the child and his or her parents and is also the medium through which education and implementation of the treatment plan takes place. These three functions of the medical interview are described by Lazare (21) in his conceptual model for the medical interview and are especially apropos in the evaluation and treatment of children with disorders of arousal.

Polysomnography

The role of polysomnography in the evaluation of disorders of arousal is limited. As described previously, sleep macro architecture in children with disorders of arousal is not very different from the sleep of age-matched controls. Some

Table 15.3   Sleep History

Circadian

  Sleep log × 2 weeks (time in bed, sleep onset, wake time) for weekday/weekend
  24-hour daily schedule (school, work, meals, play)
  Amount of light in room
  Seasonal variations

Sleep Environment

  Describe bedroom (What is in it? Who is there? How much natural light is there? Television? Radio?)

Sleep Onset

  How does child fall asleep?
  Who is present at sleep onset and what do they do?
  Are there curtain calls, fears, hypnagogic hallucinations, sleep-onset paralysis, restless legs?
  Head banging? Bodyrocking?

(continued)

Table 15.3 *Continued*

Arousals

Time of night?	Frequency?
Triggers?	Associated with injury?
Description of arousal?	How it terminates?
Level of agitation/ambulation?	How does child return to sleep?
Associated with eating/drinking?	Recall the next day?
Level of consciousness?	Age of onset?
Duration?	

Other Sleep Behavior

Seizures, enuresis, diaphoresis, restlessness, snoring, cough, choking, apnea, periodic movements of sleep, vomiting, nightmares, bruxism

Waking Behavior

Hypnopompic hallucinations, paralysis, headaches

Daytime Sleep

Naps, cataplexy, excessive daytime sleepiness

Drugs

Caffeine, OTC, legal/illegal

Medical Review of Systems

Neurologic: Headaches, attention-deficit disorder, seizures, tics, mental retardation, cataplexy, neuromuscular disease

Psychiatric: Depression, anxiety, dissociative disorders, conduct disorder, panic disorder, physical/sexual abuse, posttraumatic stress disorder, hallucinations

Ear, nose, throat: Ear infections, ear effusions, nasal airway obstruction, sinusitis, streptococci infections, swallowing problems

Cardio respiratory: Asthma, cough, heart disease, pneumonia

Gastrointestinal: Vomiting, diarrhea, constipation, pain

Growth: Failure to thrive

Allergies: Milk, seasonal, asthma, eczema

Acute medical illness

Family History

Sleep apnea/snoring

Arousals (sleepwalking, confusional arousals, night terrors, restless legs/periodic movements)

Psychiatric disease (depression)

Social issues (stress at home, divorce, family violence, drug/ETOH use)

Narcolepsy, hypersomnolence

Restless leg syndrome

Table 15.4   Characteristics of Disorders of Arousal and Seizures during Sleep Nightmares

	Disorder of Arousal	Seizures during Sleep	Nightmare
Time of night	60 to 90 minutes after sleep onset	Anytime, often at sleep onset or offset	Middle to last third of sleep period
Behavior	Variable	Stereotypical	Frightened but awake
Level of consciousness	Unarousable or confused	Unarousable	Awake
Memory of event	None	None	Vivid
Family history	Positive	Variable	Negative
Prevalence	Common	Uncommon	Very common
Sleep stage	Slow wave sleep	NREM → REM	REM
Daytime sleepiness	No	Yes	No

differences in sleep have been reported in the sleep of children with disorders of arousal, such as hypersynchronous delta (18), preceding the arousal. However, these are nonspecific findings, which are also seen in children undergoing polysomnography for other reasons and are not specific enough to be useful in the clinical evaluation of children with disorders of arousal. The primary role of polysomnography in the evaluation of children with disorders of arousal is to rule out other sleep disorders, such as obstructive sleep apnea, gastro-esophageal reflux, nocturnal psychogenic dissociative states, or seizures during sleep, which may both trigger and mimic the disorder of arousal.

If seizures during sleep are suspected as the cause of the awakenings because of the history of the stereotypical nature of the arousals, the timing of the arousals throughout the sleep period, or an increased likelihood of seizures because of concomitant neurologic problems, further diagnostic studies should be obtained. In most clinical settings, sleep-related seizures can best be evaluated with a sleep-deprived EEG or an overnight study in an EEG telemetry unit. These children should be evaluated in a sleep laboratory only if the sleep lab is experienced in the diagnosis and treatment of sleep-related seizures.

Treatment of Children with Disorders of Arousal

The most appropriate treatment for the child with an unusual nocturnal arousal depends on the diagnoses. Before considering a treatment strategy, a comprehensive sleep evaluation as described in this chapter must have been completed. If disorders of arousal are thought to be the most likely cause of the awakenings, the treatment should focus on education of the child and the parents, reassurance, and safety.

Education of parents and their children about the benign, self-limited nature of disorders of arousal is always the starting point of treatment. It is often helpful to discuss the pathophysiology of disorders of arousal in a manner understandable to both the child and parents. One analogy that has proven useful for doing this is to compare the brain during sleep to the transmission of an automobile. In this analogy, the transition out of slow wave sleep at the end of the first NREM-REM cycle is likened to the shifting of gears in an automobile with a manual transmission. A child with a disorder of arousal transitions from slow wave sleep to the next sleep stage like an automobile with a slipping clutch. In such a setting, the automobile travels smoothly while in gear and has a bumpy ride only when the gears are shifted. This is similar to a child with a disorder of arousal who generally sleeps well for most of the night but has difficulty in transitioning from slow wave sleep to the next sleep stage. However, once the shift has occurred, he or she is able to sleep quietly again.

Demystifying the symptoms should always be part of the education of the parent and child about disorders of arousal. Often parents misunderstand the problem and fear that disorders of arousal are symptoms of psychological distress. Though it is true that psychological stressors may be factors in the appearance of disorders of arousal, they are rarely the only cause. Parents sometimes worry that their child has sustained some terrible trauma, such as sexual abuse that is underpinning the sleep symptoms, and are often greatly relieved to hear that in most cases disorders of arousal have no psychological causes.

The child's *safety* is a paramount concern in managing children with disorders of arousal. The disorders of arousal are not dangerous per se, but during an event a child can put himself or herself into harm's way by walking out of the house during winter or by running through a plate glass door. In most cases, these concerns can be addressed using a simple, commonsense approach. The child should not sleep on the top bunk, obstructions should be removed from the room, double cylinder locks may need to be installed on the doors of the house, or a security system that alerts the parents that a door or window has been opened may need to be installed.

Sleep extension and regularizing the child's sleep schedule is often a good place to begin the treatment for disorders of arousal after educating, demystificating, and ensuring for the child's safety if there is any suggestion that either sleep deprivation or an irregular sleep-wake schedule is a factor. Both are very common problems in American children and may be causally related to the arousals; correcting them may lead to resolution of the arousals.

Scheduled awakenings were first suggested by Lask (22) as a treatment for disorders of arousal, and though it is not clear why this intervention is helpful, several case reports have described its efficacy (23–24). The recommended treatment is simple enough; the child is awakened 15 minutes before the time of the usual arousal. The child needs to open his or her eyes and at least mumble a response before being allowed to return to sleep. Parents continue this intervention nightly for one month. In some cases, this simple intervention has been effective. However, it should be noted that in some cases, these scheduled awakenings actually trigger an arousal.

Relaxation/mental imagery and biofeedback have both been described in several case series reports as being useful treatments for disorders of arousal (25). Though it is not clear why this intervention is effective, it has been suggested that changing the child's frame of mind at sleep onset may be important in decreasing the frequency of or response to the arousals. Unfortunately, none of these behavioral interventions has been subjected to the rigors of a careful efficacy trial comparing them with each other or with placebo.

Medication has also been described as an effective treatment of disorders of arousal in several case series reports. Clonazepam (26) has been the most widely used medication for treatment of disorders of arousal. However, there is a general hesitancy by many clinicians to begin pharmacotherapy for disorders of arousal in children because, in most cases, the events are benign and self-limited and have no direct adverse impact on the child. However, in a child with frequent, disruptive, or potentially dangerous arousals, medication may be a good short-term strategy while other nonpharmacologic modalities are initiated.

Psychotherapy or counseling is an important intervention for the child who has evidence of significant psychological distress. This is true of any child in whom these problems are discovered if these factors are considered to be having an adverse impact on the child's or family's life. However, children are rarely able to compartmentalize their emotional lives as well as adults do, so it is uncommon for the only manifestation of significant psychological difficulties to be the nocturnal awakenings.

Summary

To the casual observer, disorders of arousal appear to represent a paradox during which an individual appears to engage in waking behavior while still asleep. With the understanding that sleep and wake are not always mutually exclusive states of being, the paradox disappears. The concept of mixed state or state dissociation provides an explanation for these events that is simple, reasonable, and founded in the current understanding of the neurophysiology of sleep. Disorders of arousal are common problems, especially in young children, and can usually be fully evaluated and treated by a knowledgeable sleep clinician without the use of high technology.

SLEEP ENURESIS

Developmental Basis of Enuresis

Control of urination during wake and sleep is a developmentally acquired skill that follows a predictable sequence in children (27). During infancy, urination is purely reflexive, occurring when the bladder is full. Between 12 and 18 months of age, children first become aware of the sensation of a wet diaper. At this age, they are able to communicate by words or actions that they have voided. Between 18 months and 2 years of age, the peripherally generated signal of a full bladder is recognized centrally and children become aware of the sensation of a full bladder before they have voided. At this age, children are able to communicate that they are about to urinate. However, often this realization occurs only moments before the voiding begins. Beginning at 18 months to 3 years of age, children are not only aware of the sensation of a full bladder but also are able to centrally inhibit urination during wakefulness leading to daytime dryness. These are the developmental skills necessary for a child to be toilet trained during the day. It is after children have acquired these prerequisite neuromotor skills that they can be trained to remain dry during the night. Between 2 years and 6 years of age, children become able to centrally inhibit urination during sleep as well as during wakefulness and/or to arouse from sleep from the sensation of a full bladder. Either of these skills can facilitate the child's being consistently dry at night. Antidiuretic hormone (ADH) secretion during sleep leads to an increase in the concentration of urine and hence a decrease in the volume of urine production during sleep, which, in conjunction with an increasing bladder capacity as the child gets older, allows most children to be consistently dry at night by 6 years of age. The failure to gain these skills by age 6 is termed *nocturnal enuresis* and affects about 15% of boys and 10% of girls. As with all developmental skills, there is a wide range in time as to when normal children acquire these skills. Enuresis in childhood has a spontaneous cure rate of 10% by year (28). By 15 years of age, the prevalence of enuresis is about 1%.

Genetics

Nocturnal enuresis has an inherited component. Studies of twins show a concordance for monozygotic twins of 43% to 68% and for dizygotic twins 19% to 36%. If one parent had enuresis, the prevalence in his or her children is 41%, and if both parents were enuretic, prevalence increases to 70%. In families where neither parent has enuresis, the prevalence in the children is 15% (29). Though the mechanisms of the genetic component of enuresis have not been fully evaluated, it is presumed to be the result of a failure in arousal from sleep to the sensation of a full bladder or from the delayed acquisition of the central inhibition of urination during sleep.

Primary and Secondary Enuresis

In the pediatric literature, enuresis is classified as primary in children who have never been dry for six months and secondary in children who had been previously dry for greater than six months and then began wetting again (28). In the more recent urologic literature, enuresis is classified as monosymptomatic or polysymptomatic (30). *Monosymptomatic enuresis* is defined as the isolated symptom of nocturnal enuresis, and *polysymptomatic enuresis* is defined as the presence of daytime urologic symptoms such as frequency, urgency, and dysuria in addition to the nocturnal symptom of enuresis. Both classification schema attempt to distinguish children who fail to achieve nocturnal dryness because of a delay in the acquisition of a developmental skill from those who have some underlying pathology that leads to the enuresis, which presumably needs to be corrected before the enuresis will be resolved. Enuresis may be the final common pathway of a number of medical problems affecting the genitourinary, cardiorespiratory, gastrointestinal, endocrine, and neurologic systems. The evaluation of the mechanism by which problems in these organ systems leads to nocturnal enuresis can usually be done with a clinical history and a routine urinalysis and urine culture. The evaluation of these problems should be performed within the context of a primary care medical assessment and rarely requires a formal urologic evaluation. In a child who presents to a sleep specialist for enuresis, the history of obstructive sleep apnea should be sought and appropriate testing performed if the history is suggestive. The mechanism by which obstructive sleep apnea leads to enuresis is not known, but the enuresis often does resolve once the obstructive sleep apnea is corrected.

A small number of children with nocturnal enuresis do not have the normal rise in ADH secretion during sleep (31). ADH is a hypothalamically synthesized neuropeptide whose secretion from the posterior pituitary gland is augmented during sleep. In children without this rise in ADH, the volume of urine production during sleep exceeds the capacity of the bladder. If these children fail to arouse from the sensation of a full bladder, they wet the bed. These children have been shown to improve when provided with desmopressin, an ADH analog, at bedtime. However, the majority of children with nocturnal enuresis have a normal ADH secretion and do not warrant long-term hormonal therapy.

Early polysomnographic studies with nocturnal enuresis suggested that the wetting episodes were state dependent and occurred predominately during the transition of slow wave sleep. However, subsequent studies have demonstrated that enuresis occurs during all stages of non-REM and REM sleep and occasionally during brief periods of wakefulness during sleep (32).

Caffeine intake in the later afternoon and evening and/or excessive fluid intake in the evening can both lead to a high urine volume during sleep that may result in either nocturnal enuresis or an awakening from sleep to void. Enuresis has been associated with psychological distress in children, but it is clear that the nature of the association is not a simple causal one. Children do not compartmentalize their emotional lives very well, so a child with significant psychological distress is not likely to present solely with the symptoms of nocturnal enuresis. If, however, in the evaluation of a child with enuresis, significant problems in psychosocial interactions are uncovered that are interfering with the child's life, these problems should be addressed but should not be interpreted as the result, or the cause, of the nocturnal enuresis. Parents should be questioned as to whether coercive or punitive toilet-training practices have been used in the past, and if so, they need to be strongly counseled to discontinue such practices.

Treatment

Pharmacologic and nonpharmacologic treatments are available for enuresis. The vast majority of children will benefit from and experience success using a nonpharmacologic approach (32–35). The role of the behavioral clinician in the treatment of nocturnal enuresis includes the following steps:

1. *Ensuring that a thorough evaluation for organic causes* of enuresis has been completed. In most cases, this requires a focused history, urinalysis, and urine culture performed by the primary care provider. Formal urologic consultation is rarely required.

2. *Assessment of the family to ascertain that coercive or punitive toilet training practices* are not being used. Parents generally recognize these practices are inappropriate and may not be forthcoming about their use unless questioned specifically about them. The use of diapers or pull-ups after age 6 may be viewed by children as punitive, and in families where diapers are being used, this needs to be explicitly discussed.

3. *Avoidance of caffeine and/or excessive fluid intake in the evening* is a simple commonsense place to begin the treatment of enuresis. However, care must be taken that parents do not use this recommendation in a punitive way.

4. *Education and demystification* of the symptoms in terms that are understandable to both the parents and their children.

5. *Lifting, the awakening of the child several hours after sleep onset,* may be an effective short-term intervention for enuresis but rarely leads to long-term control of the problem. Consequently, this approach is not routinely recommended.

The following dialog with the accompanying diagram (Figure 15.3) addressing both child and parent has been a useful tool for the education and demystification of enuresis and provides positive expectations for change. This dialog describes the brain-bladder connection in terms that are physiologically accurate but can be understood by most 5-year-old children. This technique is based on the two most successful behavioral approaches to enuresis: (1) the wet alarm and (2) relaxation and mental imagery.

Do you know why the bed gets wet at night? (No)

I didn't think so. Most kids and parents who come to see me for this kind of problem don't know, so let me explain. This is a picture of your body [Figure 15.3], and I'd like to explain how a part of it works.

Here are the kidneys. Their job is to be the washing machine for the blood. They clean the blood, and what is left over after the blood is cleaned is the water your body doesn't need, or urine (pee). Your kidneys are working all the time, day and night, cleaning your blood and making the pee.

Once the pee is made, it comes down these pipes or tubes to the bladder.

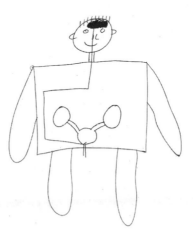

Figure 15.3   Schematic Drawing of the Body Illustrating the Physiology of Voiding.

The bladder is a big muscle that is like a storage tank that holds the pee.

At the bottom of the bladder is another pipe or tube that lets the pee out (to the vagina/to the penis).

Now here is a really important part. It is called the gate or door. The gate has a very important job. When the gate is closed, the pee stays in the bladder; when the gate opens, the pee can come out.

When you were little, your gate would open whenever your bladder was full. But now that you are growing up, you are learning to control your gate most of the time.

This is how you do it. Your gate is connected to your brain by a nerve that is like a telephone wire.

Your brain is your body's super computer; it controls everything your body does. It controls your arms and legs, your walking and talking and everything, even how you are listening so well and smiling right now. It also controls your gate.

During the day, your brain and your gate are already friends and they talk to each other, and that is why you stay dry all day.

Your brain keeps your gate closed, and that keeps the pee in. As your bladder fills up with pee and gets full, the gate sends a message up to your brain.

If we could listen in on their conversation, it might sound something like this:

> "Brain, this is the gate calling. I'm full, so you need to find me a bathroom so I can let this pee out."

Then your brain might say:

> "Gate, I hear you. You stay closed, and I will find a bathroom."

Then your brain gets your body to the bathroom and when you are in the bathroom, the brain sends a message back down to your gate:

> "Gate, this is the brain. We are at the bathroom now. You can let that pee out in the toilet where it belongs."

Then you open the gate, and the pee goes out into the toilet where it belongs.

Your brain and your gate are able to talk like this with each other automatically, and you don't even know it is happening until you need to go pee.

But at night, sometimes the brain and bladder get into an accidental bad habit of not talking and listening to each other. Now your brain doesn't sleep at night. It keeps you breathing, it keeps your heart beating, and it keeps you from falling out of bed.

Now during the night, your gate starts off closed, and your bladder slowly fills up with pee. When the bladder gets really full, the gate sends a message up to your brain to let the brain know. If your brain isn't listening, the gate sends another message up. If your brain still doesn't listen, the gate sometimes just opens up and lets the pee out. That is when the bed gets wet.

So, what we need to do is to help your brain remember to listen to your gate all night, just like it listens to your gate during the day. Because when your brain is listening to your gate all night long, you will *stay dry all night long.*

Sometimes some kids just get dry from learning this and telling their brain and bladder gate what to do, and other times some kids use a reminder alarm.

One way we can help your brain remember to listen to your gate is to use the reminder alarm. This is how it works (take out wet alarm and show it to the child). When a tiny drop of pee gets on this (touch a wet finger to the sensing device), it buzzes. That buzz is an extra reminder to your brain to, quick, close your gate.

Now this is what you should do every night before you go to bed. Look at your picture (Figure 15.3) and remind your gate to talk to your brain all night long, just like it does during the day. If while you are sleeping a tiny little drop of pee leaks out of your bladder, the reminder alarm will go off. That will be a reminder to your brain that your bladder is full and your gate is starting to open.

When you hear the buzzer, it is a signal to your brain to, quick, close your gate and to get up and go to the bathroom and let the pee out into the toilet where it belongs. Some kids like to get their mom and dad to help with this part. Once you let the pee out in the toilet, then put on some dry underwear and/or pajamas and get back in bed and remind your gate to stay shut until you wake up in the morning.

I would also like you to keep a chart/monthly calendar so you can show me each time how well you are doing. This is how to fill in the chart.

This is a dry-wet ruler.

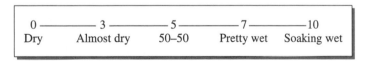

It is a ruler that measures how dry your bed is in the morning. It will be your job to use it. Every morning please mark in this chart *how dry* the bed is, 0 if the bed is completely dry, 3 if it is almost dry, and up to 10 if it is soaking wet.

This dialogue is meant as a jumping-off point. It should be modified to fit the style of the health care provider and meet the needs of the child and parent. Some generalizations about this technique:

1. It is directed toward the child and must engage the child to be effective.

2. The health care provider is seen as a coach whose job is to help the child to achieve a developmental milestone.

3. It can be used in conjunction with star charts and positive reinforcement.

4. The parents should be present to hear the explanation, but their role is primarily supportive.
   a. Help to take care of laundry
   b. Provide encouragement to the child but not pressure

5. If the child is still using nighttime diapers, make sure it is okay with both parent and child that they are not to be used. (One approach is to ask the child in the parents' presence if it is okay if he or she doesn't wear diapers anymore. Assuming the child says yes, tell him or her it is a deal and shake on it. Then direct your attention to the parent and confirm that it is okay.)

At the follow-up visit two to four weeks later, the child and health care provider review the calendar to assess progress and discuss how the program is progressing. It is useful to review the child's understanding of the technique by having the child draw the diagram and explain how his or her body is able to stay dry.

In our experience, this approach is successful in more than 75% of children. In those who are not successful, a decision needs to be made by the child, the parents, and the health care provider on what to do next. Our approach is to be empathetic with the disappointment the child and parent are feeling but reassuring that the problem is a temporary one that will improve over time. We also develop a strategy for dealing with the symptom, involving both parent and child, which focuses on minimizing the impact of the symptom on the child's life. The strategy may involve intermittent or occasional chronic use of desmopressin for special events such as sleepovers or camp. The goal of this approach is teaching the child and the parent how to gain control over a troublesome symptom.

REFERENCES

1. Laberge, L., R. E. Tremblay, F. Vitaro, and J. Montplaisir. Development of parasomnias from childhood to early adolescence. *Pediatrics* 106: 67–74, 2000.
2. Broughton, R. J. Sleep disorders: Disorders of arousal? *Science* 159: 1070–1078, 1968.
3. American Sleep Disorders Association. *The International Classification of Sleep Disorders: Diagnostic and Coding Manual.* Rochester, MN: American Sleep Disorders Association. 1990.

4. Klackenberg, G. Somnabulism in childhood-prevalence, course and behavioral correlates: A prospective longitudinal study (6–16 years). *Acta Paediatrica Scandinavica* 71: 495–499, 1982.

5. Tremblay, R. E., R. Loeber, C. Gagnon, P. Charlebois, and M. Le Blanc. Disruptive boys with stable and unstable high fighting behavior patterns during junior elementary school. *Journal of Abnormal Child Psychology* 19: 285–300, 1991.

6. Simonds, J. F. and H. Parago. Sleep behavior and disorders in children and adolescents evaluated at psychiatry clinics. *Developmental Behavioral Pediatrics* 6: 6–10, 1984.

7. Dahl, R. E. and J. Puig-Antich. Sleep disturbance in children and adolescent psychiatric disorders. *Pediatrician* 167: 32–37, 1990.

8. Jones, B. Basic mechanisms of sleep-wake states. In M. H. Kryger, T. Roth, and W. C. Dement, eds. *Principles and Practice of Sleep Medicine* (2nd Edition). Philadelphia, PA: W.B. Saunders Company, 1994: 145–162.

9. Chase, M., R. McCarley, A. Rechtschaffen, and T. Roth, eds. *Basics of Sleep Behavior.* Los Angeles, CA: UCLA Sleep Research Society. 1993: 17–78.

10. Hobson, J. A. and A. B. Schiebel. The brainstem core: Sensorimotor integration and behavioral state control. *Neurosciences Research Program Bulletin* 18(1): 1–173, 1980, February.

11. Hobson, J. A. and A. B. Steriade. Neuronal basis of behavioral state control. In F. Bloom, ed. *Handbook of Physiology* (Volume 4, Section 1). Bethesda, MD: American Physiological Society. 1986: 701–823.

12. Hobson, J., R. Lydic, and H. Baghdoyan. Evolving concepts of sleep cycle generation: From brain centers to neuronal populations. *Behavioral and Brain Sciences* 9: 371–448, 1986.

13. Rechtschaffen, A. and A. Kales. *A Manual of Standardized Terminology: Techniques and Scoring System for Sleep States of Human Subjects.* Los Angeles: UCLA Brain Information Service/Brain Research Institute. 1968.

14. Mahowald, M. W. and C. H. Schenck. Dissociated states of wakefulness and sleep. *Neurology* 42: 44–52, 1992.

15. Harrington, M., B. Rusak, and R. Mistlberger. Anatomy and physiology of the mammalian circadian system. In M. H. Kryger, T. Roth, and W. C. Dement, eds. *Principles and Practice of Sleep Medicine* (2nd Edition). Philadelphia, PA: W.B. Saunders Company. 1994: 334–345.

16. Gaudreau, H. and S. Joncas. Dynamics of slow wave activity during the NREM sleep of sleepwalkers and control subjects. *Sleep* 23: 755–760, 2000.

17. Espa, F., B. Ondze, P. Deglise, and A. Besset. Sleep architecture, slow wave activity and sleep spindles in adult patients with sleepwalking and sleep terrors. *Clinical Neurophysiology* 111: 929–939, 2000.

18. Guilleminault, C. and D. Poyares. Sleep and wakefulness in somnambulism: A spectral analysis study. *Journal of Psychosomatic Research* 51: 411–416, 2001.

19. Zuconi, M. and A. Oldani. Arousal fluctuation in nonrapid eye movement parasomnias: The role of cyclic alternating pattern as a measure of sleep instability. *Journal of Clinical Neurophysiology* 12: 147–154, 1995.

20. Smirne, S. and L. Ferini-Strambi. Clinical applications of cyclic alternating pattern. In G. Comi and C. Lucking, eds. *Clinical Neurophysiology: From Reception to Perception.* Philadelphia, PA: Elsevier Science. 1999: 109–112.

21. Lazare, M. and S. Putnam. Three functions of the medical interview. In M. Lipkin, S. Putnam, and A. Lazore, eds. *The Medical Interview: Clinical Care, Education, and Research.* New York, NY: Springer. 1995: 3–19.

22. Lask, B. Novel and nontoxic treatment for night terrors. *British Medical Journal* 297: 592, 1988.

23. Tobin, J. Treatment of somnambulism with anticipatory awakening. *Journal of Pediatrics* 122: 426–427, 1993.

24. Frank, C. and A. Spirito. The use of scheduled awakenings to eliminate childhood sleepwalking. *Journal of Pediatric Psychology* 22: 345–353, 1997.

25. Kohen, D., M. Mahowald, and G. Rosen. Sleep terrors disorder in children: The role of self hypnosis in management. *American Journal of Clinical Hypnosis* 4: 233–244, 1992.

26. Mahowald, M. and C. Schenck. NREM parasomnias. *Neurology Clinics of North America* 14: 675–696, 1996.

27. Gross, R. T. and S. M. Dornbusch. Enuresis. In M. D. Levine, W. B. Carey, A. C. Crocker, and R. T. Gross, eds. *Developmental-Behavioral Pediatrics.* Philadelphia, PA: W.B. Saunders Company. 1983: 575–586.

28. Lawless, R. Nocturnal enuresis: Current concepts. *Pediatrics in Review* 22: 399–406, 2001.

29. Bakin, H. The Genetics of Enuresis. *Clinics in Developmental Medicine* 48–49, 1973.

30. Cayan, S., E. Doruk, M. Bozlu, E. Akbay, D. Apaydin, E. Ulusoy, et al. Is routine urinary tract investigation necessary for children with monosymptomatic primary nocturnal enuresis? *Urology* 58: 598–602, 2001.

31. Riillig, S., U. B. Knudsen, J. P. Norgaard, E. B. Pederson, and J. C. Djurhuus. Abnormal diurnal rhythm of plasma vasopressin and urinary output in patients with enuresis. *American Journal of Physiology* 256: 664–671, 1989.

32. Neveus, T., A. Stenberg, G. Lackgren, T. Tuveno, and J. Helta. Sleep in children with enuresis: A polysomnographic study. *Sleep* 103: 1193–1197, 1999.

33. Olness, K. The use of self-hypnosis in the treatment of childhood nocturnal enuresis: A report of forty patients. *Clinical Pediatrics* 14: 273, 1975.

34. Kohen, D. P., S. O. Calwell, A. Heimel, and K. N. Olness. The use of relaxation-mental imagery (self-hypnosis) in the management of 505 pediatric behavioral encounters. *Journal of Developmental and Behavioral Pediatrics* 5: 21–25, 1984.

35. Kohen, D. P. A hypnotherapeutic approach to enuresis. In C. Hammond and D. Corydon, eds. *Handbook of Hypnotic Suggestions and Metaphors.* New York, NY: W.W. Norton and Company. 1990: 489–493.

Chapter 16

EFFICACY OF BEHAVIORAL INTERVENTIONS FOR PEDIATRIC SLEEP DISTURBANCE

BRETT R. KUHN AND AMY J. ELLIOTT

Disturbed sleep has been consistently identified among the most common concerns presented in clinical settings for children (1–6). Recent evidence indicates that a good night's sleep plays a critical role in early brain development, human learning, and memory consolidation (7–9), while disrupted sleep has been linked to behavior problems and poor emotional regulation (10–12). Although some pediatric sleep disorders demand medical attention (e.g., obstructive sleep apnea, narcolepsy), the majority require clinical assessment and intervention skills that specialists in behavioral medicine are ideally suited to provide.

Principles of behavior (e.g., reinforcement, extinction, shaping) that are successful in reducing daytime behavior problems are also highly effective in managing many forms of pediatric sleep disturbance (13). This should not be surprising, given the role early conditioning and parental sleep practices (e.g., whether infant is put into crib awake or already asleep) play in predicting children who become "good" versus "poor" sleepers (14–16). In fact, no fewer than five recent review articles identify behavioral interventions as the treatment of choice for pediatric sleep disturbance (17–21). This chapter evaluates the efficacy of behavioral and educational treatments for common pediatric sleep disturbances, namely bedtime resistance and night waking, parasomnias, and sleep schedule disorders using previously defined criteria to establish "efficacy" in the field of psychology.

In 1996, an American Psychological Association task group developed specific criteria, frequently referred to as the *Chambless criteria,* to evaluate psychological treatments based on the weight of the empirical support behind an intervention (22). These criteria have been systematically applied to numerous mental health conditions for both children and adults (e.g., elimination disorders, recurrent abdominal pain, panic disorder) and have become the gold standard for evaluating the efficacy of an intervention.

The Chambless criteria outline the type of support necessary for a research study to be considered *well established* or *probably efficacious* (see Table 16.1). The primary distinction between these two categories is that a *well-established* intervention has been shown to produce benefits that exceed another treatment or placebo condition that controlled for attention and expectancy variables. In addition, for an intervention to be considered *well established,* similar treatment results must be obtained by at least two independent research teams. The research may be either group or single-case experimental design; however, many more single-case studies are required for an intervention to be classified as *well established* versus *probably efficacious* (nine versus three case studies). Finally, we included a category of *promising* interventions that was recently added to the Chambless criteria by the Society of Pediatric Psychology Task Force (23). These interventions have shown some initial empirical support and make sense conceptually but lack the methodological rigor necessary to meet the standards of the Chambless criteria (see Table 16.1). The *promising* category was included because interventions that hold promise may encourage further research in the area or promote the development of novel interventions. This additional category is consistent with other review articles evaluating the efficacy of interventions for given disorders (24–25).

This focus on the integrity and rigor of the methodology applied in research studies has spawned debate over the clinical utility of a classification system, such as the Chambless criteria (22, 26). In fact, a distinction is now drawn between the results obtained from applied treatment research conducted in a controlled experimental environment and a "real-world" setting (efficacy vs. effectiveness). The term *efficacy* is used to describe results obtained from well-controlled treatment studies that show whether a treatment was beneficial for a specific problem (26). Typically, efficacy studies involve one or more control or comparison treatments, are single-blinded (in that the patients do not know whether they have been assigned to an experimental, comparison, or control condition), and use treatment manuals to increase the interval validity of the treatment given. In treatment efficacy research, outcomes are typically assessed on a short-term basis and focus on changes in a specific behavioral variable. In contrast, research on treatment effectiveness is conducted in real-world settings with fewer controls to account for potential confounding variables, and outcomes are typically assessed over a longer period of time (27). Chambless and Hollon (28) recommend emphasizing efficacy studies to evaluate the benefit of a given treatment, followed by research on clinical and cost effectiveness in different settings with divergent populations. This article primarily concentrates on efficacy

Table 16.1   Criteria for Empirically Validated Treatments

Well-Established Treatments[a]

  I. At least two good between-group design experiments demonstrating efficacy in one or more of the following ways:

    A. Superior to pill or psychological placebo or to another treatment

    B. Equivalent to an already established treatment in experiments with adequate sample sizes

OR

  II. A large series of single case design experiments ($n \geq 9$) demonstrating efficacy. These experiments must have:

    C. Used good experimental designs and

    D. Compared the intervention to another treatment as in I.A

 III. Experiments must be conducted with treatment manuals or treatment protocols specified in article.

 IV. Characteristics of the client samples must be clearly specified.

  V. Effects must have been demonstrated by at least two different investigators or investigating teams.

Probably Efficacious Treatments[a]

  I. Two experiments showing the treatment is more effective than a waiting-list control group

OR

  II. One or more experiments meeting the Well-Established Treatment Criteria I, III, and IV, but not V

OR

 III. A small series of single case design experiments ($n \geq 3$) otherwise meeting Well-Established Treatment

Promising Treatments[b]

  I. At least one well-controlled experimental study and another less rigorously controlled study by a separate investigator

OR

  II. Two or more well-controlled studies with small numbers

OR

 III. Two or more well-controlled studies by the same investigator

---

[a] From Chambless, D. L., W. C. Sanderson, V. Shoham, et al. An update on empirically validated therapies. *Clinical Psychologist* 49: 5–18, 1996.

[b] From Spirito, A. Introduction to special series on empirically supported treatments in pediatric psychology. *Journal of Pediatric Psychology* 24: 87–90, 1999.

research targeting pediatric sleep disturbances by using the Chambless classification criteria and includes information on effect sizes and clinical significance, as is appropriate (29).

BEDTIME RESISTANCE AND FREQUENT NIGHT WAKING

The hallmark of pediatric sleep disturbance in young children involves bedtime resistance and frequent night waking (18). This particular form of sleep disturbance is considered problematic by parents of 20% to 30% of young children (30–33). The clinical dyad of bedtime disturbance and frequent night waking are usually considered together because they often coexist (34–35), and treatments that target one symptom appear to generalize to the other (36). These findings may be explained by the fact that sleep initiation is required not just at bedtime, but also following brief nighttime awakenings that are part of a child's normal sleep cycle (15). Therefore, children who rely on "nonadaptive" sleep associations (e.g., feeding, rocking, parental presence) that the child cannot recreate by himself or herself will require assistance several times per night (37). Fehlings et al. identified nonadaptive sleep associations as the single most important factor associated with sleeping through the night (38). In fact, they reported that children who initiated sleep in the presence of nonadaptive sleep associations were 22 times more likely to display night awakenings than children who initiated sleep with adaptive sleep associations.

Two recent reviews of the empirical literature also came to the conclusion that research most strongly supports the use of behavioral interventions for young children with bedtime difficulties and frequent night wakings (19, 21). Ramchandani and colleagues' review of the literature included nine studies that used randomized group designs that employed medication, behavioral interventions, and nondirective education. Because only randomized group studies were included, the review ignored a multitude of well-designed within-subject studies that present strong internal validity. The authors concluded that drug treatments may provide an effective short-term option; however, behavioral interventions are more likely to yield both short-term and long-term effects for persistent childhood sleep problems. The Mindell article reviewed 41 within-subject and between-group studies of psychological (primarily behavioral) interventions for bedtime refusal and night wakings in young children. She concluded that extinction (ignoring) and parent education on prevention qualify as *well-established* treatments, while graduated extinction and scheduled awakenings should be considered as "probably efficacious" treatments (see Table 16.2 for a description of interventions). Because Mindell (19)

Table 16.2 Description of Behavioral Interventions for Bedtime Resistance and Night Waking

Extinction (Systematic Ignoring)

As applied to pediatric sleep disturbance, extinction usually involves placing the child in bed and then ignoring inappropriate child behavior (e.g., unreasonable requests, crying) until morning. Exceptions to ignoring are made in the possibility of illness or danger to the child. Extinction relies on the removal of reinforcement (e.g., parental presence, attention) maintaining problem child behaviors that interfere with sleep.

Graduated Extinction (Graduated Systematic Ignoring)

This procedure involves gradually reducing parental attention to inappropriate bedtime behaviors to allow the child to fall asleep without parental assistance. Two variations of graduated extinction have been described: (1) parents ignore inappropriate child behaviors (as in extinction) for progressively longer periods of time (e.g., 5, 10, 15 minutes) before briefly responding or checking on the child, or (2) parents respond immediately to child requests or crying, but gradually decrease the duration (e.g., 10, 7, 5 minutes) that they interact with the child. The goal of both versions is to systematically reduce parental attention, allowing inappropriate child behaviors to extinguish while promoting independent sleep onset.

Extinction with Parental Presence

This approach calls for the parent to sleep in the child's bedroom, but in a different bed, for one week. After placing the child in bed, the parent ignores the child (extinction) until he or she falls asleep. After one week, the parent resumes sleeping in a separate room.

Positive Routines

Establishing a positive bedtime routine involves temporarily delaying the bedtime to more closely coincide with the child's natural sleep onset time. Next, parents institute a positive, relaxing, and enjoyable prebedtime routine. Each activity in the routine is followed by parental praise and encouragement, signaling transition to the next activity. Once the behavioral chain is well established and the child is falling asleep quickly, the bedtime is slowly moved earlier in the evening until reaching the preestablished bedtime goal.

Faded Bedtime

The child's bedtime is delayed approximately 30 minutes later than the typical sleep onset time. If the child does not fall to sleep quickly (e.g., within 15 to 30 minutes), a response cost procedure is implemented during which the child is taken out of bed and kept awake for 30 to 60 minutes before being allowed to return to bed. This procedure continues until the child falls to sleep quickly. If the child falls to sleep quickly, the bedtime is set 30 minutes earlier the next night. The bedtime is continually "faded" according to these criteria until reaching the agreed-on bedtime goal. The sleep is also scheduled and restricted as the child is awakened at the same time each day and not allowed to sleep outside prescribed sleep times.

(continued)

Table 16.2   *Continued*

Scheduled Awakenings

After establishing a baseline of spontaneous nighttime wakings, parents schedule pre-emptive awakenings 15 to 30 minutes before the usual time of the child's spontaneous wakings. On each scheduled awakening, the child is provided with the "usual" parenting responses (e.g., feeding, rocking, soothing) as if the child had awakened spontaneously. The period of time between scheduled awakenings is systematically increased (e.g., by 30 minutes) so the child sleeps longer between scheduled awakenings or until the child is sleeping through the night.

Early Intervention/Parent Education

A variety of behavioral interventions have been used in an educative manner to promote the early establishment of healthy sleep patterns. Strategies typically target sleep routines, parental handling during sleep initiation, and parental response during night awakenings. The one consistent recommendation has been to place infants in their cribs tired but still awake to promote independent sleep skills at bedtime and to allow infants to return to sleep after waking.

published a comprehensive review of this area, we keep our coverage brief, focusing more on studies published since that review.

"Well-Established" Interventions

Extinction

Extinction has been evaluated in more clinical outcome studies than any other single treatment for pediatric sleep disturbance. The procedure is easy for parents to understand, and the underlying operant theory is well established. Specifically, termination of the reinforcement contingency that maintains a given response (e.g., crying) reduces or eliminates the potential occurrence of that response over time (39). The earliest reports of using extinction to target bedtime problems consist of uncontrolled case studies (40–41). These early reports were followed by numerous controlled, within-subject designs (42–44) and larger between-group experimental studies (45–50). The procedure has now been shown to be efficacious in five large-scale studies by four separate investigatory teams. Consequently, extinction clearly meets criteria as a *well-established* intervention for bedtime disturbance and frequent night waking (19). The primary drawback of extinction is the potential occurrence of post-extinction response bursts and spontaneous recovery of the problematic response (51–52). France (53) presents recent evidence suggesting that response bursts may be more frequent in children undergoing extinction (unmodified), compared to graduated extinction or extinction with parental presence (see Table 16.2). Parents who are unaware of the potential of response bursts may inadvertently resume reinforcing (e.g., attending) the problem behavior, creating an intermittent reinforcement schedule, and thereby increasing resistance to future extinction procedures (54).

Graduated Extinction

Graduated extinction was first described by Douglas and Richman (55) and later popularized by Ferber (56) in his popular self-help book titled *Solve Your Child's Sleep Problems.* Many parents have expressed concern and dissatisfaction with unmodified extinction (47, 57–58). Parents report that the opportunity to check on their child between intervals of crying makes the procedure easier to tolerate, which may produce higher rates of treatment integrity (48, 59). Different versions of the checking procedure have been described, but all rely on extinction combined with occasional parental "checks" that are usually faded over time. Lawton (54) found successful results with "decremental" graduated extinction (20), in which parents responded immediately but systematically reduced the duration of parental attention by one-seventh every four days over the 28-day intervention. The most common version, however, is "incremental" graduated extinction, which involves ignoring inappropriate child behavior for successively longer periods of time (e.g., 5, 10, 15 min) across successive checks within the same night (36, 60) or across successive nights (61).

With the addition of two recent studies, there are now three randomized, well-controlled group experiments to support the efficacy of graduated extinction (48, 59, 62). Because these studies were published by three separate investigator teams, there is now sufficient support for incremental graduated extinction as a *well-established* treatment for bedtime resistance and frequent night waking.

There is some indication that incremental increases between the checks may not be critical to successful outcomes. A slight modification, termed the *quick check* or *minimal check* (20, 63), is virtually identical to incremental gradual extinction except that the time periods between parental checks are maintained at a constant interval (e.g., every 10 minutes). This version has produced successful outcomes in one uncontrolled clinical outcome study (64), one multiple baseline study (53), and one group comparison study (65). Many professionals strongly advocate these checking procedures as a more "friendly" alternative to unmodified extinction. Recent data, however, suggest that compared with unmodified extinction, checking procedures may result in more, not less, crying and infant distress (53). This may be because the mere appearance of the parent at regular intervals is sufficient to reinforce the very behavior (i.e., crying) that parents are trying to extinguish.

Early Intervention/Parent Education

Providing early intervention services in an effort to prevent sleep disturbances from occurring presents an enticing alternative to treating problems after they are already firmly established. One small-scale study (66) and three large-scale studies attest to the efficacy of early intervention (67–69). After reviewing the empirical data, Mindell (19) aptly concluded that parent education as a prevention strategy meets criteria as a *well-established* intervention. Interestingly, the most impressive prevention study conducted to date is yet to be published. Symon and colleagues (70) randomly assigned 268 infants to early intervention or control at 2 to 3 weeks of age. The intervention required only 45 minutes of contact time and focused on teaching parental handling skills to promote infant independent sleep achievement skills. By 6 weeks of age, infants in the intervention group averaged nearly nine hours more sleep per week than control infants. Group differences persisted through 12 weeks, and collection of long-term data is currently underway. These data may help address the primary weakness of existing studies in this area, which has been failure to collect follow-up data to establish the true "preventive" nature of early intervention.

"Probably Efficacious" Interventions

Scheduled Awakenings

Scheduled awakenings were first described by McGarr and Hovel (71) in a single-case, reversal design. The procedure has since been evaluated in two multiple-baseline studies (72–73) and one large group comparison study (47). Overall, scheduled awakenings appear to systematically increase the length of children's sleep periods while eliminating spontaneous waking and excessive crying. Rickert and Johnson (47) compared scheduled awakening with unmodified extinction and found that, while both techniques were effective in reducing night wakings, extinction produced the most rapid results. Scheduled awakenings present a viable option for those children who, through inadvertent shaping, have become resistant to extinction-based procedures or engage in gagging, vomiting, or self-injurious behaviors during spontaneous awakenings (18). The primary disadvantage with this procedure is the length of treatment time required before a child sleeps through the night (74) because parents can expect to carry out scheduled awakenings for several weeks or more. Another constraint of scheduled awakenings is that the protocol does not address bedtime resistance or teach children sleep initiation skills. In fact, the most comprehensive study of scheduled awakenings specifically excluded children who presented with bedtime resistance because the authors felt the protocol was not appropriate for this problem (47). This limitation may compromise the external validity of scheduled awakenings, given the strong association between bedtime resistance and frequent nighttime awakenings found in clinically referred children.

"Promising" Interventions

Extinction with Parental Presence

This more recent modification to extinction is based on the assumption that children experience bedtime problems because of separation anxiety (20). The parental presence protocol calls for the parent to remain in the child's bedroom for the first week while "feigning sleep" and ignoring inappropriate child behaviors (extinction). The basic concept underlying the intervention is that the child's awareness of parental presence will be reassuring and promote quick sleep onset. Parents may also find the procedure more acceptable, leading to better adherence than unmodified extinction. Parental presence has proven efficacious in one large group study, showing results comparable to the quick check procedure in eliminating children's bedtime disturbance (65). France and Blampied (53) recently conducted a multiple baseline evaluation of extinction, extinction with minimal check, and extinction with parental presence. They concluded that parental presence produced rapid resolution of night waking and crying with fewer postextinction response bursts, making it the "treatment of choice" (53).

Positive Routines/Faded Bedtime with Response Cost

Positive routines and faded bedtime are similar strategies that both rely heavily on stimulus control as the primary agent of behavior change. Critics of behavioral reductive procedures point out that extinction-based procedures may reduce or eliminate inappropriate behaviors; however, they fail to teach or reinforce adaptive replacement behaviors. Positive bedtime routines can be conceptualized in part as a differential reinforcement procedure designed to teach children appropriate prebedtime behaviors and sleep onset skills. The procedure involves temporarily delaying bedtime to ensure rapid sleep initiation, then establishing appropriate cues for sleep onset (e.g., consistent prebedtime routine) that are chained and paired with positive parent-child interactions. Positive routines reportedly prevent long bouts of crying, reduce bedtime struggles, and alleviate parental anxiety. In contrast to extinction-based approaches, which can be difficult for parents to carry out, the positive routines protocol has been deemed an "errorless" procedure (75).

Positive bedtime routines were first used to eliminate bedtime tantrum behaviors of three children in a within-subject, A-B-C design (76). Intervention was effective in gaining voluntary bedtime compliance in all three cases. Like many studies in this area, the authors collected behavioral data (e.g., bedtime resistance) but did not address the children's actual sleep patterns (76). Two large group studies also reported beneficial results with positive routines (59, 77). One of these studies (59) used a well-defined protocol and randomized group design, placing positive routines in the "promising intervention" category.

Piazza and Fisher (78–79) used a variation of positive routines to eliminate severe sleep disturbances and increase appropriate sleep in children. Faded bedtime, both with and without response cost, has been evaluated in five treatment outcome studies employing well-controlled, within-subject designs (78–82). All but one study targeted sleep disturbances in children with developmental disabilities; however, many novel and promising interventions are established first through controlled single-subject research employing difficult populations before emerging into mainstream clinical practice (e.g., toilet training). The one published study that targeted sleep disturbance in a nondisabled toddler used a within-subject reversal design (82).

Faded bedtime and positive routines share the common components of temporarily delaying the bedtime and bedtime fading. However, as Piazza (79) points out, positive routines require a wider repertoire of responses from the parent, such as instituting a particular routine, praising each component of the routine, and repeatedly returning the child to bed if he or she comes out. At this point, bedtime fading with response cost may be the most promising alternative to extinction-based procedures and is a prime target for a randomized large group comparison study. The procedure closely resembles a combination of two behavioral interventions, sleep restriction and stimulus control instructions, which have the strongest treatment efficacy for chronic adult insomnia (83).

Beyond Descriptive Comparisons

One weakness in using descriptive criteria such as Chambless et al. (22, 26) when evaluating treatment efficacy is the overreliance on statistical significance to select outcomes. Larger samples usually produce a greater likelihood of statistical significance; however, statistical significance cannot be used to conclude that an intervention yields more powerful or clinically meaningful results. Consequently, treatment effect sizes have been recommended for inclusion in reviews of empirically supported interventions rather than sole reliance on statistical significance (29).

Compared to research on adult insomnia, the area of pediatric sleep disorders is still in its relative "infancy" (84). While dozens of published intervention studies exist for insomnia with relatively consistent outcome variables (e.g., sleep latency, number of awakenings, total sleep time; 85), the pediatric sleep literature consists of only a handful of randomized group studies with little consistency in outcome variables.

We identified randomized or partially randomized treatment outcome studies from the pediatric sleep literature; however, effect sizes could not be calculated for several studies because they either used multiple interventions (45, 86), pooled data from more than one intervention group (64–65), or failed to report statistical outcome data (62). We were, however, able to calculate effect sizes from four randomized group studies (47–48, 50, 59) that evaluated the efficacy of four separate behavioral interventions (extinction, graduated extinction, scheduled awakenings, positive routines) across six outcome measures (frequency and duration of awakenings, frequency and duration of bedtime tantrums, "good bedtimes," "good nighttimes"). Effect sizes varied considerably depending on the study, the outcome variables assessed, and the time of measurement (see Table 16.3). Based on direct comparison studies,

Table 16.3   Treatment Effect Sizes for RTC Studies of Behavioral Interventions for Bedtime Resistance/Night Waking

Study	Extinction	Graduated Extinction	Scheduled Awakenings	Positive Routines
Rickert & Johnson, 1988[a]				
Number of awakenings	$d = 2.31$		$d = 1.11$	
Adams & Rickert, 1989[a]				
Frequency bedtime tantrums		$d = .75$		$d = .88$
Duration bedtime tantrums		$d = 1.50$		$d = 1.83$
Seymour, Brock, During, & Poole, 1989[b]				
Number of awakenings	$d = .68$			
Minutes awake	$d = 1.00$			
Reid, Walter, & O'Leary, 1999[c]				
Good bedtimes[d]	$d = 2.63$	$d = 1.93$		
Good nighttimes[e]	$d = 1.29$	$d = 2.03$		

[a] Six weeks posttreatment.
[b] Four weeks posttreatment.
[c] Three weeks posttreatment.
[d] Settled alone in less than 10 minutes.
[e] Slept through night without sleeping with or waking the parents.

Note: All studies employed a RTC design; therefore, between-group effect sizes were computed on posttreatment scores.

extinction, graduated extinction, and positive routines were found to produce comparable results, with combined average effect sizes of $d = 1.58$, 1.55, and 1.35, respectively. It should be noted that for most outcome variables, the six behavioral interventions approached or surpassed $d = .80$ (see Table 16.3), which has been denoted to indicate a large treatment effect (87).

CIRCADIAN RHYTHM DISORDERS

Circadian rhythm disorders involve a misalignment between an individual's sleep pattern and the sleep pattern that is desired or considered the societal norm (88). Although there are six circadian rhythm disorders described in the literature, this discussion focuses on the three most commonly encountered in childhood and adolescence: advanced sleep phase syndrome, delayed sleep phase syndrome, and irregular sleep-wake pattern.

Advanced sleep phase syndrome (ASPS) is believed to be most common in infants, toddlers, and elderly individuals (89–90). In ASPS, the major sleep episode is advanced in relation to the desired clock time, resulting in symptoms of compelling evening sleepiness, early sleep onset, and an awakening that is earlier than desired (88). There are few reports of ASPS in the literature, and although there is one report of phase advance chronotherapy being successful in an older adult (91), we found no published treatment studies targeting children or adolescents. Clinical practice recommendations typically involved delaying the bedtime in 15-minute increments with corresponding delays in naptimes and mealtimes, along with increased light exposure in the evening and decreased exposure in the morning (92).

The most common circadian sleep disturbance among older children and adolescents is delayed sleep phase syndrome (DSPS, 93–94). In DSPS, the major sleep episode is delayed in relation to the desired clock time, which results in symptoms of sleep onset insomnia and/or difficulty in awakening at the desired time (88). DSPS was initially described with reference to adults; however, four older adolescents were included in the original group of 30 patients. Many participants in this seminal article reported that their sleep difficulties began in childhood or adolescence (95). More recent reports have also identified early age of onset (96–97). Children and adolescents with DSPS show increased risk of behavior problems and depression, have difficulty adjusting to school life, and may demonstrate poor class attendance or school refusal (94, 98–99). DSPS appears to be multiply determined, with psychosocial, genetic, and biological factors all weighing heavily in the etiology (100–103).

Behavioral treatments for DSPS have typically included one or more of three primary components: stabilization of the sleep schedule, gradual realignment to

a desired sleep schedule (phase-advance or phase-delay chronotherapy), and re
wards or behavioral contracts to facilitate maintenance of treatment effects.
While controlled laboratory research indicates that the circadian timing system
can be reset with careful control over light exposure, sleep scheduling, and motivation for adherence (104), there are few data to support these commonly recommended treatments for circadian rhythm disorders in pediatric populations.
In fact, there is currently not a single intervention for DSPS that has sufficient
empirical support to be classified by Chambless criteria.

The behavioral literature primarily focuses on obtaining appropriate sleep
schedules by either advancing or systematically delaying the sleep phase until
the desired sleep-wake schedule is achieved. Ferber has advocated using phase
advance with younger children with DSPS, which involves gradually advancing
the waking time, followed by a gradual advance of the child's bedtime (95,
105–106), but there has been no research evaluating this approach with children.
Attempts to phase advance have failed with adolescents and adults with DSPS
(94, 107–108).

Phase-delay chronotherapy (109) involves first stabilizing the child's sleep
schedule, then "lengthening" the day by delaying both bedtime and wake time by
three hours each day over successive days until the desired sleep phase is
reached. During schedule realignment, unscheduled napping should be avoided,
and mealtimes, physical activities, and light exposure should be appropriately
adapted within scheduled wake times. Once the desired sleep-wake schedule is
achieved, bedtimes and wake times must be closely adhered to throughout the
week or children will drift back to their previous sleep-wake schedule. As opposed to phase advancing, incremental phase delays capitalize on human beings'
natural circadian drift, due to an endogenous period that is slightly longer than
24 hours (110). Although chronotherapy has been primarily used with adults
(111), there are a few published studies that have targeted child participants
(112–114). Dahl, Pelham, and Wierson (112) used chronotherapy and a behavioral intervention (extinction) to treat the sleep problems of a 10-year-old girl diagnosed with DSPS and attention deficit-hyperactivity disorder (ADHD). The
intervention package, which took one week to implement, produced an increase
in total sleep time from 7.2 to 9.0 hours per night. Pre- and postintervention behavioral measures and teacher ratings indicated significant improvement in peer
interactions, increased productivity on a timed arithmetic task, and increased
completion of academic seatwork. Although ADHD symptomatology persisted,
the improvement in sleep reportedly produced a significant reduction in the
severity of symptoms and clinical impairment.

The only study to involve numerous participants employed a combination
of treatment protocols in an attempt to establish a step-by-step treatment protocol for DSPS. Okawa et al. (113) successfully treated 13 of 20 adolescents

with chronotherapy, regulation of the lighting environment, methyl cobalamin, and/or melatonin. These researchers advocated the use of bright light exposure before implementing other pharmacological or behavioral treatments because the environmental light-dark cycle is the primary mechanism responsible for entraining the human circadian system to a 24-hour day (111). Despite the fact that chronotherapy has received widespread billing as a treatment for DSPS, there has been surprisingly little research on the procedure since it was first introduced in 1981, and the field has turned its attention more toward melatonin and timed light exposure (89).

Thorpy and colleagues (94) devised an interesting alternative to daily progressive chronotherapy that they proposed was less disruptive to participants' weekly school schedules. Sleep deprivation with phase advance (SDPA) involves keeping a regular sleep schedule for six days, followed by one night of total sleep deprivation on the weekend. Bedtime on the following night is advanced 90 minutes earlier than the previous six days, and the new sleep schedule is then maintained for the next six days. The process is repeated on successive weekends until the desired schedule is attained. SDPA "appeared to be helpful" for the group of adolescents described; however, the protocol still awaits formal empirical evaluation.

Irregular sleep-wake patterns consist of temporally disorganized and variable episodes of sleeping and waking behavior (88). Irregular sleep schedules appear to occur more frequently in young children with inconsistent bedtimes and wake times and adolescents who demonstrate large discrepancies between their weekday and weekend sleep schedule (92). Mindell successfully treated a 2-year-old blind child with an irregular sleep schedule (115). A strict sleep and feeding schedule was introduced to increase the likelihood the child would be tired at bedtime and fall asleep quickly. Although this procedure did not systematically advance the bedtime, the same effect was achieved. This report was an uncontrolled pre- and posttreatment study, but observable effects of the schedule were immediate and lasting. The authors postulated that imposing strict schedule changes is likely to be more successful in young children who still have polyphasic sleep patterns. Finally, Pizza and colleagues (114) used chronotherapy to effectively treat an 8-year-old female with developmental disabilities and a disrupted sleep-wake schedule characterized by irregular sleep onset times, variable wake times, inappropriate day sleep, and reduced total sleep time. Immediate improvements in the child's sleep pattern were observed after chronotherapy was introduced, achieving an age-appropriate bedtime within 11 days. Four-month follow-up data indicated that the improvements were maintained. These results suggest that the utility of phase delay chronotherapy may extend beyond delayed sleep phase syndrome to other sleep schedule disturbances.

PARASOMNIAS

Parasomnia is a general term used to describe a group of undesirable behaviors that occur during sleep or are exacerbated by sleep (88). Parasomnias involve disorders of arousal, partial arousal, or sleep stage transition. The most common forms of parasomnia include sleepwalking, sleep terrors, nightmares, and rhythmic movement disorder (RMD). Because there is very little outcome research attesting to the efficacy of behavioral interventions for parasomnias in children, much of this section focuses on clinical approaches, which need to be subjected to empirical study. The clinical evaluation and differential diagnoses of parasomnias, including indications for overnight polysomnography, are well described elsewhere and are not the focus of this chapter (116–117).

Sleep Terrors and Sleepwalking

Sleepwalking (somnambulism) and sleep terrors (pavor nocturnus) constitute non-REM (NREM) parasomnias that are considered partial arousal disorders because their underlying process reflects incomplete arousal from sleep (116). In fact, many children who experience sleep terrors develop sleepwalking at an older age (118–119). Sleepwalking (somnambulism) consists of a series of complex behaviors initiated from slow wave sleep that result in walking during sleep. Sleep terrors are also characterized by a sudden arousal from slow wave sleep, but the behavioral presentation typically consists of a piercing scream or cry accompanied by autonomic and behavioral manifestations of intense fear (88). Sleepwalking and sleep terrors, while topographically different, fall within the spectrum of partial arousal disorders because they share a number of clinical characteristics, including age of onset, timing of the event within the sleep cycle, behavioral characteristics, genetics, and pathophysiology (120).

Partial arousal parasomnias usually occur during the first few hours of sleep, toward the end of the first sleep cycle as the child transitions out of slow wave (i.e., deep) sleep. Genetic factors are thought to be highly predisposing, but expression of the trait may be influenced by environmental factors (118, 121–123). For example, event frequency appears to rise in the presence of any factor that amplifies a child's "pressure" to achieve sleep or maintain deep sleep (e.g., late bedtime). Hypothalamic regulation of the homeostatic sleep process produces mounting "pressure" or drive to fall to sleep and maintain slow wave sleep as the child remains awake for longer periods (124–125). There are several findings that link partial arousal events to increased homeostatic sleep pressure. First, sleepwalking and sleep terrors occur most frequently during early to middle childhood when slow wave (deep) sleep is predominant, and the events are usually outgrown during puberty when slow wave sleep sharply declines. Second, recent evidence indicates that short-term sleep deprivation effectively induces somnambulistic events in adults with a history of sleepwalking (126). Third, children with primary sleep disorders (e.g., obstructive sleep apnea) and behavioral sleep disorders (e.g., bedtime resistance, sleep onset delay, frequent night wakings) appear to display increases in parasomnia activity due to sleep fragmentation or compromised sleep time (127). Fourth, insufficient sleep resulting from an irregular sleep schedule, staying up late, giving up a daily nap, or waking early in the morning appears to increase the frequency of events (128). Finally, there is preliminary evidence that simply increasing a child's total sleep time can substantially reduce sleepwalking and sleep terrors in children (129).

A review of the literature reveals that clinical recommendations have focused more on reassuring parents and ensuring the child's safety, rather than treating the disorder itself. There is, however, one promising behavioral strategy to directly intervene instead of simply waiting for the child to "outgrow" the parasomnia.

Promising Interventions

Scheduled awakenings involve the parent's waking the child 15 to 30 minutes before an expected partial arousal event. Although initially used to treat nighttime awakenings, scheduled awakenings gained popularity as an intervention for parasomnias after the publication of uncontrolled reports proclaiming the elimination of sleepwalking (130) and sleep terrors (131). More recently, two multiple baseline studies reported success with the use of scheduled awakenings to treat partial arousal parasomnias (132–133). Because the literature consists of only two controlled single-subject studies and no comparison studies, scheduled awakenings falls under the classification of *promising* intervention.

The mechanism underlying scheduled awakening's utility in decreasing partial arousal parasomnias in children is unclear. One possibility is that the awakenings alter the child's sleep patterns to eliminate the disruption in slow wave sleep (130, 132). Alternatively, scheduled awakenings may condition the child for self-arousal just before an event, thereby avoiding it altogether. Finally, it could be that scheduled awakenings indirectly reduce partial arousal events by increasing the child's total sleep time. As mentioned previously, scheduled awakenings are used for children with frequent nighttime awakenings and have been found to systematically increase the length of children's sleep periods. Durand and Mindell (132) noted an unexpected and unexplained increase in total sleep time for all three of their participants after implementing scheduled awakenings, which presented an unfortunate confound of the independent variable.

Behavioral clinicians interested in using scheduled awakenings will find little guidance in how to implement the intervention. Procedural details have varied considerably across investigators in terms of the timing of awakenings, the degree of arousal produced, the duration of treatment, and the rate of treatment tapering. For example, the degree of arousal has varied from getting children to merely open their eyes (132) to waking children fully for five minutes (130). Differences in the length of time that parents are asked to continue the procedure have varied as well. Some discontinued waking the child immediately after one parasomnia-free night (130), whereas others continued the intervention for one month (133). While it is possible that one variation works more effectively, the literature does not support any definitive statements about procedural permutations at this time.

Nightmares

Nightmares are frightening dreams that usually awaken the sleeper from REM sleep (88). They typically involve an episode of sudden awakening from sleep with intense anxiety or fear of harm. One way nightmares can be distinguished from sleep terrors is that on awakening, the child is usually alert with little confusion or disorientation. Furthermore, most children seek parental reassurance, describe vivid details of the frightening images, and have difficulty returning to sleep. The timing of events is also important because in contrast to sleep terrors, which occur during the first half of the night with slow wave NREM sleep, nightmares take place during REM sleep, which is more prominent during the latter half of the night.

Frequent, disturbing nightmares have been linked to psychopathology and poor "well-being" in adults (134–136). Studies with children, however, have produced mixed results (137–138). Some contend that nightmares serve as a barometer of the child's overall level of adjustment (139). Certainly, there are reports of nightmares being triggered by traumatic events (140–142), and nightmares are common among children involved in automobile accidents or who experience severe burn injuries (143–145). Blum and Carey (146) suggested that nightmares may even be prompted by a child's attempts to master normal developmental milestones such as toilet training or starting school. Other potential nightmare precipitants include illness, use of certain medications (e.g., sedative/hypnotics, beta-blockers, amphetamines), and withdrawal from alcohol or medication (e.g., benzodiazepines; 147–148).

The clinical approach for children who experience occasional nightmares usually involves nothing more than education that nightmares are an unavoidable part of growing up and reassurance that they do not necessarily signify emotional disturbance. Nightmares that occur frequently or contain extremely disturbing content may warrant professional attention. Surprisingly, there is no solid research to guide professionals in their efforts to assist children who experience frequent or disturbing nightmares.

Rather than viewing nightmares as reflecting intrapsychic struggles, Halliday (139) contends that nightmares should be treated as behaviors that are responsive to environmental contingencies, calling for closer scrutiny to external, precipitating, and maintaining factors. Further studies are needed to support a behavioral conceptualization of nightmare events with children. To date, the empirical literature on behavioral interventions for children with nightmares consists of two nonrandomized group studies (149–150), one quasi-experimental case report, and a handful of nonexperimental case descriptions (152–155). Two of the more frequently cited studies did not even directly measure nightmare frequency as an outcome (151, 154). Consequently, the current state of the empirical research fails to support a single intervention as *promising,* according to our adopted criteria.

Wile (149) published the largest, albeit uncontrolled, group study with 25 children between the ages of 6 and 14 years. Group 1 comprised 11 children who were taught to "think of positive dreams in the place of nightmares." Group 2 consisted of 11 children who were provided therapeutic suggestion (e.g., "I am going to sleep quietly tonight"), while Group 3 included three children who were encouraged to engage in dream-relevant content coping tasks during the day. Although termed *indirect suggestion,* this intervention obviously consisted of in vivo exposure. One child who had nightmares of black horses after seeing a dead black horse was taken to visit horses and encouraged to learn about them, while another child who dreamt of skeletons coming out of the closet was taken to a museum of natural history to see numerous skeletons. The median time for the nightmares to disappear was three months for Group 1, five months for Group 2, and two months for Group 3. Although Wile (149) comprises the largest study to date, the method of subject assignment was not described, no statistical tests were employed, there was no control group, and there were only three children in the third group. Nonetheless, the study pioneered systematic evaluation of focused interventions to reduce nightmares in children, which was a radical departure from the Freudian era in which dreams were considered symbolic discharges of repressed sexual conflict.

The first and only controlled group study to date was recently published by Krakow and colleagues (150), who are well known for their work with adult nightmare sufferers (156–159). Nineteen adolescent females (ages 13 to 18 years) with chronic nightmares were assigned to wait-list control or to active intervention consisting of a six-hour workshop on imagery rehearsal therapy (IRT). The IRT intervention consisted of three steps:

1. Self-selecting a nightmare
2. Changing the nightmare "anyway you wish"
3. Rehearsing the new version 5 to 20 minutes each day

At three months, retrospective report indicated that nightmare frequency decreased significantly in the treatment group with no change in the control group. The authors recognized the limitations of their study, including the small sample size, nonrandomized assignment of subjects, use of a selective population (residential facility), and instruments that are not standardized for use with adolescents. In addition, nightmare frequency was measured via retrospective report, which has been shown to be significantly less reliable than daily nightmare logs (160).

Notably missing in the literature is a unifying theoretical rationale and behavioral conceptualization to explain the effectiveness of interventions that target nightmares. One hypothesis underlying dream rescripting approaches is that these interventions encourage people to restructure their dream content during waking hours, which may be systematically exposing the person to a "feared stimulus." The role of exposure and desensitization in reducing fears and anxieties is well known. Exposure-based interventions (e.g., systematic desensitization, in vivo exposure, imaginal desensitization, emotive imagery) have long been the mainstay of behavioral interventions for anxiety disorders including fears, phobias, obsessive-compulsive disorder, and posttraumatic stress disorder. In fact, exposure therapy has more empirical evidence than any other intervention for the treatment of trauma-related symptoms (161). Numerous studies have employed exposure-based strategies to reduce nightmare frequency and distress in adults (162–173). It could be argued that most studies targeting children with nightmares have contained a strong element of exposure to fear-related stimuli or distressing nightmare content, including those using dream rescripting techniques and eye movement desensitization (149–155, 174).

Researchers interested in pediatric sleep should find the treatment of nightmares a ripe area to make their "mark." There are several important points to take into account. First, accurate identification and measurement of nightmares in young children are challenging. Unlike the behavioral manifestations of sleepwalking, night terrors, and enuresis, nightmare episodes may not be accompanied by external manifestations that are readily apparent to parents sleeping in another room (175). Second, the existing literature contains differences in the operational definition of nightmares, which leads to uncertainty about the epidemiology, etiology diagnosis, and treatment of nightmares in children (139). The pediatric sleep literature is fraught with examples of confusion concerning nightmare and sleep terrors (176–177). For example, the Kellerman (178) study uses the terms *night terrors* and *nightmares* interchangeably in text, leading some authors to cite the study as targeting sleep terrors (179) while others cite it in support for the treatment of nightmares (139). Roberts (174) also used the two terms interchangeably and purportedly treated *nightmares;* however, the clinical description was more consistent with sleep terrors because the events usually occurred within an hour of the child's falling to sleep, the child engaged in motor movements during the events, and "at no time was she able to remember the content of her dreams" (174). Finally, nightmares as "frightening dreams that awaken the child from REM sleep" should be clearly distinguished from a child's verbal report of "nightmares" following normal nighttime awakenings that are then reinforced (e.g., serve as the child's "admission ticket" into the parents' bed; 180).

In summary, there is surprisingly little quality research supporting clinical interventions for children who experience frequent or disturbing nightmares. The empirical support that does exist suggests that exposure-based therapies may be a fertile area for future research.

Rhythmic Movement Disorder

Rhythmic Movement Disorder (RMD) is a sleep-wake transition disorder that comprises a group of stereotyped, repetitive movements involving large muscles, usually of the head and neck (88). Although the movements typically occur immediately before sleep onset and into light sleep, recent polysomnographic (PSG) studies have documented the behavior during REM sleep when muscle activity is normally absent (181–182). Episodes typically last from 5 to 30 minutes, but they can persist for hours. Children usually engage in the movements before sleep onset, then again during the night when required to fall back to sleep following normal awakenings.

The topography of the rhythmic movements varies along a broad spectrum (e.g., head banging, head rolling, and body rocking; 117). Head banging (jactatio capitis nocturna) is the most commonly recognized form, characterized by repeated lifting of the head (or upper torso) and forcible (or even violent) banging of the head into the pillow, the mattress, headboard, or wall.

As a group, the quality of sleep in children with RMD does not appear to differ from other children (183). The majority do not cry even with violent activity; in fact, many children appear to find pleasure in the activity and may protest if the behavior is prevented (184). Paradoxically, it is the disturbed sleep of family members that often prompts referral. The movements can become noisy as the child hits the bed frame or the headboard knocks against the wall. Additionally, the movements can be accompanied by loud humming or chanting. One exasperated mother attending our sleep clinic admitted to getting so "fed up" with the noise that she once moved her son out onto the porch to sleep the remainder of the night. The vast majority of children who exhibit rhythmic movements show onset before 2 years of age, and for most there is rapid remission by 4 years of age (88, 183). There are documented reports of RMD in adults (182, 185–189); however, the rhythmic activity nearly always begins in infancy or early childhood (181).

The etiology of RMD is unknown. Given the high prevalence in infancy, it likely represents a normal tendency toward rhythmic activities that develops into a learned pattern of self-regulating behavior (190–192). We propose that RMD is best conceptualized as a stereotypic movement or habit disorder because the essential feature represents "motor behavior that is repetitive, often seemingly driven, and nonfunctional" (193). Although a formal functional analysis of RMD has never been reported, two functional conceptualizations might explain why RMD has been described as difficult to treat. Rhythmic movement, like many habit disorders, could be maintained through automatic reinforcement rather than attention or escape (194–195). This might explain why teaching parents to simply "ignore" the child when engaging in rhythmic behavior is generally not effective. This conceptualization, however, fails to explain why the rhythmic activity is limited to the presleep period and is not seen in other contexts during the day. Another possibility is that over time, rhythmic movements become highly conditioned with sleep initiation and are reinforced by sleep itself. In this case, extinction programs would be difficult to apply because the reinforcing property (e.g., falling to sleep) is not easily removed (196).

The diagnosis of RMD can be challenging in certain cases, yet relatively straightforward in others. Habit behaviors such as RMD can often be distinguished from organically based movements because the former can be produced voluntarily, can be temporarily suppressed, and can be modified by distractions or special attention (197). Medical etiology should always be ruled out, especially when RMD presents for the first time after early childhood (198). Accurate diagnosis can be greatly aided by having parents videotape the nocturnal events or through split-screen video-polysomnographic analysis (199).

On reviewing the treatment literature, considerable confusion concerning the definition of RMD is quickly discovered. Many studies cited to have targeted RMD actually addressed daytime self-injurious behavior, usually in individuals with mental disabilities (200–202). Using a consistent definition and diagnostic criteria of RMD, such as the one used by the *International Classification of Sleep Disorders* (88), will be a critical step toward advancing the scientific literature in this area.

No randomized group treatment studies have been published. In addition, no two studies have evaluated the same treatment protocol, leaving the area without a single *promising* intervention. The entire literature on behavioral interventions for RMD in children consists of eight published articles that base their results on anecdotal reports, uncontrolled (e.g., A-B design) single-subject studies, and quasi-experimental single-subject designs. Although the state of the empirical literature cannot be construed to provide strong support for using behavioral interventions, the case for using psychopharmacological agents is even weaker. The medication literature consists entirely of uncontrolled anecdotal reports with no measures of RMD activity at pre- or posttreatment. In contrast, there are a handful of published quasi-experimental designs that collected pre- and posttreatment frequency data to show that behavioral interventions can produce rapid and substantial reductions in RMD with durable and lasting effects (196, 203–206). Linscheid and colleagues (207) probably provide the best model for researchers interested in the area. The authors operationally defined rhythmic behavior, used direct behavioral observations with interobserver reliability, and employed an interval recording system to assess frequency. Unfortunately, the study lacked a true research design to provide stronger support for their overcorrection intervention.

While there are no *well-established* or *probably efficacious* interventions for RMD at this time, we do feel there is an intervention package that should be tested in future research studies. The most systematic and comprehensive research on behavioral treatment of habit disorders has been with a multicomponent procedure termed *habit reversal* (208). As originally conceptualized, habit reversal contains four separate components (awareness training, competing response training, motivation enhancement, generalization); however, simplified versions have been found effective (195). Habit reversal has been effective with numerous behaviors that range greatly in topography, including vocal and motor tics, hair pulling, stuttering, thumb sucking, and fingernail biting (209–210). Although there are no published treatment outcome studies evaluating the use of habit reversal for RMD, the majority of successful intervention studies employing behavioral interventions for RMD have incorporated one or more habit reversal components.

Several studies for RMD incorporated immediate detection and feedback for the presence of rhythmic behavior (e.g., awareness training) by using verbal prompts from all night observers, a contingent light signal, or audible alarms attached to the bed or headboard (203 207). Because rhythmic movement is often highly conditioned to the sleep onset process, many recommend teaching the child replacement behaviors (e.g., competing response training). While some studies explicitly taught alternative sleep initiation behaviors, children in other studies appeared to develop these replacement behaviors on their own such as learning to sleep on their back rather than front, mild rocking from side-to-side as opposed to violent head banging, or "grinding" their head into the pillow rather than banging it (203, 205, 207). Strauss (205) used a positive practice procedure to teach a 7-year-old girl to repeatedly stop her head just before striking the bed, then lie down calmly. Contingency management (e.g., motivation enhancement) using star charts, tangibles, or financial rewards has been used to reinforce alternative sleep-initiation behaviors or the cessation of rhythmic behavior (203, 205, 211). Mild punishments such as response cost have also been used, including waking the child or having the child walk around for a brief time before being allowed to return to bed (196, 204). Finally, two studies used professionals to deliver the intervention in a hospital setting before teaching parents to use the protocol at home (i.e., generalization; 196, 207).

CONCLUSION

The past decade has witnessed heightened interest and increased recognition of the impact that sleep has on children's development, learning, mood, and behavior. Clinical services for pediatric sleep disorders are increasingly being established across the country (212), and the field of pediatric sleep medicine has witnessed a recent proliferation of activity, including the publication of review articles (17–21), clinical practice guidelines (213–214), and self-help books for parents (74, 215). On reviewing the empirical foundation supporting all this activity, we believe many readers will agree that the field is still in its relative "infancy." With the exception of bedtime refusal and night waking, there are few empirically supported interventions for pediatric sleep problems. The field is dominated by uncontrolled case reports that far outnumber experimental studies. The majority of the randomized studies that have been conducted recruited subjects through newspaper advertisement, limiting the external validity of the findings to clinical populations. In general, sample sizes have been small and the recording periods have been short-term with only a few studies collecting follow-up data. Unlike the area of adult insomnia, there has been little agreement in outcome variables. Some studies included behavioral outcome variables (e.g., duration of crying or screaming, frequency of coming out of the bedroom) while others included sleep-related variables (e.g., sleep latency, frequency/duration of awakenings, total sleep time). A select number of studies have incorporated both behavioral and sleep-related variables, but other major studies have included neither. The literature is also rife with confusion surrounding the definition of certain disorders (e.g., nightmares versus sleep terrors, rhythmic movement disorder versus self-injurious behavior), which has resulted in certain interventions being recommended for the "wrong" sleep disorder. The use of formal diagnostic criteria, such as those published by the American Sleep Disorders Association (now the American Academy of Sleep Medicine; 88) should help resolve much of this inconsistency.

For interested researchers in the field, Reid et al. (48) provides a nice model to follow when designing a treatment outcome study. The authors employed randomized assignment with detailed entry criteria, used a scripted treatment manual, included multiple outcome measures, and collected follow-up data. Reid et al. (48) also collected data on treatment integrity, treatment satisfaction, and side effects of the treatment. Additional studies are needed to allow professionals to truly follow a consumer-driven model and turn the decision concerning appropriate intervention over to parents after fully describing the various treatment options, their efficacy, advantages, disadvantages, and potential side effects (57).

In conclusion, we hope this critical review will provide guidance to clinicians working with families and encouragement and direction to researchers in the field. While some readers may view the empirical glass as "half empty," we see a rapidly developing field that provides abundant opportunities to establish a scientific basis for promising interventions or to create novel interventions for children and adolescents with disturbed sleep.

REFERENCES

1. Arndorfer, R. E., K. D. Allen, and L. Aljazireh. Behavioral health needs in pediatric medicine and the acceptability of behavioral solutions: Implications for behavioral psychologists. *Behavior Therapy* 30: 137–148, 1999.

2. Ford, D. E. and D. B. Kamerow. Epidemiologic study of sleep disturbances and psychiatric disorders: An opportunity for prevention? *Journal of the American Medical Association* 262: 1479–1484, 1989.

3. Lavigne, J. V., R. Arend, D. Rosenbaum, et al. Sleep and behavior problems among preschoolers. *Journal of Developmental and Behavioral Pediatrics* 20: 164–169, 1999.

4. Keren, M., R. Feldman, and S. Tyano. Diagnoses and interactive patterns of infants referred to a community-based infant mental health clinic. *Journal of the American Academy of Child and Adolescent Psychiatry* 40: 27–35, 2001.

5. Meisbov, G. B., C. S. Schroeder, and L. Wesson. Parental concerns about their children. In M. Roberts, G. Koocher, D. Routh, and D. Willis, eds. *Readings in Pediatric Psychology.* New York, NY: Plenum Press. 1993: 307–317.

6. Mindell, J. A., M. L. Moline, S. M. Zendell, L. W. Brown, and J. M. Fry. Pediatricians and sleep disorders: Training and practice. *Pediatrics* 94: 194–200, 1994.

7. Frank, M. G., N. P. Issa, and M. P. Stryker. Sleep enhances plasticity in the developing visual cortex. *Neuron* 30: 275–287, 2001.

8. Gais, S., W. Plihal, U. Wagner, and J. Born. Early sleep triggers memory for early visual discrimination skills. *Nature Neuroscience* 3: 1335–1339, 2000.

9. Stickgold, R., L. James, and J. A. Hobson. Visual discrimination learning requires sleep after training. *Nature Neuroscience* 3: 1237–1238, 2000.

10. Dahl, R. E. The regulation of sleep and arousal: Development and psychopathology. *Development and Psychopathology* 8: 3–27, 1996.

11. Minde, K., A. Faucon, and S. Falkner. Sleep problems in toddlers: Effects of treatment on their daytime behavior. *Journal of the American Academy of Child and Adolescent Psychiatry* 33: 1114–1121, 1994.

12. Sadeh, A., A. Raviv, and R. Gruber. *Sleep and Neurobehavioral Functioning in School-Age Children.* Paper presented at Satellite Symposium: Development and Sleep, 14th Congress of the European Sleep Research Society, Madrid, Spain. 1998, September.

13. Douglas, J. Training parents to manage their child's sleep problem. In C. E. Schaefer and J. M. Briesmeister, eds. *Handbook of Parent Training: Parents as Co-Therapists for Children's Behavior Problems.* New York, NY: John Wiley & Sons. 1989: 13–37.

14. Adair, R., H. Bauchner, B. Philipp, S. Levenson, and B. Zuckerman. Night waking during infancy: Role of parental presence at bedtime. *Pediatrics* 87: 500–504, 1991.

15. Anders, T. F., L. F. Halpern, and J. Hua. Sleeping through the night: A developmental perspective. *Pediatrics* 90: 554–560, 1992.

16. Van Tassel, E. B. The relative influence of child and environmental characteristics on sleep disturbances in the first and second years of life. *Journal of Developmental and Behavioral Pediatrics* 6: 81–85, 1985.

17. Anders, T. F. and L. A. Eiben. Pediatric sleep disorders: A review of the past 10 years. *Journal of the American Academy of Child and Adolescent Psychiatry* 36: 9–20, 1997.

18. Kuhn, B. R. and D. Weidinger. Interventions for infant and toddler sleep disturbance: A review. *Child and Family Behavior Therapy* 22: 33–50, 2000.

19. Mindell, J. A. Empirically supported treatments in pediatric psychology: Bedtime refusal and night wakings in young children. *Journal of Pediatric Psychology* 24: 465–481, 1999.

20. Owens, J. L., K. G. France, and L. Wiggs. Behavioral and cognitive-behavioral interventions for sleep disorders in infants and children: A review. *Sleep Medicine Reviews* 3: 281–302, 1999.

21. Ramchandani, P., L. Wiggs, V. Webb, and G. Stores. A systematic review of treatments for settling problems and night waking in young children. *British Medical Journal* 320(7229): 209–213, 2000.

22. Chambless, D. L., W. C. Sanderson, V. Shoham, et al. An update on empirically validated therapies. *Clinical Psychologist* 49: 5–18, 1996.

23. Spirito, A. Introduction to special series on empirically supported treatments in pediatric psychology. *Journal of Pediatric Psychology* 24: 87–90, 1999.

24. Janicke, D. M. and J. W. Finney. Empirically supported treatments in pediatric psychology: Recurrent abdominal pain. *Journal of Pediatric Psychology* 24: 115–127, 1999.

25. Mellon, M. W. and M. L. McGrath. Empirically supported treatments in pediatric psychology: Nocturnal enuresis. *Journal of Pediatric Psychology* 25: 193–214, 2000.

26. Chambless, D. L., M. J. Baker, D. H. Baucom, et al. Update on empirically validated therapies. II. *Clinical Psychologist* 51: 3–16, 1998.

27. Nathan, P. E., S. P. Stuart, and S. L. Dolan. Research on psychotherapy efficacy and effectiveness: Between Scylla and Charybdis? *Psychological Bulletin* 126: 964–981, 2000.

28. Chambless, D. L. and S. D. Hollon. Defining empirically supported therapies. *Journal of Consulting and Clinical Psychology* 66: 7–18, 1998.

29. Drotar, D. Enhancing reviews of psychological treatments with pediatric populations: Thoughts on next steps. *Journal of Pediatric Psychology* 27: 167–176, 2002.

30. Armstrong, K. L., R. A. Quinn, and M. R. Dadds. The sleep patterns of normal children. *Medical Journal of Australia* 161: 202–206, 1994.

31. Blader, J. C., H. S. Koplewicz, H. Abikoff, and C. Foley. Sleep problems of elementary school children. A community survey. *Archives of Pediatric and Adolescent Medicine* 151: 473–480, 1997.

32. Richman, N., J. Stevenson, and P. J. Graham. *Pre-School to School: A Behavioural Study* (Volume 228). New York, NY: Academic Press. 1982.

33. Lozoff, B., A. W. Wolf, and N. S. Davis. Sleep problems seen in pediatric practice. *Pediatrics* 75: 477–483, 1985.

34. Richman, N. A community survey of characteristics of one- to two-year-olds with sleep disruptions. *Journal of the American Academy of Child Psychiatry* 20: 281–291, 1981.

35. Richman, N., J. E. Stevenson, and P. J. Graham. Prevalence of behaviour problems in 3-year-old children: An epidemiological study in a London borough. *Journal of Child Psychology and Psychiatry* 16: 277–287, 1975.

36. Mindell, J. A. and V. M. Durand. Treatment of childhood sleep disorders: Generalization across disorders and effects on family members. Special issue: Interventions in pediatric psychology. *Journal of Pediatric Psychology* 18: 731–750, 1993.

37. Goodlin-Jones, B. L., M. M. Burnham, E. E. Gaylor, and T. F. Anders. Night waking, sleep-wake organization, and self-soothing in the first year of life. *Journal of Developmental and Behavioral Pediatrics* 22: 226–233, 2001.

38. Fehlings, D. Frequent night awakenings in infants and preschool children referred to a sleep disorders clinic: The role of non-adaptive sleep associations. *Children's Health Care* 30: 43–55, 2001.

39. Lerman, D. C. and B. A. Iwata. Developing a technology for the use of operant extinction in clinical settings: An examination of basic and applied research. *Journal of Applied Behavior Analysis* 29: 345–382, 1996.

40. Williams, C. D. The elimination of tantrum behavior by extinction procedures. *Journal of Abnormal and Social Psychology* 59: 269, 1959.

41. Wright, L., J. Woodcock, and R. Scott. Treatment of sleep disturbance in a young child by conditioning. *Southern Medical Journal* 63: 174–176, 1970.

42. Rapoff, M. A., E. R. Christophersen, and K. E. Rapoff. The management of common childhood bedtime problems by pediatric nurse practitioners. *Journal of Pediatric Psychology* 7: 179–196, 1982.

43. Chadez, L. H. and P. S. Nurius. Stopping bedtime crying: Treating the child and the parents. *Journal of Clinical Child Psychology* 16: 212–217, 1987.

44. France, K. G. and S. M. Hudson. Behavior management of infant sleep disturbance. *Journal of Applied Behavior Analysis* 23: 91–98, 1990.

45. France, K. G., N. M. Blampied, and P. Wilkinson. Treatment of infant sleep disturbance by trimeprazine in combination with extinction. *Journal of Developmental and Behavioral Pediatrics* 12: 308–314, 1991.

46. France, K. G. Behavior characteristics and security in sleep-disturbed infants treated with extinction. *Journal of Pediatric Psychology* 17: 467–475, 1992.

47. Rickert, V. I. and C. M. Johnson. Reducing nocturnal awakening and crying episodes in infants and young children: A comparison between scheduled awakenings and systematic ignoring. *Pediatrics* 81: 203–212, 1988.

48. Reid, M. J., A. L. Walter, and S. G. O'Leary. Treatment of young children's bedtime refusal and nighttime wakings: A comparison of "standard" and graduated ignoring procedures. *Journal of Abnormal Child Psychology* 27: 5–16, 1999.

49. Seymour, F. W., G. Bayfield, P. Brock, and M. During. Management of night-waking in young children. *Australian Journal of Family Therapy* 4: 217–223, 1983.

50. Seymour, F. W., P. Brock, M. During, and G. Poole. Reducing sleep disruptions in young children: Evaluation of therapist-guided and written information approaches: A brief report. *Journal of Child Psychology and Psychiatry* 30: 913–918, 1989.

51. Lerman, D. C., M. E. Kelley, C. M. Van Camp, and H. S. Roane. Effects of reinforcement magnitude on spontaneous recovery. *Journal of Applied Behavior Analysis* 32: 197–200, 1999.

52. Lerman, D. C., B. A. Iwata, and M. D. Wallace. Side effects of extinction: Prevalence of bursting and aggression during the treatment of self-injurious behavior. *Journal of Applied Behavior Analysis* 32: 1–8, 1999.

53. France, K. G. and N. M. Blampied. *Modifications of Systematic Ignoring in the Management of Infant Sleep Disturbance: Efficacy and Infant Distress*. Manuscript submitted for publication.

54. Lawton, C., K. G. France, and N. M. Blampied. Treatment of infant sleep disturbance by graduated extinction. *Child and Family Behavior Therapy* 13: 39–56, 1991.

55. Douglas, J. and N. Richman. *My Child Won't Sleep.* Harmondsworth, England: Penguin Books. 1984.

56. Ferber, R. *Solve Your Child's Sleep Problems.* New York, NY: Simon & Schuster. 1985.

57. France, K. G. Handling parents' concerns regarding the behavioural treatment of infant sleep disturbance. *Behaviour Change* 11: 101–109, 1994.

58. Seymour, F. W. Parent management of sleep difficulties in young children. *Behaviour Change* 4: 39–48, 1987.

59. Adams, L. A. and V. I. Rickert. Reducing bedtime tantrums: Comparison between positive routines and graduated extinction. *Pediatrics* 84: 756–761, 1989.

60. Durand, V. M. and J. A. Mindell. Behavioral treatment of multiple childhood sleep disorders: Effects on child and family. *Behavior Modification* 14: 37–49, 1990.

61. Rolider, A. and R. Van Houten. Training parents to use extinction to eliminate nighttime crying by gradually increasing the criteria for ignoring crying. *Education and Treatment of Children* 7: 119–124, 1984.

62. Hiscock, H. and M. Wake. Randomised controlled trial of behavioural infant sleep intervention to improve infant sleep and maternal mood. *British Medical Journal* 324(7345): 1062, 2002.

63. Schaefer, C. E. and M. R. Petronko. *Teach Your Baby to Sleep through the Night.* New York, NY: G.P. Putnam's Sons. 1987.

64. Pritchard, A. and P. Appleton. Management of sleep problems in pre-school children. *Early Child Development and Care* 34: 227–240, 1988.

65. Sadeh, A. Assessment of intervention for infant night waking: Parental reports and activity-based home monitoring. *Journal of Consulting and Clinical Psychology* 62: 63–68, 1994.

66. Pinilla, T. and L. L. Birch. Help me make it through the night: Behavioral entrainment of breast-fed infants' sleep patterns [see comments]. *Pediatrics* 91: 436–444, 1993.

67. Wolfson, A., P. Lacks, and A. Futterman. Effects of parent training on infant sleeping patterns, parents' stress, and perceived parental competence. *Journal of Consulting and Clinical Psychology* 60: 41–48, 1992.

68. Adair, R., B. Zuckerman, H. Bauchner, B. Philipp, and S. Levenson. Reducing night waking in infancy: A primary care intervention. *Pediatrics* 89: 585–588, 1992.

69. Kerr, S. M., S. A. Jowett, and L. N. Smith. Preventing sleep problems in infants: A randomized controlled trial. *Journal of Advanced Nursing* 24: 938–942, 1996.

70. Symon, B. G., J. Martin, and J. Marley. *A Randomized, Controlled Trial of Protocol for Improving Sleep Performance in Newborn Infants.* Paper presented at the Annual Scientific Meeting of the Royal Australian College of General Practitioners, Adelaide, Australia. 1999, October.

71. McGarr, R. J. and M. F. Hovell. In search of the sand man: Shaping an infant to sleep. *Education and Treatment of Children* 3: 173–182, 1980.

72. Johnson, C. M. and M. Lerner. Amelioration of infant sleep disturbances: II. Effects of scheduled awakenings by compliant parents. *Infant Mental Health Journal* 6: 21–30, 1985.

73. Johnson, C. M., S. Bradley-Johnson, and J. M. Stack. Decreasing the frequency of infants' nocturnal crying with the use of scheduled awakenings. *Family Practice Research Journal* 1: 98–104, 1981.

74. Mindell, J. A. *Sleeping through the Night: How Infants, Toddlers, and Their Parents Can Get a Good Night's Sleep.* New York, NY: HarperPerennial/HarperCollins. 1997.

75. Durand, V. M. *Sleep Better! A Guide to Improving the Sleep for Children with Special Needs.* New York, NY: Paul H. Brookes. 1998.

76. Milan, M. A., Z. P. Mitchell, M. I. Berger, and D. F. Pierson. Positive routines: A rapid alternative to extinction for elimination of bedtime tantrum behavior. *Child Behavior Therapy* 3: 13–25, 1981.

77. Galbraith, L. and K. E. Hewitt. Behavioural treatment for sleep disturbance. *Health Visit* 66: 169–171, 1993.

78. Piazza, C. C. and W. W. Fisher. A faded bedtime with response cost protocol for treatment of multiple sleep problems in children. *Journal of Applied Behavior Analysis* 24: 129–140, 1991.

79. Piazza, C. C. and W. W. Fisher. Bedtime fading in the treatment of pediatric insomnia. *Journal of Behavior Therapy and Experimental Psychiatry* 22: 53–56, 1991.

80. Piazza, C. C., W. W. Fisher, and H. Moser. Behavioral treatment of sleep dysfunction in patients with the Rett syndrome. *Brain and Development* 13: 232–237, 1991.

81. Piazza, C. C., W. W. Fisher, and M. Sherer. Treatment of multiple sleep problems in children with developmental disabilities: Faded bedtime with response cost versus bedtime scheduling. *Developmental Medicine and Child Neurology* 39: 414–418, 1997.

82. Ashbaugh, R. and S. Peck. Treatment of sleep problems in a toddler: A replication of the faded bedtime with response cost protocol. *Journal of Applied Behavior Analysis* 31: 127–129, 1998.

83. Morin, C. M., J. P. Culbert, and S. M. Schwartz. Nonpharmacological interventions for insomnia: A meta-analysis of treatment efficacy. *American Journal of Psychiatry* 151: 1172–1180, 1994.

84. Dahl, R. Pediatric sleep disorders: "A field in its infancy (but growing)." *Sleep Medicine Reviews* 3: 263–264, 1999.

85. Smith, M. T., M. L. Perlis, A. Park, et al. Comparative meta-analysis of pharmacotherapy and behavior therapy for persistent insomnia. *American Journal of Psychiatry* 159: 5–11, 2002.

86. Scott, G. and M. P. Richards. Night waking in infants: Effects of providing advice and support for parents. *Journal of Child Psychology and Psychiatry* 31: 551–567, 1990.

87. Cohen, J. *Statistical Power Analysis for the Behavioral Sciences.* New York, NY: Academic Press. 1977.

88. American Sleep Disorders Association. *The International Classification of Sleep Disorders, Revised: Diagnostic and Coding Manual.* Rochester, MN: American Sleep Disorders Association. 1997.

89. Burns, R. E., M. J. Sateia, and J. T. Lee-Chiong. Basic principles of chronobiology and disorders and circadian sleep-wake rhythm. In J. T. Lee-Chiong, M. J. Sateia, and M. A. Carskadon, eds. *Sleep Medicine.* Philadelphia, PA: Hanley and Belfus, Inc. 2002: 245–254.

90. Ferber, R. Circadian and schedule disturbances. In C. Guilleminault, ed. *Sleep and Its Disorders in Children.* New York, NY: Raven Press. 1987: 165–175.

91. Moldofsky, H., S. Musisi, and E. A. Phillipson. Treatment of a case of advanced sleep phase syndrome by phase advance chronotherapy. *Sleep* 9: 61–65, 1986.

92. Ferber, R. Circadian rhythm sleep disorders in childhood. In R. Ferber and M. H. Kryger, eds. *Principles and Practice of Sleep Medicine in the Child.* Philadelphia, PA: W.B. Saunders Company. 1995: 91–98.

93. Baker, S. K. and P. C. Zee. Circadian disorders of the sleep-wake cycle. In M. H. Kryger, T. Roth, and W. C. Dement, eds. *Principles and Practices of Sleep Medicine* (3rd Edition). Philadelphia, PA: W.B. Saunders Company. 2000: 606–614.

94. Thorpy, M. J., E. Korman, A. J. Spielman, and P. B. Glovinsky. Delayed sleep phase syndrome in adolescents. *Journal of Adolescent Health Care* 9: 22–27, 1988.

95. Weitzman, E. D., C. A. Czeisler, R. M. Coleman, et al. Delayed sleep phase syndrome: A chronobiological disorder with sleep-onset insomnia. *Archives of General Psychiatry* 38: 737–746, 1981.

96. Dagan, Y. and M. Eisenstein. Circadian rhythm sleep disorders: Toward a more precise definition and diagnosis. *Chronobiology International* 16: 213–222, 1999.

97. Yamadera, H., K. Takahashi, and M. Okawa. A multicenter study of sleep-wake rhythm disorders: Clinical features of sleep-wake rhythm disorders. *Psychiatry and Clinical Neurosciences* 50: 195–201, 1996.

98. Ohta, T., T. Iwata, Y. Kayukawa, and T. Okada. Daily activity and persistent sleep-wake schedule disorders. *Progress in Neuro-Psychopharmacology and Biological Psychiatry* 16: 529–537, 1992.

99. Tomoda, A., T. Miike, K. Yonamine, K. Adachi, and S. Shiraishi. Disturbed circadian core body temperature rhythm and sleep disturbance in school refusal children and adolescents. *Biological Psychiatry* 41: 810–813, 1997.

100. Takahashi, Y., H. Hohjoh, and K. Matsuura. Predisposing factors in delayed sleep phase syndrome. *Psychiatry and Clinical Neurosciences* 54: 356–358, 2000.

101. Hohjoh, H., Y. Takahashi, Y. Hatta, et al. Possible association of human leucocyte antigen DR1 with delayed sleep phase syndrome. *Psychiatry and Clinical Neurosciences* 53: 527–529, 1999.

102. Carskadon, M. A., C. Vieira, and C. Acebo. Association between puberty and delayed phase preference. *Sleep* 16: 258–262, 1993.

103. Wolfson, A. R. Sleeping patterns of children and adolescents: Developmental trends, disruptions, and adaptations. *Child and Adolescent Psychiatric Clinics of North America* 5: 549–568, 1996.

104. Carskadon, M. A. When worlds collide: Adolescent need for sleep versus societal demands. *Phi Delta Kappan* January: 348–353, 1999.

105. Ferber, R. A. Delayed sleep phase syndrome versus motivated sleep phase delay in adolescents. *Sleep Research* 12: 239, 1983.

106. Ferber, R. Sleep schedule-dependent causes of insomnia and sleepiness in middle childhood and adolescence. *Pediatrician* 17: 13–20, 1990.

107. Alvarez, B., M. J. Dahlitz, J. Vignau, and J. D. Parkes. The delayed sleep phase syndrome: Clinical and investigative findings in 14 subjects. *Journal of Neurology, Neurosurgery, and Psychiatry* 55: 665–670, 1992.

108. Regestein, Q. R. Treating insomnia: A practical guide for managing chronic sleeplessness, circa 1975. *Comprehensive Psychiatry* 17: 517–526, 1976.

109. Czeisler, C. A., G. S. Richardson, R. M. Coleman, et al. Chronotherapy: Resetting the circadian clocks of patients with delayed sleep phase insomnia. *Sleep* 4: 1–21, 1981.

110. Campbell, S. S., D. Dawson, and J. Zulley. When the human circadian system is caught napping: Evidence for endogenous rhythms close to 24 hours. *Sleep* 16: 638–640, 1993.

111. Campbell, S. S., P. J. Murphy, C. J. van den Heuvel, M. L. Roberts, and T. N. Stauble. Etiology and treatment of intrinsic circadian rhythm sleep disorders. *Sleep Medicine Reviews* 3: 179–200, 1999.

112. Dahl, R. E., W. E. Pelham, and M. Wierson. The role of sleep disturbances in attention deficit disorder symptoms: A case study. *Journal of Pediatric Psychology* 16: 229–239, 1991.

113. Okawa, M., M. Uchiyama, S. Ozaki, K. Shibui, and H. Ichikawa. Circadian rhythm sleep disorders in adolescents: Clinical trials of combined treatments based on chronobiology. *Psychiatry and Clinical Neurosciences* 52: 483–490, 1998.

114. Piazza, C. C., L. P. Hagopian, C. R. Hughes, and W. W. Fisher. Using chronotherapy to treat severe sleep problems: A case study. *American Journal on Mental Retardation* 102: 358–366, 1998.

115. Mindell, J. A., R. Goldberg, and J. M. Fry. Treatment of a circadian rhythm disturbance in a 2-year-old blind child. *Journal of Visual Impairment and Blindness* 90: 162–166, 1996.

116. Rosen, G. M., R. Ferber, and M. W. Mahowald. Evaluation of parasomnias in children. *Child and Adolescent Psychiatric Clinics of North America* 5: 601–616, 1996.

117. Mahowald, M. W. and M. J. Thorpy. Nonarousal parasomnias in the child. In R. Ferber and M. Kryger, eds. *Principles and Practice of Sleep Medicine in the Child*. Philadelphia, PA: W.B. Saunders Company. 1995: 115–123.

118. Kales, A., C. R. Soldatos, E. O. Bixler, et al. Hereditary factors in sleepwalking and night terrors. *British Journal of Psychiatry* 137: 111–118, 1980.

119. Klackenberg, G. Incidence of parasomnias in children in a general population. In C. Guilleminault, ed. *Sleep and Its Disorders in Children.* New York, NY: Raven Press. 1987: 99–113.

120. Broughton, R. J. Sleep disorders: Disorders of arousal? *Science* 159(819): 1070–1078, 1968.

121. Abe, K., M. Amatomi, and N. Oda. Sleepwalking and recurrent sleeptalking in children of childhood sleepwalkers. *American Journal of Psychiatry* 141: 800–801, 1984.

122. Bakwin, H. Sleep-walking in twins. *Lancet* 2(670): 446–447, 1970.

123. Berlin, R. M. and U. Qayyum. Sleepwalking: Diagnosis and treatment through the life cycle. *Psychosomatics* 27: 755–760, 1986.

124. Hirshkowitz, M., C. A. Moore, and G. Minhoto. The basics of sleep. In M. R. Pressman and W. C. Orr, eds. *Understanding Sleep: The Evaluation and Treatment of Sleep Disorders.* Washington, DC: American Psychological Press. 1997: 11–34.

125. Sack, R. L. Shift work and jet lag. In J. T. Lee-Chiong, M. J. Sateia, and M. A. Carskadon, eds. *Sleep Medicine.* Philadelphia, PA: Hanley and Belfus, Inc. 2002: 255–263.

126. Joncas, S., A. Zadra, J. Paquet, and J. Montplaisir. The value of sleep deprivation as a diagnostic tool in adult sleepwalkers. *Neurology* 58: 936–940, 2002.

127. Mehlenbeck, R., A. Spirito, J. Owens, and J. Boergers. The clinical presentation of childhood partial arousal parasomnias. *Sleep Medicine* 1: 307–312, 2000.

128. Rosen, G., M. W. Mahowald, and R. Ferber. Sleepwalking, confusional arousals, and sleep terrors in the child. In R. Ferber and M. Kryger, eds. *Principles and Practice of Sleep Medicine in the Child.* Philadelphia, PA: W.B. Saunders Company. 1995: 99–106.

129. Kuhn, B. R. Increasing sleep time effectively reduces sleepwalking and sleep terrors in children. *Sleep* 24(Suppl.): A209–A210, 2001.

130. Tobin, J. D., Jr. Treatment of somnambulism with anticipatory awakening. *Journal of Pediatrics* 122: 426–427, 1993.

131. Lask, B. Novel and non-toxic treatment for night terrors. *British Medical Journal* 297: 6648, 1988.

132. Durand, V. M. and J. A. Mindell. Behavioral intervention for childhood sleep terrors. *Behavior Therapy* 30: 705–715, 1999.

133. Frank, N. C., A. Spirito, L. Stark, and J. Owens-Stively. The use of scheduled awakenings to eliminate childhood sleepwalking. *Journal of Pediatric Psychology* 22: 345–353, 1997.

134. Levin, R. and G. Fireman. Nightmare prevalence, nightmare distress, and self-reported psychological disturbance. *Sleep* 25: 205–212, 2002.

135. Hublin, C., J. Kaprio, M. Partinen, and M. Koskenvuo. Nightmares: Familial aggregation and association with psychiatric disorders in a nationwide twin cohort. *American Journal of Medical Genetics* 88: 329–336, 1999.

136. Zadra, A. and D. C. Donderi. Nightmares and bad dreams: Their prevalence and relationship to well-being. *Journal of Abnormal Psychology* 109: 273–281, 2000.

137. Hawkins, C. and T. I. Williams. Nightmares, life events and behaviour problems in preschool children: Child care. *Health and Development* 18: 117–128, 1992.

138. Nielsen, T. A., L. Laberge, J. Paquet, R. E. Tremblay, F. Vitaro, and J. Montplaisir. Development of disturbing dreams during adolescence and their relation to anxiety symptoms. *Sleep* 23: 727–736, 2000.

139. Halliday, G. Treating nightmares in children. In C. E. Schaefer, ed. *Clinical Handbook of Sleep Disorders in Children*. Northvale, NJ: Jason Aronson. 1995: 149–176.

140. Terr, L. C. Psychic trauma in children: Observations following the Chowchilla school-bus kidnapping. *American Journal of Psychiatry* 138: 14–19, 1981.

141. Terr, L. C. Chowchilla revisited: The effects of psychic trauma four years after a school-bus kidnapping. *American Journal of Psychiatry* 140: 1543–1550, 1983.

142. Wood, J. M., R. R. Bootzin, D. Rosenhan, Nolen Hoeksema, S., et al. Effects of the 1989 San Francisco earthquake on frequency and content of nightmares. *Journal of Abnormal Psychology* 101: 219–224, 1992.

143. Kravitz, M., B. J. McCoy, D. M. Tompkins, et al. Sleep disorders in children after burn injury [see comments]. *Journal of Burn Care Rehabilitation* 14: 83–90, 1993.

144. Stoddard, F. J. Body image development in the burned child. *Journal of the American Academy of Child Psychiatry* 21: 502–507, 1982.

145. Ellis, A., G. Stores, and R. Mayou. Psychological consequences of road traffic accidents in children. *European Child and Adolescent Psychiatry* 7: 61–68, 1998.

146. Blum, N. J. and W. B. Carey. Sleep problems among infants and young children. *Pediatrics in Review* 17: 87–92, 1996.

147. Thompson, D. F. and D. R. Pierce. Drug-induced nightmares. *Annals of Pharmacotherapy* 33: 93–98, 1999.

148. Pagel, J. F. Nightmares and disorders of dreaming. *American Family Physician* 61: 2037–2042, 2000.

149. Wile, I. Auto-suggested dreams as factor in therapy. *American Journal of Orthopsychiatry* 4: 449–463, 1934.

150. Krakow, B., D. Sandoval, R. Schrader, et al. Treatment of chronic nightmares in adjudicated adolescent girls in a residential facility. *Journal of Adolescent Health Care* 29: 94–100, 2001.

151. Palace, E. M. and C. Johnston. Treatment of recurrent nightmares by the dream reorganization approach. *Journal of Behavior Therapy and Experimental Psychiatry* 20: 219–226, 1989.

152. Handler, L. The amelioration of nightmares in children. *Psychotherapy: Theory, Research and Practice* 9: 54–56, 1972.

153. Cavior, N. and A. M. Deutsch. Systematic desensitization to reduce dream-induced anxiety. *Journal of Nervous and Mental Diseases* 161: 433–435, 1975.

154. Kellerman, J. Rapid treatment of nocturnal anxiety in children. *Journal of Behavior Therapy and Experimental Psychiatry* 11: 9–11, 1980.

155. Pellicer, X. Eye movement desensitization treatment of a child's nightmares: A case report. *Journal of Behavior Therapy and Experimental Psychiatry* 24: 73–75, 1993.

156. Krakow, B., M. Hollifield, L. Johnston, et al. Imagery rehearsal therapy for chronic nightmares in sexual assault survivors with posttraumatic stress disorder: A randomized controlled trial. *Journal of the American Medical Association* 286: 537–545, 2001.

157. Krakow, B., R. Kellner, D. Pathak, and L. Lambert. Imagery rehearsal treatment for chronic nightmares. *Behavioural Research and Therapy* 33: 837–843, 1995.

158. Kellner, R., J. Neidhardt, B. Krakow, and D. Pathak. Changes in chronic nightmares after one session of desensitization or rehearsal instructions. *American Journal of Psychiatry* 149: 659–663, 1992.

159. Neidhardt, J., B. Krakow, R. Kellner, and D. Pathak. The beneficial effects of one treatment session and recording of nightmares on chronic nightmare sufferers. *Sleep* 15: 470–473, 1992.

160. Wood, J. M. and R. R. Bootzin. The prevalence of nightmares and their independence from anxiety. *Journal of Abnormal Psychology* 99: 64–68, 1990.

161. Rothbaum, B. O. and A. C. Schwartz. Exposure therapy for posttraumatic stress disorder. *American Journal of Psychotherapy* 56: 59–75, 2002.

162. Burgess, M., M. Gill, and I. Marks. Postal self-exposure treatment of recurrent nightmares. Randomised controlled trial. *British Journal of Psychiatry* 172: 257–262, 1998.

163. Burgess, M., I. M. Marks, and M. Gill. Postal self-exposure treatment of recurrent nightmares. *British Journal Psychiatry* 165: 388–391, 1994.

164. Cautela, J. Behavior therapy and the need for behavioral assessment. *Psychotherapy* 5: 175–179, 1968.

165. Cellucci, A. and P. Lawrence. Systematic desensitization to reduce dream anxiety. *Journal of Nervous and Mental Disease* 161: 433–435, 1978.

166. Eccles, A., A. Wilde, and W. L. Marshall. In vivo desensitization in the treatment of recurrent nightmares. *Journal of Behavior Therapy and Experimental Psychiatry* 19: 285–288, 1988.

167. Geer, J. H. and I. Silverman. Treatment of a recurrent nightmare by behavior-modification procedures: A case study. *Journal of Abnormal Psychology* 72: 188–190, 1967.

168. Haynes, S. and D. Mooney. Nightmares: Etiological, theoretical, and behavioral treatment considerations. *Psychological Record* 25: 225–236, 1975.

169. Marks, I., K. Lovell, H. Noshirvani, M. Livanou, and S. Thrasher. Treatment of posttraumatic stress disorder by exposure and/or cognitive restructuring: A controlled study. *Archives of General Psychiatry* 55: 317–325, 1998.

170. Miller, W. R. and M. DiPilato. Treatment of nightmares via relaxation and desensitization: A controlled evaluation. *Journal of Consulting and Clinical Psychology* 51: 870–877, 1983.

171. Schindler, F. Treatment by systematic desensitization of a recurring nightmare of a real life trauma. *Journal of Behavior Therapy and Experimental Psychiatry* 11: 53–54, 1980.

172. Shorkey, C. and D. Himle. Systematic desensitization treatment of a recurring nightmare and related insomnia. *Journal of Behavior Therapy and Experimental Psychiatry* 5: 97–98, 1974.

173. Silverman, I. and J. H. Geer. The elimination of a recurrent nightmare by desensitization of a related phobia. *Behavioural Research and Therapy* 6: 109–111, 1968.

174. Roberts, R. N. and S. B. Gordon. Reducing childhood nightmares subsequent to a burn trauma. *Child Behavior Therapy* 1: 373, 1979.

175. Castiglia, P. T. Nightmares. *Journal of Pediatric Health Care* 7: 125–126, 1993.

176. Sperling, M. Pavor nocturnus. *Journal of the American Psychoanalytic Association* 6: 79–94, 1958.

177. Maskey, S. Sleep disorders. Simple treatment for night terrors. *British Medical Journal* 306(6890): 1478, 1993.

178. Kellerman, J. Behavioral treatment of night terrors in a child with acute leukemia. *Journal of Nervous and Mental Diseases* 167: 182–185, 1979.

179. Mindell, J. A. Sleep disorders in children. *Health Psychology* 12: 151–162, 1993.

180. Kuhn, B. R. Behavioral treatment of sleep disorders: Pediatric parasomnias. *Sleep Review* 2: 29–32, 2001.

181. Kohyama, J., F. Matsukura, K. Kimura, and N. Tachibana. Rhythmic movement disorder: Polysomnographic study and summary of reported cases. *Brain and Development* 24: 33–38, 2002.

182. Kempenaers, C., E. Bouillon, and J. Mendlewicz. A rhythmic movement disorder in REM sleep: A case report. *Sleep* 17: 274–279, 1994.

183. Klackenberg, G. Rhythmic movements in infancy and early childhood. *Acta Paediatrica Scandinavica* 224(Suppl.): 74–83, 1971.

184. Kravitz, H., V. Rosenthal, Z. Teplitz, J. B. Murphy, and R. E. Lesser. A study of headbanging in infants and children. *Diseases of the Nervous System* 21: 203–208, 1960.

185. Thorpy, M. J. and A. J. Spielman. Persistent jactatio nocturna. *Neurology* 34(Suppl. 1): 208–209, 1984.

186. Rosenberg, C. Elimination of a rhythmic movement disorder with hypnosis: A case report. *Sleep* 18: 608–609, 1995.

187. Chisholm, T. and R. L. Morehouse. Adult headbanging: Sleep studies and treatment [see comments]. *Sleep* 19: 343–346, 1996.

188. Manni, R. and A. Tartara. Clonazepam treatment of rhythmic movement disorders [letter to editor]. *Sleep* 20: 812, 1997.

189. Alves, R. S., F. Aloe, A. B. Silva, and S. M. Tavares. Jactatio capitis nocturna with persistence in adulthood: Case report. *Arquiros de Neuro-Psiquiatria* 56: 655–657, 1998.

190. Leung, A. K. and W. L. Robson. Head banging. *Journal of the Singapore Paediatric Society* 32: 14–17, 1990.

191. Dahl, R. E. The pharmacologic treatment of sleep disorders. *Psychiatric Clinics of North America* 15: 161–178, 1992.

192. Thorpy, M. J. Rhythmic movement disorder. In M. J. Thorpy, ed. *Handbook of Sleep Disorders*. New York, NY: Marcel Dekker, Inc. 1990: 609–629.

193. American Psychiatric Association. *Diagnostic and Statistical Manual of Mental Disorders* (4th Edition). Washington, DC: 1994.

194. Miltenberger, R. G., E. S. Long, J. T. Rapp, V. A. Lumley, and A. E. Elliott. Evaluating the function of hair pulling: A preliminary investigation. *Behavior Therapy* 29: 211–219, 1998.

195. Miltenberger, R. G., R. W. Fuqua, and D. W. Woods. Applying behavior analysis to clinical problems: Review and analysis of habit reversal. *Journal of Applied Behavior Analysis* 31: 447–469, 1998.

196. Golding, K. Nocturnal headbanging as a settling habit: The behavioural treatment of a 4-year old boy. *Clinical Child Psychology and Psychiatry* 3: 25–30, 1998.

197. Christophersen, E. R. *Pediatric Compliance: A Guide for the Primary Care Physician.* New York, NY: Plenum. 1994.

198. Thorpy, M. J. and P. B. Glovinsky. Parasomnias. *Psychiatric Clinics of North America* 10: 623–639, 1987.

199. Dyken, M. E., D. C. Lin Dyken, and T. Yamada. Diagnosing rhythmic movement disorder with video-polysomnography. *Pediatric Neurology* 16: 37–41, 1997.

200. Prochaska, J. Remote-control aversive stimulation in the treatment of head banging in a retardate child. *Journal of Behavior Therapy and Experimental Psychiatry* 5: 285–289, 1974.

201. DeCatanzaro, D. A., and G. Baldwin. Effective treatment of self-injurious behavior through a forced arm exercise. *American Journal of Mental Deficiency* 82: 433–439, 1978.

202. Tarpley, H. D. and S. R. Schroeder. Comparison of DRO and DRI on rate of suppression of self-injurious behavior. *American Journal of Mental Deficiency* 84: 188–194, 1979.

203. Balaschak, B. A. and D. I. Mostofsky. Treatment of nocturnal headbanging by behavioral contractions. *Journal of Behavior Therapy and Experimental Psychiatry* 11: 117–120, 1980.

204. Lindsay, S. J., P. M. Salkovskis, and K. Stoll. Rhythmical body movement in sleep: A brief review and treatment study. *Behaviour Research and Therapy* 20: 523–526, 1982.

205. Strauss, C. C., A. Rubinoff, and B. M. Atkeson. Elimination of nocturnal headbanging in a normal seven-year-old girl using overcorrection plus rewards. *Journal of Behavior Therapy and Experimental Psychiatry* 14: 269–273, 1983.

206. Martin, R. D. and J. B. Conway. Aversive stimulation to eliminate infant nocturnal rocking. *Journal of Behavior Therapy and Experimental Psychiatry* 7: 200–201, 1976.

207. Linscheid, T. R., A. P. Copeland, D. M. Jacobstein, and J. L. Smith. Overcorrection treatment for nighttime self-injurious behavior in two normal children. *Journal of Pediatric Psychology* 6: 29–35, 1981.

208. Azrin, N. H. and R. G. Nunn. Habit-reversal: A method of eliminating nervous habits and tics. *Behavioural Research and Therapy* 11: 619–628, 1973.

209. Woods, D. W. and R. G. Miltenberger. Habit reversal: A review of applications and variations. *Journal of Behavior Therapy and Experimental Psychiatry* 26: 123–131, 1995.

210. Woods, D. W. and R. G. Miltenberger. A review of habit reversal with childhood habit disorders. *Education and Treatment of Children* 19: 197–214, 1996.

211. Bramble, D. Two cases of severe head-banging parasomnias in peripubertal males resulting from otitis media in toddlerhood. *Child Care, Health and Development* 21: 247–253, 1995.

212. Owens, J. and J. A. Mindell. Clinical sleep services for children: Clinical and administrative considerations. *Sleep Medicine* 3: 291–294, 2002.

213. Stores, G. *A Clinical Guide to Sleep Disorders in Children and Adolescents.* Cambridge, England: Cambridge University Press. 2001.

214. Ferber, R. and M. Kryger, eds. *Principles and Practice of Sleep Medicine in the Child.* Philadelphia, PA: W.B. Saunders Company. 1995.

215. Sadeh, A. *Sleeping like a Baby: A Sensitive and Sensible Approach to Solving Your Child's Sleep Problems.* London, England: Yale University Press. 2001.

Author Index

Subject Index